ITI Treatment Guide
Volume 11

ITI Treatment Guide

Editors:
D. Wismeijer, S. Barter, N. Donos

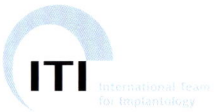

Authors:
G. Gallucci, C. Evans, A. Tahmaseb

Volume 11

Digital Workflows
in Implant Dentistry

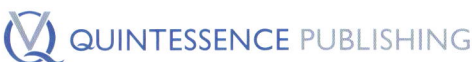

Berlin, Barcelona, Chicago, Istanbul, London, Mexico City,
Milan, Moscow, Paris, Prague, Seoul, Tokyo, Warsaw

German National Library CIP Data

The German National Library has listed this publication in the German National Bibliography. Detailed bibliographical data are available at http://dnb.ddb.de.

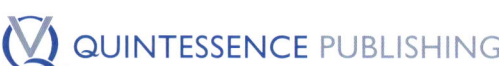

© 2019 Quintessenz Verlags-GmbH
Ifenpfad 2 – 4, 12107 Berlin, Germany
www.quintessenz.de

Illustrations: Ute Drewes, Basel (CH),
www.drewes.ch
Copyediting: Triacom Dental, Barendorf (DE),
www.triacom.com
Graphic concept: Wirz Corporate AG, Zürich (CH)
Production: Juliane Richter, Berlin (DE)
Printing: Aumüller Druck GmbH & Co. KG,
Regensburg (DE),
www.aumueller-druck.de

Printed in Germany
ISBN: 978-3-86867-385-2

The ITI Mission is ...

"... to serve the dental profession by providing a growing global network for life-long learning in implant dentistry through comprehensive quality education and innovative research to the benefit of the patient."

Preface

Since the first Treatment Guide appeared in 2007, the field of implant dentistry has progressed significantly in terms of implant design, surgical techniques, and materials, as well as abutment design and restorative materials. In recent years, however, one of the changes that is having far-reaching effects on how we practice implant dentistry has been the introduction of digital workflows—with the associated benefits as well as the challenges they pose to practitioners.

At the 6th ITI Consensus Conference in Amsterdam in 2018, progress in digital technology was examined by one of the working groups that looked into, in partic-ular, computer-aided implant surgery, implant impres-sion techniques, the accuracy of linear measurement of cone-beam CT images, and the accuracy of static com-puter-aided implant surgery.

The fruits of these discussions have been integrated in this volume. In 14 chapters that include 13 clinical cases, the authors have covered a broad spectrum of technol-ogies, procedures, and approaches, as well as offering recommendations and taking a look at developments currently in the pipeline.

S. Barter   N. Donos   D. Wismeijer

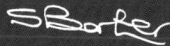

Acknowledgments

The authors would like to express their gratitude to Dr. Friedrich Buck for his excellent support in the preparation and coordination of this Treatment Guide. We would also like to thank Ms. Ute Drewes for the professional illustrations, Ms. Juliane Richter (Quintessence Publishing) for the typesetting and for coordinating the production workflow, Mr. Per N. Döhler for the language editing, as well as Mr. Stephen Barter for additional editorial assistance.

Editors and Authors

Editors:

Daniel Wismeijer
    DMD, Professor
    Head of the Department of Oral Implantology and
    Prosthetic Dentistry
    Section of Implantology and Prosthetic Dentistry
    Academic Center for Dentistry Amsterdam (ACTA)
    Free University
    Gustav Mahlerlaan 3004
    1081 LA Amsterdam
    Netherlands
    Email: d.wismeijer@acta.nl

Stephen Barter
    BDS, MSurgDent RCS
    Specialist in Oral Surgery
    Hon Senior Clinical Lecturer/Consultant Oral Surgeon
    Centre for Oral Clinical Research
    Institute of Dentistry
    Barts and The London School of Medicine and
    Dentistry, Queen Mary University of London (QMUL)
    Turner Street
    London E1 2AD
    United Kingdom
    Email: s.barter@gmx.com

Nikolaos Donos
    DDS, MS, FHEA, FDSRC, PhD
    Professor, Head and Chair, Periodontology and
    Implant Dentistry,
    Head of Clinical Research
    Institute of Dentistry, Queen Mary University of
    London,
    Institute of Dentistry, Barts and The London School
    of Medicine and Dentistry
    Turner Street
    London E1 2AD
    United Kingdom
    Email: n.donos@qmul.ac.uk

Authors:

German O. Gallucci
    DDS, Dr med dent (DMSc), PhD
    Raymond J. and Elva Pomfret Nagle Associate
    Professor of Restorative Dentistry
    Chair, Department of Restorative Sciences and
    Biomaterial Sciences
    Harvard School of Dental Medicine
    188 Longwood Avenue
    Boston, MA 02115
    USA
    Email: german_gallucci@hsdm.harvard.edu

Christopher Evans
    BDSc Hons (Qld), MDSc (Melb); MRACDS (Pros), FPFA
    Suite 4, 1st Floor, 232 Bay St
    Brighton, VIC 3186
    Australia
    Email: chris@evansprosthodontics.com

Ali Tahmaseb
    DDS, PhD
    Associate Professor
    Academic Centre for Dentistry Amsterdam (ACTA)
    Field of Oral Implantology and Prosthodontics
    Gustav Mahlerlaan 3004
    1081 LA Amsterdam
    Netherlands
    -and-
    Associate Professor
    Department of Oral and Maxillofacial Surgery
    Erasmus MC
    P.O. Box 2040
    3000 CA Rotterdam
    Netherlands
    Email: ali@tahmaseb.eu

Contributors

Nawal Alharbi
　BDS, MSc, PhD
　Department of Prosthetic Dental Science
　King Saud University
　Riyadh 4545, Saudi Arabia
　Email: nalharbi@ksu.edu.sa

Orlando Álvarez del Canto
　DDS, MS
　Oral Implantology
　Av. Presidente Kennedy 7100 Of. 601
　Vitacura, Santiago, 7650618, Chile
　Email: dr.alvarez@oseointegracion.cl

Jyme Charette
　DMD, MSD
　Renew Institute: Beyond Dentistry
　4938 Brownsboro Road, Suite 205
　Louisville, KY 40222, USA
　Email: jyme@renew-institute.com

Krzysztof Chmielewski
　MSc
　SmileClinic
　Karola Szymanowskiego 2
　80-280 Gdańsk, Poland
　Email: krischmielewski@me.com

André Barbisan de Souza
　DDS, MSc
　Department of Prosthodontics
　Tufts University School of Dental Medicine (TUSDM)
　One Kneeland Street, DHS-1242
　Boston, MA 02111, USA
　Email: andre.de_souza@tufts.edu

Wiebe Derksen
　DDS, MSc
　Academic Centre for Dentistry Amsterdam (ACTA)
　Oral Implantology and Restorative Dentistry
　Gustav Mahlerlaan 3004
　1081 LA Amsterdam, Netherlands
　Email: w.derksen@acta.nl

Simon Doliveux
　DDS, MMSc
　Department of Restorative Dentistry and
　Biomaterial Sciences
　Harvard School of Dental Medicine
　188 Longwood Avenue
　Boston, MA 02130, USA
　Email: simon_doliveux@hsdm.harvard.edu

Christianne Fijnheer
　MSc, MSc
　Academic Centre for Dentistry Amsterdam (ACTA)
　Oral Implantology and Restorative Dentistry
　Gustav Mahlerlaan 3004
　1081 LA Amsterdam, Netherlands
　Email: christianne.fijnheer@dentalclinics.nl

Gary Finelle
　DDS
　Dental7paris
　59 Avenue de la Bourdonnais
　75007 Paris, France
　Email: gary.finelle@dental7paris.com

Adam Hamilton
　BDSc, FRACDS, DCD
　Harvard School of Dental Medicine
　Restorative Dentistry and Biomaterials Sciences
　Division of Regenerative and Implant Sciences
　188 Longwood Avenue
　Boston, MA 02115, USA
　Email: adam_hamilton@hsdm.harvard.edu

Bassam Hassan
　DDS, MSc, PhD
　Prosthodontist
　Acibadem International Medical Centre
　Arlandaweg 10
　1043 HP Amsterdam, Netherlands
　Email: nassam.hassan@acibademimc.com

Tim Joda
Prof Dr med dent, DMD, MSc, PhD
University of Basel
Reconstructive Dentistry
University Center for Dental Medicine Basel (UZB)
Hebelstrasse 3
4056 Basel, Switzerland
Email: tim.joda@unibas.ch

Ali Murat Kökat
DDS, PhD
Prosthodontist
Professor, Istanbul Okan University
Faculty of Dentistry
Akfirat
Istanbul 34359, Turkey
Email: alimurat@outlook.com

Alejandro Lanis
DDS, MS
Oral Implantology
Assistant Professor, School of Dentistry
Pontificia Universidad Católica de Chile
Private Practice
Av. Presidente Kennedy 7100 Of. 601, Vitacura
Santiago, 7650618, Chile
Email: dr.alejandrolanis@gmail.com

Wei-Shao Lin
DDS, FACP
Diplomate of the American Board of Prosthodontics
Associate Professor, Indiana University School of
Dentistry, Department of Prosthodontics
1121 W Michigan Street, DS-S406
Indianapolis, IN 46202, USA
Email: weislin@iu.edu

Dean Morton
BDS, MS, FACP
Indiana Dental Association Professor and Chair
Department of Prosthodontics
Director, Center for Implant, Esthetic and
Innovative Dentistry
Indiana University School of Dentistry
1121 W. Michigan Street, DS-S316
Indianapolis, IN 46202, USA
Email: deamorto@iu.edu

Panos Papaspyridakos
DDS, MS, PhD
Tufts University School of Dental Medicine
Division of Postgraduate Prosthodontics
1 Kneeland Street
Boston, MA 02111, USA
Email: panpapaspyridakos@gmail.com

Waldemar D. Polido
DDS, MS, PhD
Clinical Professor and Program Director, Predoctoral
Oral and Maxillofacial Surgery
Co-Director, Center for Implant, Esthetic and
Innovative Dentistry, Indiana University School of
Dentistry
1050 Wishard Boulevard, Room 2200
Indianapolis, IN 46202, USA
Email: wdpolido@iu.edu

Gerry Raghoebar
DDS, MD, PhD
Professor
University Medical Center Groningen
Hanzeplein 1
9700 RB Groningen, Netherlands
Email: g.m.raghoebar@umcg.nl

R. H. Schepers
DDS, MD, PhD
Assistant Professor
University Medical Center Groningen
Hanzeplein 1
9700 RB Groningen, Netherlands
Email: r.h.schepers@umcg.nl

Newton Sesma
DDS, MSD, PhD
University of São Paulo School of Dentistry
Av. Prof. Lineu Prestes, 2227
São Paulo – SP, 05508-000, Brazil
Email: sesma@usp.br

Arjan Vissink
DDS, MD, PhD
Professor
University Medical Center Groningen
Hanzeplein 1
9700 RB Groningen, Netherlands
Email: a.vissink@umcg.nl

M. J. H. Witjes
DDS, MD, PhD
Associate Professor
University Medical Center Groningen
Hanzeplein 1
9700 RB Groningen, Netherlands
Email: m.j.h.witjes@umcg.nl

Table of Contents

1 <u>Introduction</u>

G. Gallucci

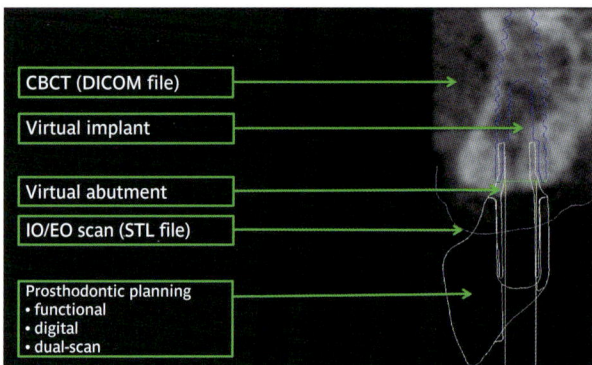

CBCT (DICOM file)

Virtual implant

Virtual abutment

IO/EO scan (STL file)

Prosthodontic planning
• functional
• digital
• dual-scan

Fig 1   Digital dataset used for planning in implant prosthodontics. CBCT: Cone-beam computed tomography. DICOM: Digital imaging and communications in medicine. IOS: Intraoral scanner. EOS: Extraoral scanner. STL: Standard tessellation language (formerly stereolithography).

The present Volume 11 of the ITI Treatment Guide explores the advances in implant dentistry made by incorporating digital dental technology (DDT). In this context, current implant prosthodontic protocols are revisited to accommodate modern technology and techniques.

This volume begins by addressing the technology and the necessary tools for the incorporation of DDT in a digital workflow, along with the clinical steps required for data acquisition. This includes imaging by cone-beam computed tomography (CBCT), intraoral scanning (IOS), extraoral scanning (EOS), and facial scanning (FS). It then turns to the different software tools needed to manipulate the digital data. A section is also dedicated to the integration of DDT into patient care by merging different datasets to virtually reconstruct the patient's orofacial anatomy.

An example dataset used in DDT for virtual implant planning incorporates several digital elements, as shown in Fig 1. Two main aspects of this dataset are the technology used for capturing orofacial structures in digital format and the software used to manipulate those digital files in order to perform virtual treatment planning, or to use computer-assisted design/computer-assisted manufacturing (CAD/CAM) technology.

1.1 Acquiring Digital Data

Different technologies are used to capture orofacial structures in a digital format. For instance, a CBCT unit is used to obtain a digital 3D rendering of the selected anatomical areas.

Chapter 2 describes in detail the imaging techniques and specifications for CBCT use in Implant Dentistry. While CBCT has the capability to capture most orofacial structures, it is mostly used to digitally replicate structures of higher density such as bone and teeth. A CBCT will produce a file in a format called DICOM (*Digital Imaging and Communications in Medicine*); this is a standard format commonly accepted in medicine.

CBCT images are often merged with IOS or EOS images obtained with a surface scanner. These types of scanners generally yield the generic STL file format (formerly known as *Stereolithography* format, now *Standard Tessellation Language* format). STL files are native to the stereolithography CAD software used by 3D systems. Unlike DICOM files, surface scanners produce a 3D representation of the surface of a scanned object. For this reason, a more detailed 3D representation of the scanned anatomical structures can be obtained when STL files are matched with a DICOM file.

Chapter 3 describes digital intraoral and extraoral scanning techniques as well as the associated technology. In addition to intraoral and extraoral scanning, the tissues of the face can be captured by a facial scanner (FS) to produce an additional dataset that can be merged with DICOM and IOS/EOS STL files, the goal being to obtain a complete virtual representation of the patient.

The current state of face scanning and an overview of the currently available technology are presented in *Chapter 4*.

1.2 Manipulating Digital Data

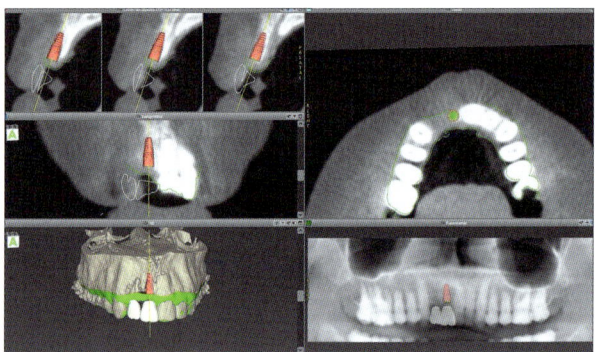

Fig 2   Virtual planning software for implant prosthodontics. Grey: DICOM. Green: STL. Red: Proposed implant. White: digital prosthetic setup. – Top left window: Cross-sectional views. Top right window: Axial view. Middle left window: Tangential view. Bottom left window: 3D reconstruction. Bottom right window: Panoramic view.

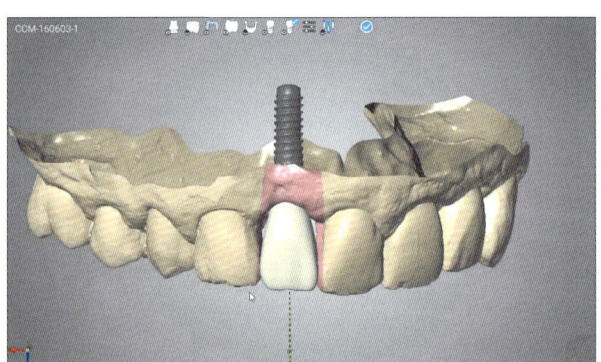

Fig 3   Screenshot of a CAD screen for an implant crown. (Courtesy of Chris Evans.)

Different software packages are available that can process digital files such as DICOM and STL for the virtual planning of implant placement, the digital design of surgical guides, or the digital fabrication of implant-supported prostheses. These software packages are divided into two main groups: (1) virtual implant-planning software and (2) CAD/CAM software. These two digital platforms can also be integrated to facilitate the free exchange of information.

Virtual planning software is used to select the ideal implant type and plan the implant's position in relation to the anatomy of the patient and the desired implant-prosthetic design. Fig 2 shows an example display of virtual planning software that has been used to plan an implant case.

Several planning steps are performed in this platform as follows:

1. Importing, segmenting, and aligning DICOM files
2. Setting the panoramic curve
3. Matching of DICOM and STL files
4. Digital tooth set-up (prosthetic planning)
5. Virtual implant selection and planning
6. Virtual abutment selection and planning
7. Virtual bone augmentation planning
8. Digital design of a surgical template for guided implant placement
9. Rendering a surgical protocol
10. Connectivity with CAD/CAM software

These steps are described in detail in **Chapters 5 to 9**.

In dentistry, CAD/CAM software is generally used for digital prosthodontics. Here, the main file format used is an STL file obtained via an IOS or EOS unit. Initially, the CAD side of the software is used to manipulate the STL file to design diagnostic models, implant abutments, a temporary implant prosthesis, and the final implant-supported prosthesis (Fig 3).

For implant-supported prostheses, the implant position is captured by an IOS or EOS image of a master cast using scanbodies (impression copings for digital surface scanning). These are geometric objects of known dimension (Fig 4) connected to the dental implant instead of the regular impression coping. The scanbody is usually constructed from PEEK material and has a dimension that can be recognized by the CAD software. Based on the scanbodies, the CAD software recognizes the implant type and spatial orientation allowing for the subsequent design of the implant prosthesis. CAD software packages offer an array of tools and commands for the virtual design of implant prostheses.

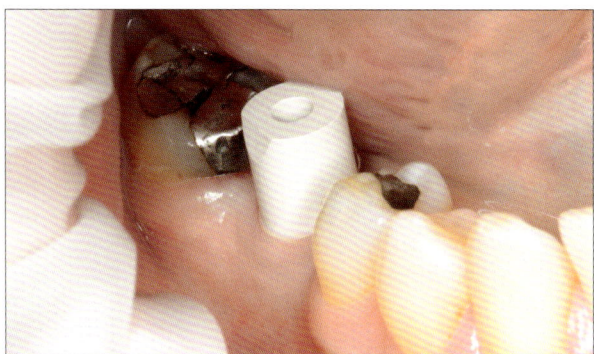

Fig 4   Scanbody in situ.

Once the CAD process is completed, a new STL file can be exported to various types of hardware to perform the CAM portion of the process. Implant-supported restorations can be manufactured by two main processes: additive or subtractive manufacturing. These steps are described in detail in **Chapters 10 and 11**.

Additive manufacturing (AM) is the process of joining materials to make objects from 3D model data, usually layer upon layer. Examples of additive 3D printing/manufacturing are:

1. Vat photopolymerization (digital light processing)
2. Powder-bed fusion (laser sintering)
3. Binder jetting (powder-bed and inkjet 3D printer)
4. Material jetting (multi-jet modeling)
5. Sheet lamination (selective deposition lamination)
6. Material extrusion (fused filament fabrication)
7. Directed energy deposition (laser metal deposition)

Subtractive manufacturing is a process by which 3D objects are constructed by successively cutting material away from a solid block of material, also known as milling or machining.

The clinical implementation of DDT in implant dentistry should optimize patient care by simplifying treatment while maintaining or improving the predictability of the outcome. Through a series of step by step clinical cases presented in **Chapter 13**, the reader will be able to consider the integration of digital protocols into their practice by understanding the technology necessary for acquiring and processing digital information and for the implementation of appropriate treatment protocols.

The progression of chapters in this volume of the ITI Treatment Guide was carefully conceived in a logical sequence to illustrate a clinical workflow. This workflow, when applied to DDT, is of paramount significance, since it will influence the treatment sequence. **Chapter 7** addresses digital workflows applied to patient care to integrate technology, techniques, and treatment sequencing with DDT to enhance patient safety and treatment reproducibility.

The authors offer clinical recommendations, assess future developments, and discuss the learning curve associated with the adoption of emerging technologies, with the associated risks and benefits. DDT is a very rapidly changing field—a field producing changes faster than the profession can absorb into clinical practice. The speed of progress is certainly fast enough to render any attempt at printed scientific literature unlikely to remain current for very long!

2 Surface Scans

C. Evans

2.1 Introduction

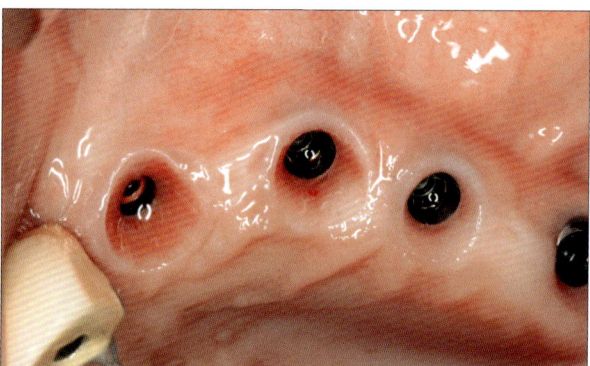

Fig 1   The mobility of the peri-implant tissues, vestibular mucosa, and frenal attachments may complicate the exact duplication of implants and related structures.

When undertaking dental implant procedures, an accurate duplication of the teeth/implants and surrounding tissues is required for both treatment planning and to enable fabrication of the prosthesis. Historically, such duplicates have taken the form of a physical stone model or working cast, which is produced from an impression of the oral cavity. Exact duplication of the structures in the oral cavity is complicated by factors such as multiple undercut surfaces due to variations in tooth morphology and axial inclination, the presence of fixed and movable soft tissues, frenal attachments, and the underlying muscles (Fig 1). The mouth is also an inherently moist environment due to the presence of saliva and crevicular fluid, which can compromise the accurate capture of shapes and contours without distortion. Inaccuracies can also arise from different properties of impression materials and issues relating to tray construction and rigidity, or patient compliance and movements.

Conventional impression materials are often hydrophilic to accommodate moisture and elastomeric to allow reversible deformation on removal from the mouth. The desired extent of the surface to be captured is determined by the type of prosthesis planned. For removable prostheses, a full-border extension of the impression will be necessary to avoid overextension of the prosthesis into the moveable tissues.

Impressions are then poured in type 3 or type 4 dental stone to provide a physical model. Inaccuracies can also occur in model production. When prosthetic reconstructions are made on immobile structures such as dental implants, inaccuracies in the dental cast as a consequence of the above-mentioned factors can result in an incorrect fit of the prosthetic framework. This in turn will result in delays, additional costs, frustration for the dentist, and patient dissatisfaction.

The introduction of the computer-aided design/computer-aided manufacture (CAD/CAM) concept to replace conventional impression/model techniques was first presented by François Duret in his thesis presented at the Université Claude Bernard, Faculté d'Odontologie, in Lyon, France in 1973, entitled "Empreinte Optique" (Optical Impression). Duret was able to complete intraoral scans using two cameras, two lasers, and a fiberoptic feed to enable the information to be transmitted to a large dental laboratory who could then manufacture a CAD/CAM restoration. This technology was subsequently refined by Werner Mörmann and Marco Brandestini in the 1980s at the University of Zürich for use in restorative dentistry and became commercially available as a CAD/CAM system for dental restorations in 1987 (Cerec; Dentsply Sirona, Bensheim, Germany). This was the first optical non-contact direct intraoral scanning system.

With the introduction of CAD/CAM in dental prosthetics, the first step in the workflow is acquiring a digital representation of the oral cavity. Digitization of the important structures by means of surface scans is considered a more straightforward technique than conventional impressions and may show less variability (Figs 2 and 3).

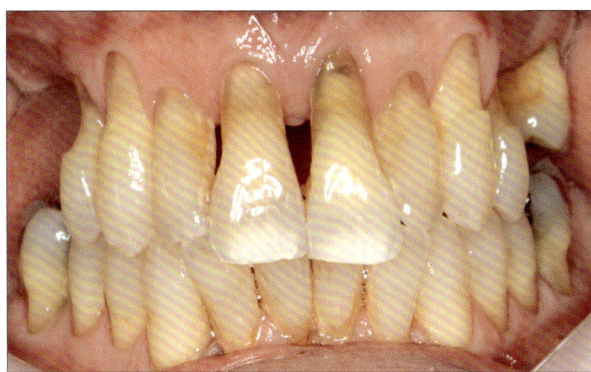

Fig 2   Clinical case with advanced gingival recession.

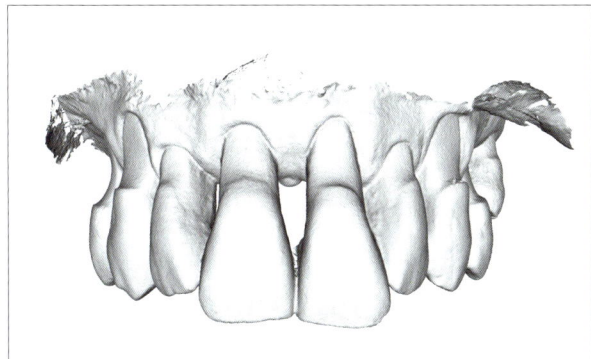

Fig 3   Surface scan of the clinical case in Fig 2.

2.2 Analog Impressions

Conventional impressions have been used for many years to capture the position of dental implants. They require an impression post to be placed onto the dental implant and a viscous impression material to set in the patient's mouth. A very high degree of dimensional accuracy is required for these materials to accurately duplicate the positions of the implants (Fig 4), and such materials have not been without limitations (Hamalian and coworkers 2011).

2.2.1   Material Accuracy

Traditionally, different types of impression material may be selected depending on the required level of accuracy for the intended dental procedure (Hamalian and coworkers 2011). The accuracy of impression materials may be affected by:

- Storage conditions
- Temperature
- Errors in mixing dosage and time
- Tray rigidity and positioning in the mouth
- Clinical technique
- Patient movement

- Setting time
- Continued chemical reaction after initial setting

Accurate surface detail is essential to avoid occlusal inaccuracies when positioning the antagonist model. Injectable low-viscosity materials are first flowed over surfaces to reduce the risk of air voids, and a heavier viscosity material is then placed in an impression tray, which supports and slightly displaces the material completely around the target structure. The time for setting will vary depending on the nature of the material. Voids or air bubbles within the impression may further reduce the accuracy of the impression.

2.2.2   Patient Comfort

Impression materials frequently require setting times in excess of four minutes. While many patients can tolerate conventional impression techniques, some patients find the procedure unpleasant, reporting a gagging feeling, excess saliva production, TMJ pain from prolonged opening, restricted access for appropriately fitting trays sizes, breathing difficulties, or an unpleasant taste.

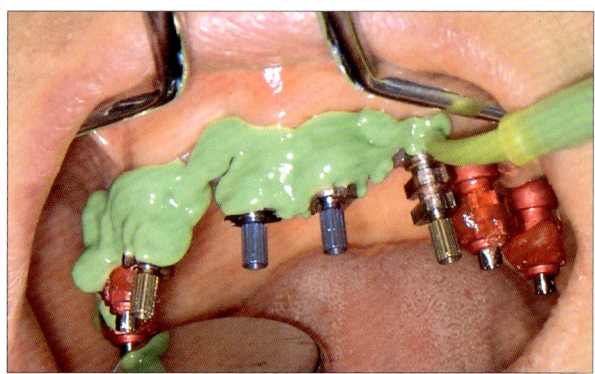

Fig 4   Conventional impression material being flowed around impression posts.

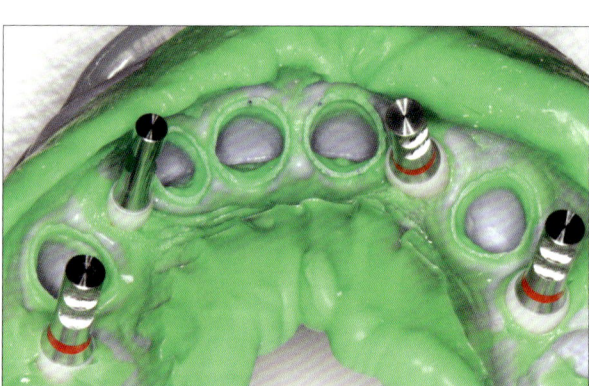

Fig 5   Impression.

2.2.3 Cast Production

When removed from the mouth, the impression material produces a "negative" of the relevant anatomy and requires a suitable dental stone to be poured in order to form a replica of the oral structures. Following removal from the patients' mouth, an appropriately matched laboratory analog is connected to the impression coping within the dental impression (Fig 5). Usually, a removable silicone material will first be placed around the implant analog to replicate the peri-implant soft tissue, and the gypsum stone is subsequently poured (Figs 6 and 7). There is a delay involved in releasing the model, as dental stone requires time for setting. The model itself is prone to dimensional errors caused by factors including:

- The mixing ratio of the dental stone
- Handling by the dental technician
- Surface abrasion and damage such as chipping and cracking
- Additionally, bubble formation can result in poor contact-point accuracy and occlusal errors (Fig 8)

(Buzayan and coworkers 2013; Holst and coworkers 2007).

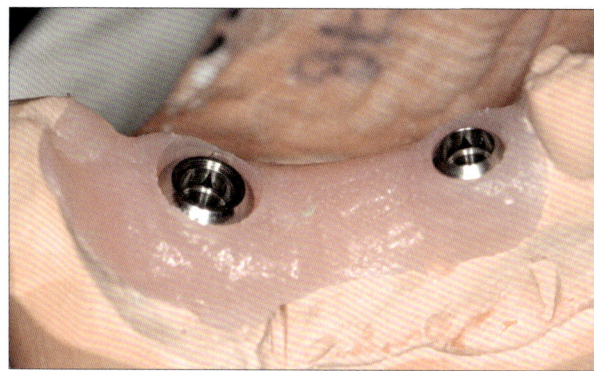

Fig 6   Stone cast with implant analogs in position, gingival mask in place.

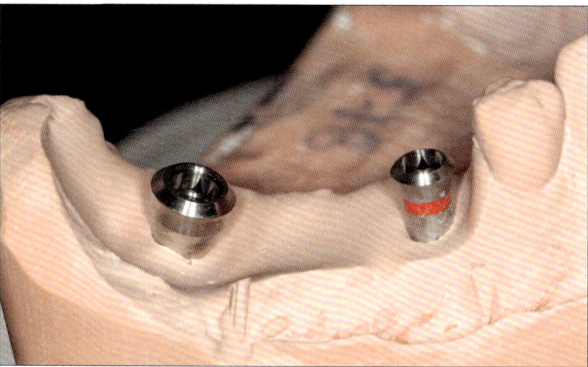

Fig 7   Stone cast with implant analogs in position, gingival mask removed.

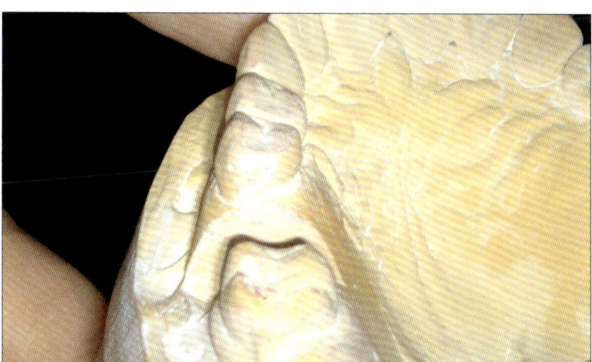

Fig 8   Stone cast showing bubbles and dragging, abrasion of the contact points, and residual plaster from articulation, all of which degrade the quality of the model.

2.3 Digital "Impressions"—Digitization of the Oral Cavity

Conventional impression techniques capture the impression coping connected to the dental implant. The production of a CAD/CAM dental prosthesis first requires the digitization of the relevant intraoral structures. A digital or "virtual" working model can then be used for the computer-aided processes.

When scanning dental implants, a geometric object of known dimensions called a scanbody (Fig 10) is connected to the dental implant instead of the conventional impression coping. The scanbody is usually constructed from PEEK material and has dimensions that can be recognized by the CAD software. A surface scan of the clinical situation is then obtained with specialized hardware, producing a digital file that can be imported into software packages for CAD/CAM.

2.3.1 File Formats

The standard file format of intraoral scanners is the STL file (Surface Tessellated Language). This file describes the surface geometry of three-dimensional objects by triangulation in binary code. The STL file format was created in 1987 by 3D Systems (Rock Hill, SC, USA) when they first developed the process of stereolithography (Wong and Hernandez 2012; Joda and coworkers 2017).

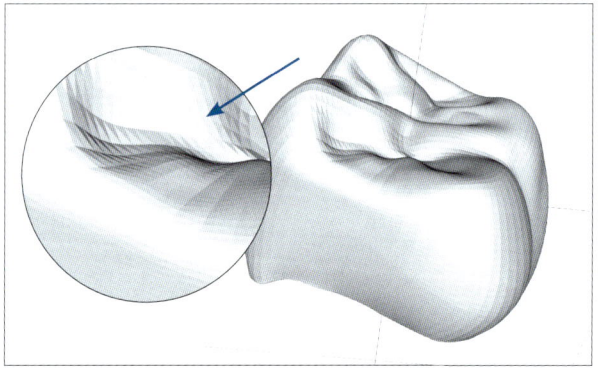

Fig 9 Following translation of the XYZ cloud points to a mesh of 3D triangles, the final contour is represented. Note the discrete appearance of meshed triangular geometry.

Digitization of the oral cavity creates a "point cloud." This is a set of data points in a three-dimensional coordinate system, usually X- Y-, and Z-coordinates, intended to represent the external surface of an object. Point clouds are usually polygon or triangle mesh models converted through a process commonly referred to as surface reconstruction to form the STL file (Fig 9).

The STL file creation links the continuous geometry of small triangles together to form the intended shape. This process can be inaccurate if the size of the mesh triangles is too large to fit the contour of the desired shape; in this case, information will be lost. Smaller triangles achieve a more realistic rendering of the object. Since the geometrical shape of a triangle has sharp edges, additional edges are sometimes added to the overall contour, which will then need to be adjusted to fit the final shape. This process can also introduce inaccuracy to the file, because an algorithm replaces the continuous contour, producing discrete steps in the surface contour.

Other files types also exist to store the data from a digital scan; some are manufacturers' proprietary systems that can only be used with the corresponding software ("closed systems"), while others may be used with multiple software packages ("open systems"). Examples include:

.PLY	Polygon File Format (also known as the Stanford Triangle Format) (Carestream; Rochester, NY, USA)
.OBJ	A simple data format used by the True Definition scanner (3M Espe; St. Paul, MN, USA); the file format is open and has been adopted by many 3D graphics applications
.DCM/.3OXZ	Both open and closed versions exist (3shape; Copenhagen, Denmark)
.RST/.DXD	(Cerec; Dentsply Sirona, Bensheim, Germany)

Reported advantages of these alternative file types over the STL file format include the storage of additional information such as color, texture, and marginal line data. While many different manufacturers employ different file systems, an open system is usually preferred to a closed system: the open system allows the surface scan file type to be used in any CAD software program without the need for file conversion, which is often limited and restricted by licensing arrangements associated with closed systems. There is also the risk of data loss or possible data-set corruption associated with file conversion packages.

The digitization of a complex intraoral morphology can be achieved via three distinct processes:

- Extraoral scanners that scan and digitize a traditional stone model produced using conventional impression techniques
- Extraoral scanners that scan and digitize a conventional impression
- Intraoral scanners, which perform non-contact optical scanning with a light emitting device to directly digitize the oral structures

2.3.2 Extraoral Scanning Systems

Following the production of the traditional gypsum stone cast with embedded analog implant replicas and removable-tissue silicone in place, a dental technician scans the model using a desktop laboratory scanner. Early-generation scanners required a contact probe to trace the contour of the stone model and develop the digital file. This has largely been replaced with non-contact optical scanners, which removes the limitation of the probe being unable to contact certain areas due to its physical size. A laboratory scanner uses a model holder that moves the cast in the path of a light-emitting device. Early-generation scanners required the model to be placed within a zone of scanning accuracy on a plasticine supporting base, but most scanners now utilize rotating model supports to enable complete visualization of surfaces and their associated undercuts.

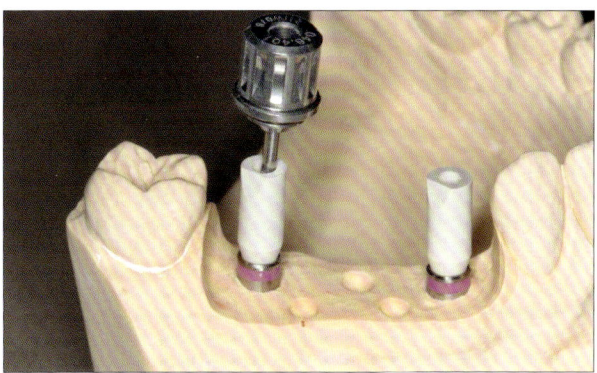

Fig 10   Scanbody connection.

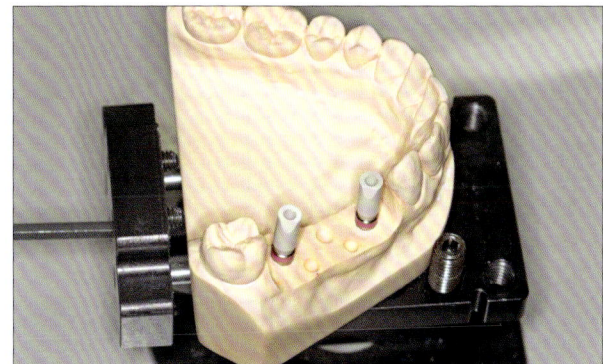

Fig 11   Model holder.

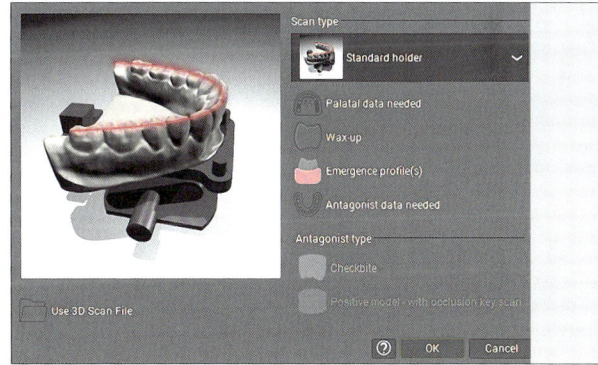

Fig 12   Setup for the laboratory scan.

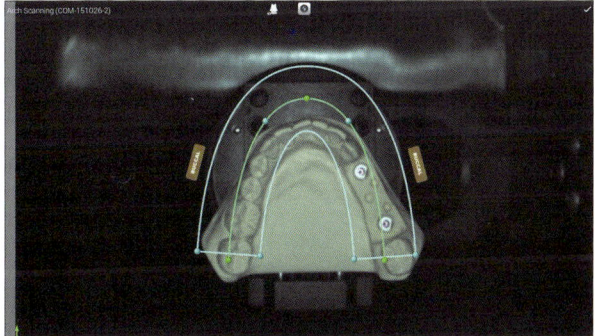

Fig 13   Preview to orient position of cast.

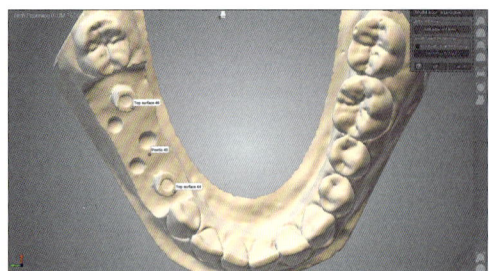

Fig 14 Implant scanbody located.

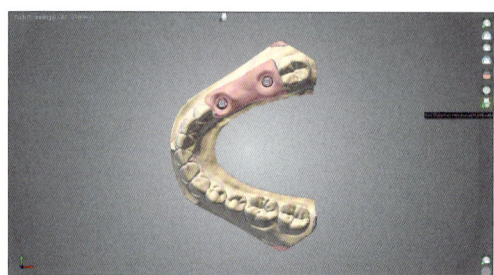

Fig 15 Virtual model ready for the CAD process.

Since the model is passed into a static light-emitting/light-receiving device, the rendering of the image is completed in a single plane. This offers the advantage of greater interpositional accuracy of the components within the model. Laboratory scanners are preferred when digitizing working casts for fabricating large frameworks used in full-arch reconstructions. The scanbodies must be placed in the cast with care to avoid damage to their fitting surfaces. The scanner software employs a strategy where the first scan pass is of the scanbodies without the removable soft tissue in place. The scanbodies are subsequently removed, and the removable silicone tissue is replaced on the cast; a second "tissue" scan is then performed. The laboratory software will remove any matched duplicate surfaces and insert a "virtual" implant into the rendered image of the cast so that a digital replica of the oral situation is created, with a removable tissue layer (Figs 10 to 15).

2.3.3 Impression Scanning

An alternative to scanning the object directly is to scan a conventional negative impression. This technique is essentially only useful for non-implant restorative cases. The impression is placed in a holder and inserted into the laboratory scanner. The impression material selected must contain a filler particle, usually titanium dioxide, to make it readable by the scanner. Limitations of the technique are found, for example in cases with long clinical crowns, perhaps due to natural teeth with periodontal attachment loss, as the full depth of contour can be obscured from the scanner head.

2.3.4 Intraoral Scanning Systems

Optical, non-contact, direct intraoral scanning systems use a "wand" containing a light-emitting device and integrated sensors to capture the intraoral form directly within the patient's mouth, generating a digital replica of the dentition and related structures. Direct digitization offers clinicians the benefit of being able to view the digital replica of the oral cavity without delay.

Examples of technologies available for intraoral scanning include:

- Active Wavefront Sampling (3M True Definition scanner; 3M Espe, St. Paul, MN, USA)
- Confocal imaging (iTero, Amsterdam, Netherlands)
- Triangulation stripe light projection (Cerec; Dentsply Sirona, Bensheim, Germany)
- Optical coherence tomography (E4D, Richardson, TX, USA)

Again, for intraoral scanning of dental implants, a scanbody is inserted into the implant (Fig 16).

The intraoral form presents a challenge to optical scanning in that the surfaces to be captured as an image are highly reflective or have a high degree of translucency. Depending on the optical scanning technique employed, powder-coating with a titanium or magnesium dioxide powder may be required to enable the scanner to capture the image (Fig 17). Some scanners do not require the application of powder to capture the scanbody's position accurately.

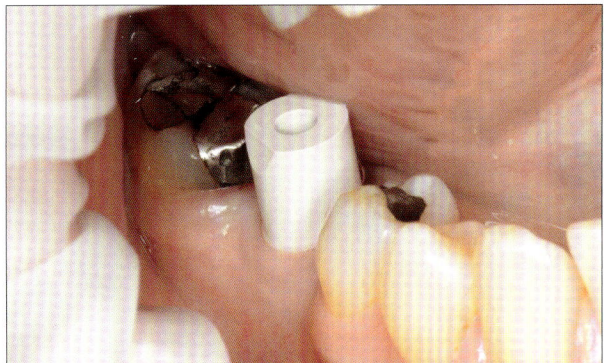

Fig 16   Scanbody in situ.

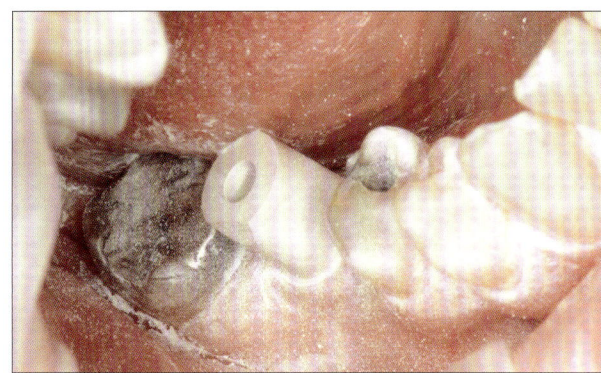

Fig 17   Scanbody following light scan-powder application.

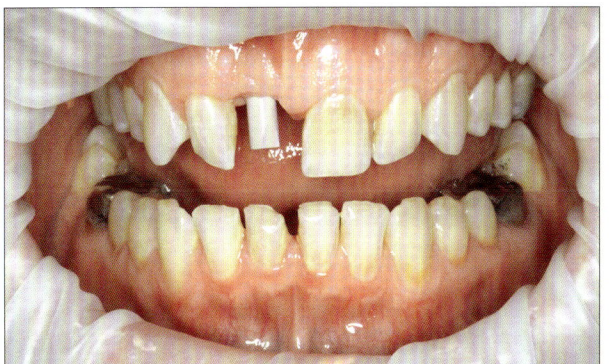

Fig 18   Retraction of the patient's lips helps provide access for the scanning device. In this case, an Optragate (Ivoclar Vivadent, Schaan, Liechtenstein) was used to maintain lip retraction.

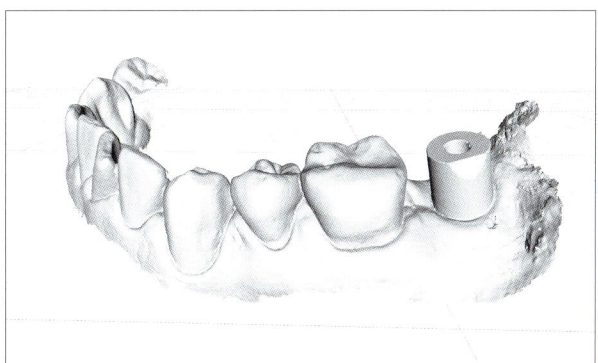

Fig 19   Surface scan ready for transfer to the CAD software.

To assist with intraoral scanning, retraction devices for lips and cheeks are often employed (Fig 18).

The data set is progressively captured in incremental images with a small field of view. The rendering of the oral cavity is constructed by the stitching together of these smaller images. To successfully merge the images, areas or objects of similarity must be found to enable the images to be successfully merged.

If multiple teeth are missing, the ability to accurately register the soft-tissue contour of the mouth can be more challenging, as the mobility of the soft tissue can prevent the scanner from recognizing sufficient points of similarity. Additionally, intraoral scanners will have a preferred path of travel and data capture that the operator should follow in order for the software algorithms to accurately reconstruct the image. Deviation from the scan path may create inaccuracies in the data captured.

When the resulting surface scan file is transferred to the CAD software, the virtual implant will be reconstructed within the image (Fig 19).

The extent of recorded information depends on the scanbody configuration, the position of the scanbody within the dental arch, and the proximity of neighboring structures (teeth and scanbodies). Studies suggest that the extent of recorded information might also depend on the scanning device itself, resulting in different values according to the precision of different systems.

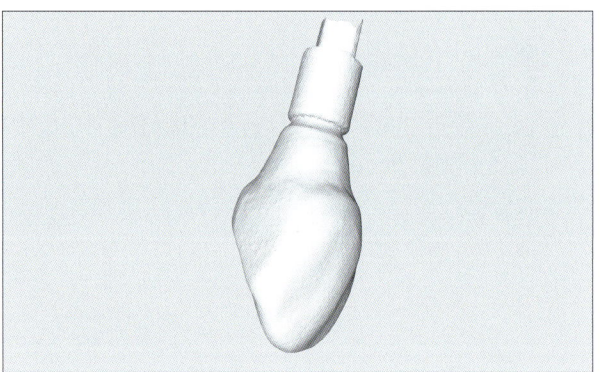

Fig 20   Scan of the provisional restoration.

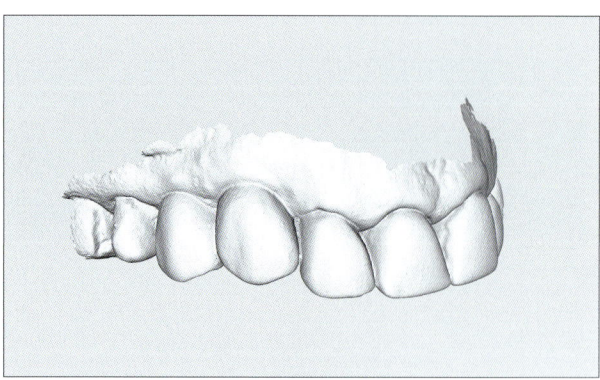

Fig 21   Scan of the provisional in place.

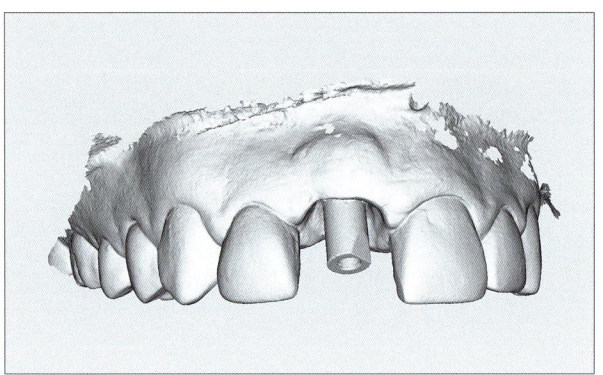

Fig 22   Surface scan of the tissue state after removal of the provisional restoration.

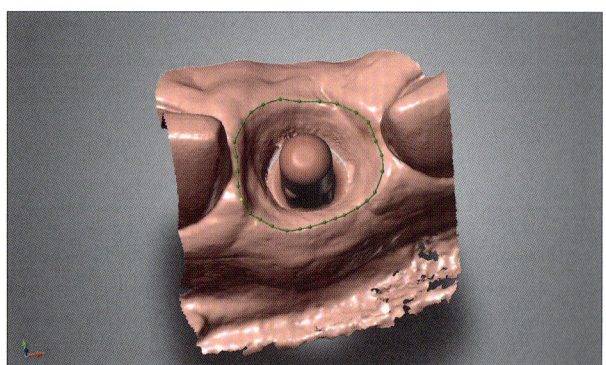

Fig 23   Customized tissue contour capture after surface scanning.

2.3.5   Emergence-Profile Scans

Tissue customization is frequently employed for implants in the esthetic zone to sculpt and shape the peri-implant mucosa prior to the delivery of a definitive restoration. With conventional impressions, this involves additional steps to create customized impression copings. With digital scanning, it is possible to directly scan the emergence profile of the customized provisional restoration (Fig 20) together with two surface scans: one with the provisional in situ (Fig 21) and one with the scanbody in place (Figs 22 and 23). Functions within the CAD software allows this emergence contour established in the provisional to be duplicated for the final restoration.

2.4 Accuracy: Trueness and Precision

Trueness and precision are often used interchangeably when describing the accuracy of digitizing the intraoral form. However, there are important differences between the two terms. Trueness is the ability of a measurement to match the actual value of the quantity being measured. However, precision is the ability of a measurement to be consistently repeated. International standards are used by manufacturing companies to allow comparison of different machines (ISO 12836:2012; ISO 12836:2015).

Since dental implants are immovable objects, implant prostheses rely on a high degree of accuracy to create a prosthesis that passively fits the implants. Any misfit in a framework for multiple implants has been shown to contribute to mechanical and biological complications (Abduo and Lyons 2013). The use of CAD/CAM technology aims to reduce the potential for misfits by reducing human intervention and the accumulation of minor fabrication errors inherent in analog workflows that include waxing, investing, casting, and polishing. For this to be realized in the CAD/CAM process, the digitization of surfaces by optical scanning must be accurate to faithfully represent the features within the oral cavity.

Unlike conventional impressions, where the material selected has inherent limitations affecting accuracy, the accuracy of detail captured is consistent and therefore the practicality of using the scanner within the mouth must be considered. Therefore, when using an intraoral scanner some physical requirements must be satisfied. If the scanning "wand" is dimensionally too large it will not effectively reach all areas of the mouth, potentially compromising the quantity and quality of the captured data (Fig 24).

Other inaccuracies in the intraoral scanning process can arise from several sources:

- In order for the scanner to capture the required areas, the light-emitting device must be able to access all areas of the dentition (Fig 25).
- Incomplete acquisition of the surface of a scanbody by the scanning device may result in failure of the software to recognize the scanbody or cause imprecise computing of the cylinder position and its geometric characteristics (Fig 26).
- Degradation in the precision of measurement of the angles between multiple scanbodies may arise from

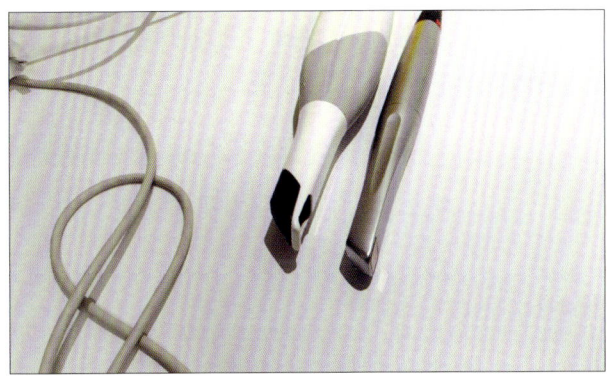

Fig 24   Two different scanner tip sizes. A larger size could limit the ability to reach certain areas of the patient's mouth.

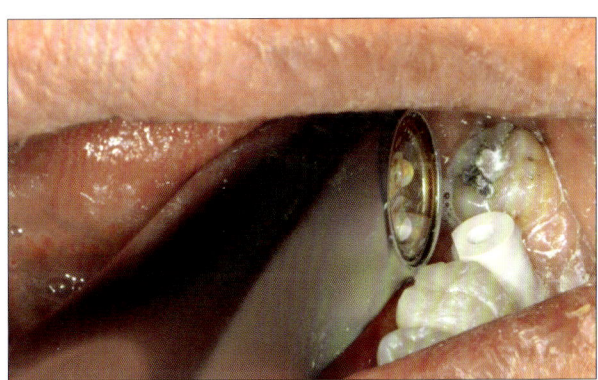

Fig 25   Positioning of the scanner tip to assist in retracting the tongue.

size differences in the scanbodies and from the algorithms used for the surface-scan reconstruction.

- Fogging or moisture contamination of the glass surface of the scanner tip can reduce the accuracy of the scan. While most systems have inbuilt heating elements within the scanner tip to reduce fogging, slow-speed evacuation is also of assistance.

2.4.1 Technique Selection

Since dental implants are immobile structures within the alveolar bone, any inaccuracy in the impression or scanning technique may result in an inadequate prosthetic fit. Intraoral scanning techniques have the potential to offer time- and cost-saving benefits to clinicians. Additionally, the peri-implant mucosal position is captured in a passive state, which allows for a more accurate location of intended cementation lines. For single-unit and short-span prostheses of up to three units, intraoral scanning is claimed to be as accurate as conventional impression techniques, but there are few studies to verify such claims (Ender and Mehl 2011; van der Meer and coworkers 2012).

When dental implants are surrounded by a deep soft-tissue collar, the length of the scanbody may be insufficiently visible through the mucosa for the optical sensor and a conventional impression followed by laboratory scanning may be advisable, as the removable tissue model may allow more accurate scanbody identification (Gimenez-Gonzalez and coworkers 2016).

Creating restorations based on sectional scans of the dental arch is possible. However, when more extensive restorative solutions are required, the clinician should make a complete-arch scan to ensure the accurate reconstruction of the clinical situation and create a restoration that harmonizes with the occlusion and functional form. Additionally, in the CAD design process, the dental technician may choose to use a "mirroring anatomy" function, which requires the contralateral tooth form(s) to be captured in the scan.

However, the lack of clearly identifiable static anatomical landmarks in the edentulous arch that can compromise the stitching together of small field of view images captured by intraoral scanners can result in positional discrepancies and inaccurate inter-implant relationships.

This may change as intraoral scanning technology improves in the future, but at present, full-arch reconstructions requiring multiple splinted implants are best captured using conventional impressions subsequently scanned with a laboratory scanner (Andriessen and coworkers 2014) (Fig 27).

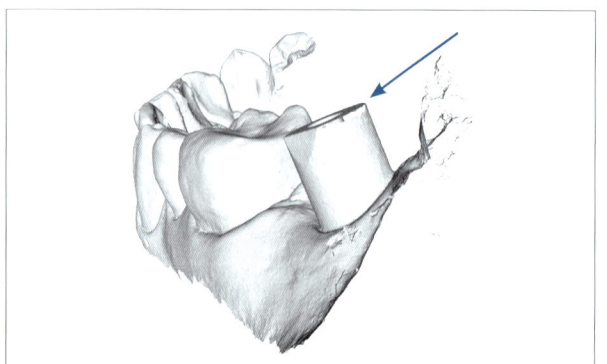

Fig 26 Void as seen on the distal surface of the scanbody. This may limit the accuracy of implant location within the CAD software. The clinician should strive to have the entire surface captured in the scan.

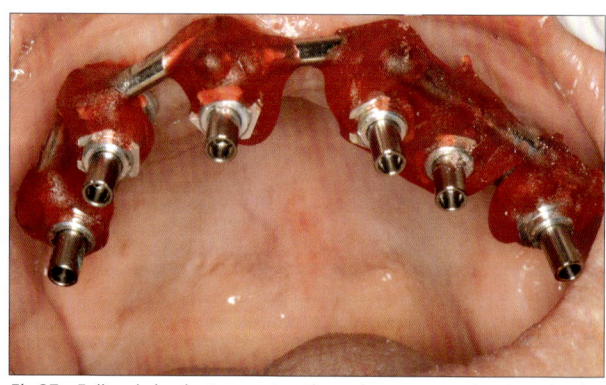

Fig 27 Full-arch implant reconstruction using a conventional analog impression where the impression copings are rigidly splinted. This provides the most accurate method of recording the implant positions in a full-arch case.

2.5 The Need for Physical Models

The dental technician may still require a model for certain stages in finalizing the prosthesis. In such situations, intraoral scanning can be used to produce models for the dental technician to complete the restoration. When a model is requested, this is usually a 3D-printed model or a stereolithographic (SLA) polyurethane die, with a holder for a repositionable laboratory analog (Figs 28 to 30).

Completely monolithic restorations are becoming increasingly popular as a means of avoiding technical complications such as fractures in a ceramic build-up, the high cost of conventional metal-ceramic restorations, and lengthy production time associated with such restorations (Joda 2017a). It is possible for monolithic restorations to be produced without the need for a working model in a direct CAD/CAM process.

Currently, monolithic materials are not suitable for use in highly aesthetic cases, where layering ceramics are required to develop appropriate translucency and staining to match the natural dentition. Additionally, when longer-span prosthetic designs are necessary or metal frameworks are used, a model is required for contact point formation and occlusal design.

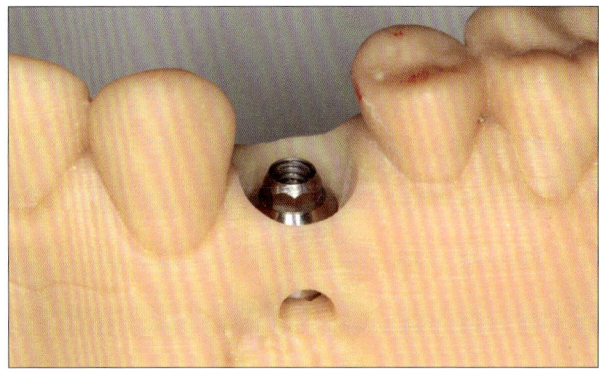

Fig 28 Abutment and repositionable analog located with a 3D-printed model. Note viewing window to confirm the repositionable analog is fully seated in the model.

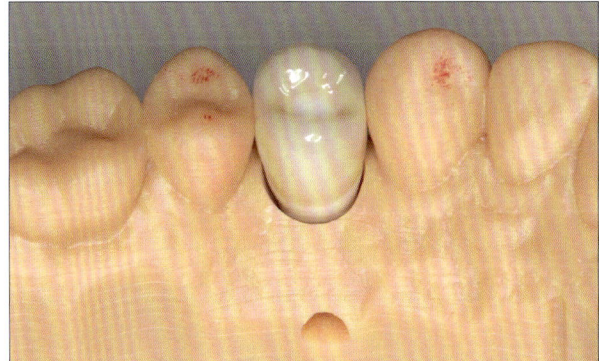

Fig 29 CAD/CAM implant restoration on 3D SLA printed model used for contact point and occlusal verification.

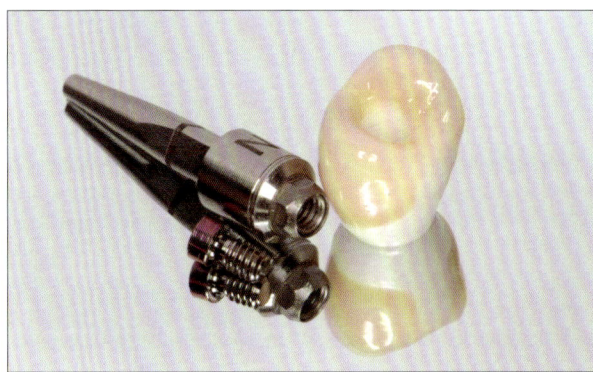

Fig 30 Repositionable analog removed from the model and layered CAD/CAM zirconia restoration.

2.6 Concluding Remarks

- Intraoral scans are possible for a wide variety of clinical situations, but at this point they are not suitable in every clinical case.
- Models and impressions can be scanned to be loaded into CAD/CAM software.
- Working in a model-free environment is possible when using monolithic restorations. However, when producing non-monolithic or layered restorations, a working model is required.

3 Facial Scanning

A. Tahmaseb, B. Hassan

The increasing availability of compact, efficient, in-office digital intraoral (IOS) scanners and cone-beam computed tomography (CBCT) scanners has been accompanied by an expanding armamentarium of software tools to visualize, analyze, and merge the datasets generated by these scanners for use in daily practice. For the first time in dental medicine, the concept of designing a "virtual patient replica" could become a reality. Three-dimensional (3D) imaging of the dentition, alveolar bone, and surrounding soft tissues constitutes what can be described as the "diagnostic triad." When combined, these may provide the digital basis for comprehensive treatment planning.

Until recently, there has been a disproportionate emphasis in implant dentistry on capturing only two elements of this triad, namely the teeth and bone, with very little regard given to the patient's external (facial) profile. However, imaging of the extraoral soft-tissue profile is relevant; it is the facial entity that is most readily visible (Rangel and coworkers 2008). A thorough and comprehensive evaluation of the facial soft-tissue profile can benefit the preoperative diagnosis with more predictable treatment outcomes and better esthetic results.

This technology has gained popularity since the introduction of the so-called "digital smile design" (DSD), which provides an opportunity to evaluate the patient's esthetics before considering the actual dental restoration. In the fields of orthodontics and orthognathic maxillofacial surgery, there has been burgeoning interest in applying facial scanning technology to plan advanced and complex cases. Predicting a patient's postsurgical profile changes has made it possible to plan complex surgery and to better manage patient expectations. Numerous articles and reviews have been published on the applications of this novel technology, assessment of accuracy, and ongoing developments (Hajeer and coworkers 2004). However, there are still many obstacles to reliability, so routine daily use in the dental surgery has not yet been realized.

3.1 Technological Evolution

One of the earliest attempts to replicate the facial profile was made in 1893, when Case used plaster of Paris to model the patient's face (Case 1893). In 1915, van Loon introduced the "cubus cranioforus," where dental casts were "fused" with plaster casts of the face in anatomically correct positions (van Loon 1915).

Irrespective of how cumbersome and time-consuming it was to create this "analog" set-up, early pioneers in the field firmly believed that esthetic considerations regarding the facial profile should guide treatment planning when deciding on the occlusal relationships of maxillary and mandibular complete dentures. In 1949, Tanner and Weiner utilized photogrammetry to study facial esthetics (Tanner and Weiner 1949). Photogrammetry consists of measurements made on photographs, something that at the time offered decisive advantages over direct facial anthropometry (measurements performed directly on the face), as a permanent record of the patient's facial profile was obtained with this technique. The technique was also less sensitive to patient movement artifacts than direct anthropometry. However, manually matching different photographs to create a facial map proved to be a tedious and time-consuming task.

In the 1980s, stereophotogrammetry was introduced as a novel technique to capture 3D information on physical objects, first employed in maxillofacial imaging for monitoring patients with facial asymmetry (Burke 1983). This technique constitutes a true 3D registration in that two or more photographs are taken either simultaneously or sequentially from different angles and arranged in a specific set-up to form a "stereo pair."

The captured pairs of photographs are then combined to create an image by providing 3D coordinates (Kau and coworkers 2007). Stereophotogrammetry is a general term used to describe a broad range of technologies for acquiring 3D surface information by different methods. An earlier version of this technology, dubbed "analog stereophotogrammetry," relied on processing conventional printed photographs that were fed into an instrument known as the "analytical stereo plotter," designed to provide a contour map exhibiting 3D coordinates of different landmarks. This technique was successfully used to map the maxillofacial region in order to study facial asymmetry (Ras and coworkers 1995). However, these analog systems or their digitized variants have now largely been abandoned.

3.2 Technological Principles of Contemporary Facial Scanning

Contemporary non-contact digital stereophotogrammetry uses diverse energy sources, optical sensors, and computer algorithms to calculate 3D measurements. However, all digital stereophotogrammetry techniques are based on the mathematical principles of trigonometry.

Based on the scanning technology used, two different image acquisition methods can be distinguished: laser scanning and structured-light projection techniques. Both techniques have their applications in dentistry, and both exhibit specific advantages and disadvantages. Laser scanning is the most widely applicable method for capturing 3D information of inanimate objects for medical and industrial applications. In prosthetic dentistry, this technique is routinely applied in the dental laboratory to digitize dental impressions or dental casts and forms the basis for designing CAD/CAM prostheses.

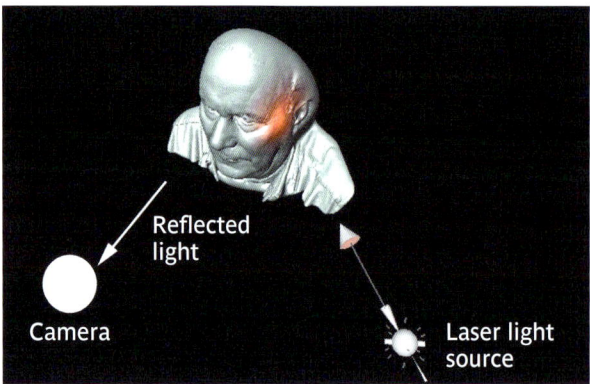

Fig 1   Laser surface scanning system: the laser light is reflected from the object and captured by a camera system.

However, the technique can also be used to obtain facial scans in vivo. The basic laser scanner set-up consists of a laser light source, an optical sensor such as a camera, and the object to be scanned—the face. The laser beam, which could be a spot or a line, is first projected onto the face. The deflected laser beam is then captured by the camera sensor, which is placed at a known distance from the laser source. The face, the camera, and the laser light source form a triangle. The distance between the laser beam and the face can be calculated by applying the principles of trigonometry. This process is repeated in a linear fashion as a laser light is swept across the face until a complete 3D point cloud (x, y, and z) of coordinates is formed (Fig 1).

Laser scanning techniques have been successfully applied to study facial esthetics (Moss and coworkers 1995). Laser technology allows rapid and highly accurate scanning of the face at a wide angle and is not sensitive to lighting conditions. Laser scanners can also be lightweight and portable, which enables the face to be scanned from multiple angles and is useful where office space is limited. Furthermore, no further post-processing or merging of images from multiple views is required. However, since the image is not captured all at once, the technique is inevitably sensitive to motion artifacts, possibly resulting in reduced geometric accuracy (Bush and Antonyshyn 1996; Ismail and coworkers 2002). Also, the potential danger of laser light to the eye means that only eye-safe lasers can be applied. Several available commercial systems (e.g., Fastscan; Polhemus, Vermont, Canada) promise universal applicability to capture the face.

Further validation is required to determine the specific indications for which this scanning technology may be applicable in implant dentistry. Table 1 describes the available technologies, their characteristics, advantages, and disadvantages.

Table 1   An overview of available facial scanning systems, their characteristics, advantages and disadvantages (taken from Hassan B, Giménez Gonzáles B, Tahmaseb A, Jacobs R, Bornstein MM. Three-dimensional facial scanning technology: applications and future trends. Forum Implantologicum. 2014; 10: 77 – 86).

Scanning technology	Commercial System	Characteristics	Advantages	Disadvantages
Laser scanning	• FastScan	• Hand-held, portable	• Non-invasive • Wide angle • Insensitive to lighting conditions • No post-processing	• Sensitive to motion artifacts • Operator experience
Structured light (active stereophotogrammetry)	• Pritidenta • Priti mirror	• Single camera system	• Photo-realistic • Rapid scanning • Non-invasive	• Narrow angle • Multiple shots • Sensitive to lighting conditions • Post-processing
Structured light (active stereophotogrammetry)	• 3dMDface	• Multiple cameras	• Photo-realistic • Extremely rapid scanning < 1 s • Non-invasive	• Expensive • Large footprint • Post-processing
Digital camera system (passive stereophotogrammetry)	• Di3D	• Multiple cameras	• Photo-realistic • Extremely rapid scanning < 1 s • Non-invasive • No white light	• Expensive • Large footprint • Post-processing

Structured light scanning, or active stereophotogrammetry technology, operates on similar principles of trigonometry, but instead of the laser, a safe (white or blue) light is projected onto the face in a specific or a random pattern. On contacting the facial surface, this light pattern (referred to as fringe) bends and twists to follow the contours of the facial profile. The camera captures the deformed light pattern and a 3D facial coordinate map is formed (Fig 2). This map is then post-processed to create a 3D surface representation of the face. Simultaneously, digital 2D photographs are captured and the 3D surface data are then combined with this 2D texture photo of the patient to provide a colored 3D surface.

In a single-scanner system, the scan is limited to a narrow angle, requiring data acquisition from multiple directions to cover the face completely. The patient is required to sit on a turning table, which could be manually or computer-controlled, to rotate and acquire snapshots of the face from multiple angles. This makes such scans prone to motion artifacts and requires further post-processing to align or merge the different views in order to obtain a single 3D mesh. The lack of automation of the digitization process remains the main disadvantage of single-camera systems (D'Apuzzo 2006).

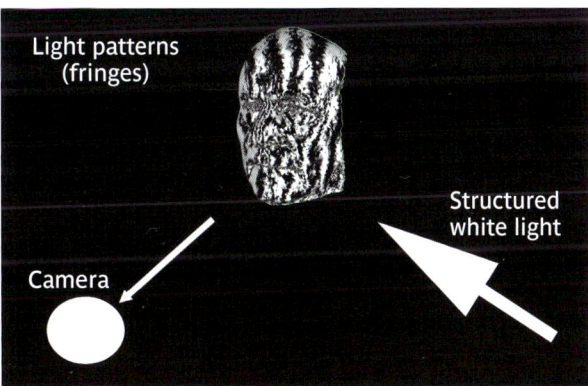

Fig 2   Structured-light scanning system: The light pattern is projected onto the face, forming light and dark patterns (fringes), which are captured by a camera system.

The use of multiple projectors and cameras to instantly capture the face at an angle of almost 180 degrees eliminates the need for the patient to be rotated on a turntable, reducing the risk of motion artifacts. Currently, this technique remains the most clinically applicable method for acquiring 3D facial surfaces in the maxillofacial region, owing to its high accuracy (within 0.5 mm) and a short scanning time of under one second. However, the acquisition costs of the system and its footprint (office space required for the machine) remain limiting factors (Lübbers and coworkers 2010). An example of such a system is the 3dMDface (3dMD, Atlanta, GA, USA), which is equipped with six cameras for capturing white-light and color photographs.

Moiré profilometry is a specific form of structured light scanning that was pioneered in the 1970s (Takasaki 1970). The term originates from moire (moiré in its French adjectival form), a type of textile, traditionally of silk but now also of cotton or synthetic fiber, with a rippled or "watered" appearance. In this technique, a grid is placed close to the face, and the light patterns are projected onto the grid and captured by the camera. While the imaging principle is similar to structured-light scanning, there are significant differences. A profilometer is a measuring instrument used to measure the profile of a surface. Moiré profilometry permits even higher resolution scanning, as it can detect small bends and twists in the light pattern that otherwise remain invisible to the sensor. Moiré profilometry also opens up the potential for real-time clinical image acquisition. The technology is widely applied outside dentistry in the aviation and biometrics industries. However, it demands a complicated set-up, expensive hardware, and extensive user experience; to date, image acquisition remains slower than with other structured-light techniques, which also makes the technology vulnerable to motion artifacts (Artopoulos and coworkers 2014).

The final form of digital stereophotogrammetry is passive stereophotogrammetry. Through simply acquiring a pair of high-resolution 2D digital photographs, a dense 3D point cloud can be virtually reconstructed using a special software algorithm. Using this approach, there is no need to use a light pattern or any other form of laser scanning. This technique has the advantage of extremely rapid scanning and an uncomplicated set-up. The procedure resembles that of taking ordinary photographs. However, multiple digital cameras need to capture multiple images (2 to 6 photographs) instantaneously, to form the stereo pair, and post-processing is required, although this is largely automated. The accuracy of one such passive stereo system (Di3D, Dimensional Imaging, Glasgow, UK) was recently found to be within clinically acceptable limits (Deli and coworkers 2013).

3.3 Applications in Prosthetic Dentistry

The main indication for facial scanning in dentistry is to improve preoperative diagnostics while providing an objective tool for treatment outcome assessment and follow-up. However, there are currently no software packages or devices available that combine all the functions described above. Most available software packages allow the capture of only one or two elements of the diagnostic triad. Ideally, one single comprehensive software package should permit all three datasets to be imported in an automated registration process. In addition, a dedicated module for prosthetic design would be desirable. The intended prosthesis, whether a tooth-supported crown or a fixed prosthesis on dental implants, could then be fabricated using this data.

However, to manipulate the acquired datasets to simulate different treatment scenarios, the surface data first needs to be post-processed. Converting the dense point cloud into a different, more manageable format requires special post-processing algorithms that are not readily available in most dental CAD software. Secondly, facial scanners must capture the visible part of the teeth (typically the labial surfaces of anterior teeth) to provide adequate reference surfaces for matching with intraoral scans of the dentition. This mandates that facial scanners be capable of capturing the labial surfaces of anterior teeth with sufficient resolution to permit image fusion with the intraoral scans of the dentition. Amongst the three currently available facial scanning technologies, the structured-light technique seems to be the most appropriate for such a demanding task, as it allows for high-resolution image capture. A few recent attempts have been reported in the literature, but with mixed results (Rangel and coworkers 2008; Rosati and coworkers 2010). However, these reports were based on idealized natural dentitions and the patients had no existing prosthesis (whether fixed or removable) in the anterior region.

Imaging the visible facial dental structures at high resolution is more complicated if the patient is edentulous or if only implants are in place. In such situations, the facial scanner must capture the labial surface of the edentulous alveolar process, existing dentures, fixed prosthetic superstructures, or impression posts/scanbodies in order to provide sufficient fiducial markers for image fusion with the intraoral scans. There are no reports at present to assess the validity of such a registration.

Similarly, the merging of acquired CBCT datasets and facial scans can prove to be equally problematic. Large patches of corresponding soft tissue areas are required to permit proper image fusion.

While CBCT is capable of portraying the external soft-tissue profile with sufficient accuracy, the quality of the 3D measurements obtained is inherently dependent on the chosen scanner system, scan settings, and reconstruction algorithms (Hassan and coworkers 2013). In addition, combining facial scans with CBCT would inevitably require a larger field of view (FoV) of the radiographic scan than the standard average of 8 × 8 cm currently utilized for planning most implant guided-surgery cases. Matching accuracy between large field-of-view CBCT datasets and 3D facial photographs has been found to be within 1.5 mm (Maal and coworkers 2008). However, the use of large-FoV CBCT scans can reduce the quality of the scan as a consequence of limiting the increased radiation exposure to the patient; the clinician also needs to consider the concomitant medico-legal requirements for interpreting large-field CBCT scan data (Horner and coworkers 2009).

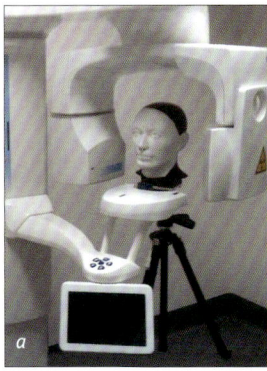

Fig 3a   An example of a CBCT unit with a built-in facial scanning system, allowing for integrated 3D clinical and radiographic imaging (Planmeca ProMax 3D combined with ProFace; Planmeca, Helsinki, Finland).

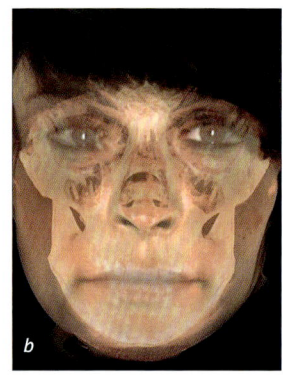

Fig 3b   Results of a combined integrated scan allowing the underlying bony tissues to be visualized together with the soft tissues of the same subject.

Novel developments include the integration of facial scanning hardware into the CBCT unit, allowing for smooth fusion and accurate registration. Such integration may overcome some of the post-processing registration challenges. However, the procedure is associated with prolonged scanning times and lower resolution than with the traditional stereophotogrammetry set-up (Figs 3a-b).

3.4 Clinical Case

The following pilot case is presented (with the informed consent of the patient) as an example of such a digital set-up:

A 70-year-old male patient presented with a malfunctioning upper, fixed long-span metal-ceramic bridge. The patient's chief complaint was the absence of posterior teeth and his inability to chew properly (Figs 4a-b and 5a-d). Following examination and diagnosis, the treatment plan called for the extraction of the remaining teeth, followed by a new implant-supported fixed dental prosthesis.

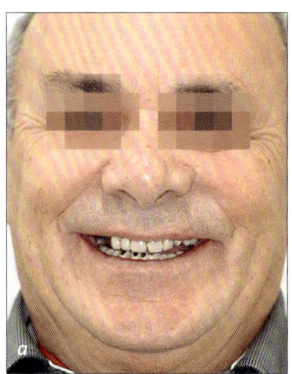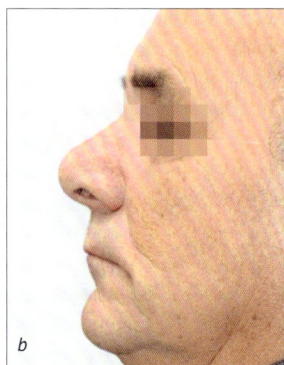

Figs 4a-b   Clinical extraoral photos of the patient.

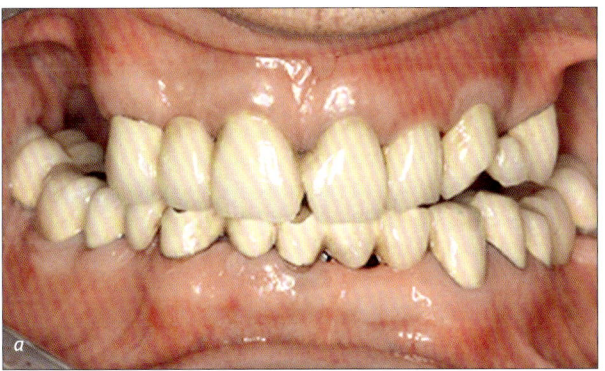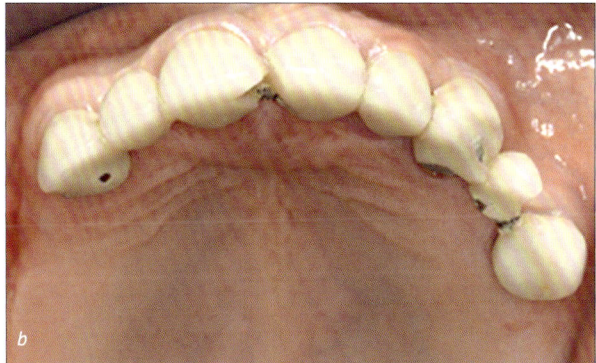

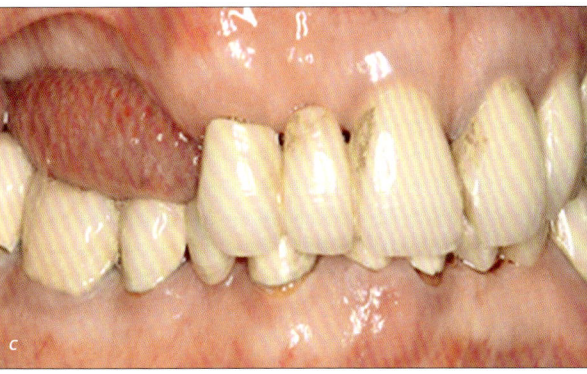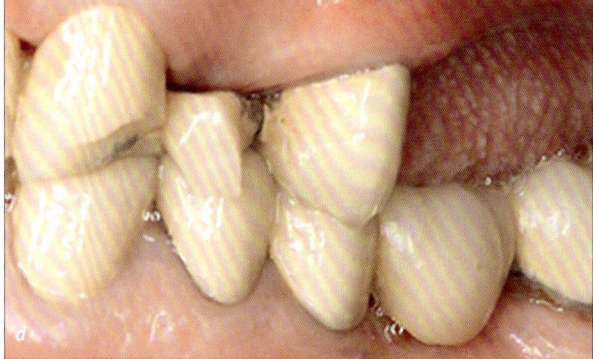

Figs 5a-d   Clinical intraoral photos of the patient (the same one as in Fig 4) demonstrating the status of the bridge in the upper jaw.

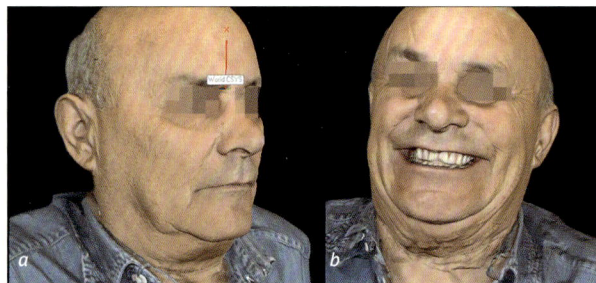

Figs 6a-b Pritidenta 3D (Pritidenta, Leinfelden, Germany) facial scan of the patient in neutral and smiling positions.

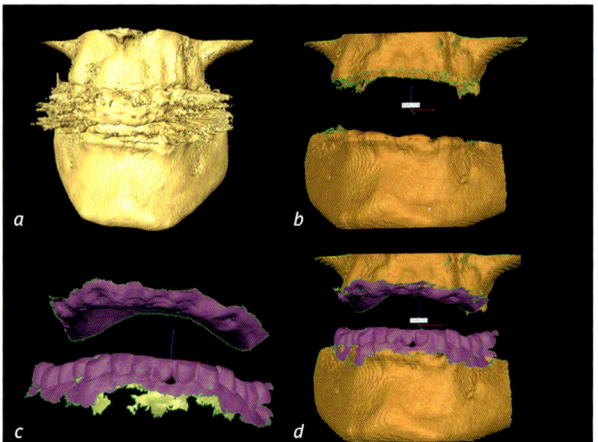

Figs 7a-d The original CBCT scan with a medium field of view (8 × 8 cm) (a). Notice the excessive streak artifacts resulting from the metal-ceramic bridge. The teeth were then digitally removed (b) and the True Definition 3D (3M ESPE, St. Paul, MN, USA) intraoral scan (c) was fitted to the CBCT scan in the anatomically correct position (d).

The patient's facial morphology was scanned using the Pritidenta 3D single-camera facial scanner (Pritidenta, Leinfelden, Germany) in both neutral and smiling expressions (Figs 6a-b). CBCT scan data were acquired using the Accuitomo 170 (FoV 8 × 8 cm, 180-degree rotation, standard resolution; Morita, Kyoto, Japan). The intraoral scans of the edentulous maxilla and the dentate mandible were obtained using a 3M True Definition scanner (3M ESPE, St. Paul, MN, USA). The intraoral scans were merged with the CBCT reconstructions of the alveolar process (Figs 7a-d).

Following removal of the remaining teeth, a 3D facial image of the edentulous patient was obtained (Fig 8). The scan data and digital occlusal records could then be exported to specialized software to design and fabricate the prosthesis. An example of such a tool is the AvaDent software (Avadent; Global Dental Science, Scottsdale, AZ, USA), which permits a fully milled provisional denture to be produced based on 3D scan data (Fig 9).

After duplication and 3D scanning of the interim prosthesis, the patient's face was scanned again with the denture in place to provide reference points for the 3D mock-up (Fig 10). The merged CBCT and intraoral scan datasets were then merged with the facial scans (Figs 11a-d).

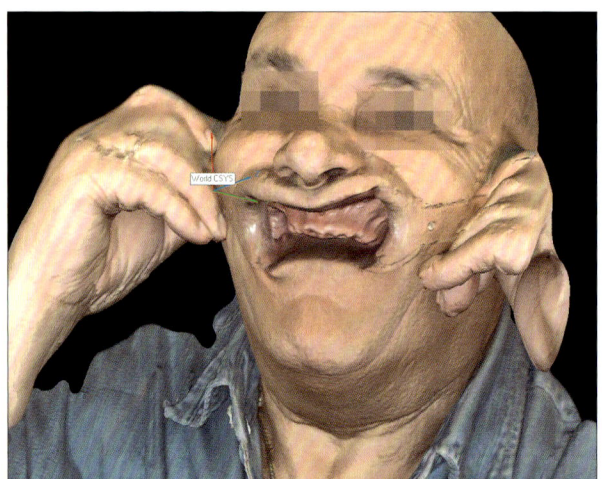

Fig 8 Pritidenta scan of the edentulous alveolar ridge. The head had to be tilted upwards to provide maximum exposure of the edentulous region.

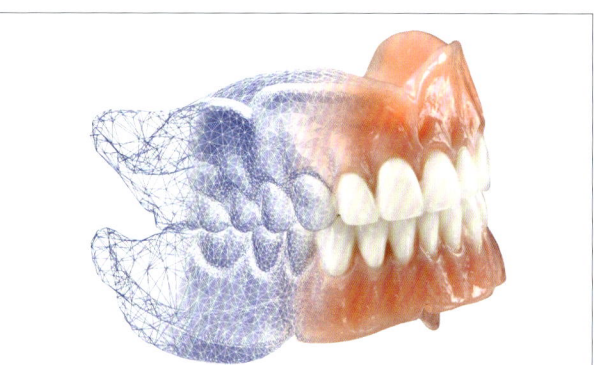

Fig 9 An example of a digitally designed and fabricated removable complete denture (Avadent; Global Dental Science, Scottsdale, AZ, USA).

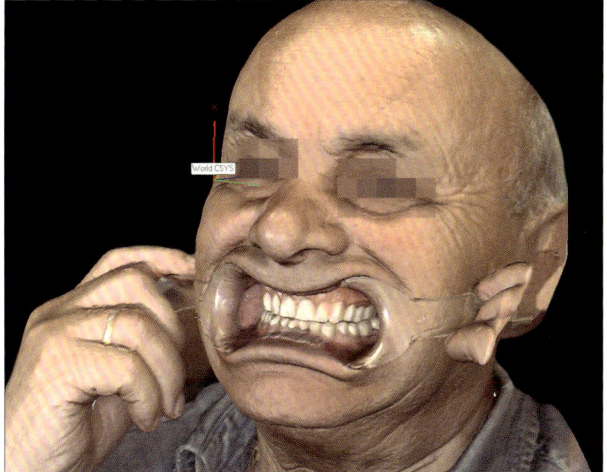

Fig 10   Pritidenta facial scan of the patient with upper interim denture. The acrylic teeth pose no challenge to the scanner.

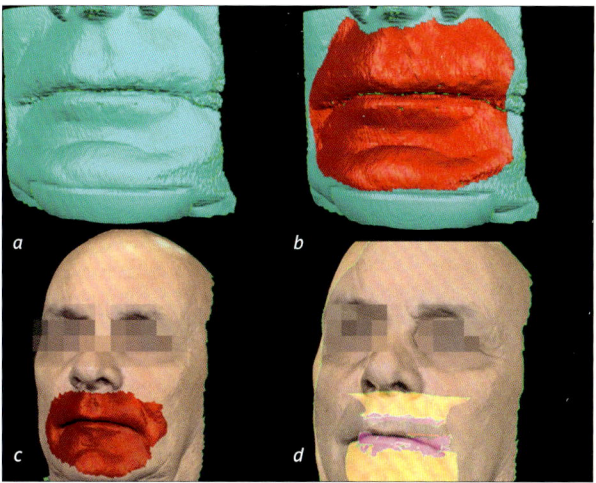

Figs 11a-d   The process of merging a CBCT scan and a facial scan. Starting from the soft-tissue reconstruction from a CBCT scan (a), a region of interest is selected (red patch in b) and a corresponding region of interest is selected on the 3D surface scan (red patch in c), leading to acceptable registration results (d—yellow: CBCT scan; purple: digital intraoral scan).

The surgery was planned using coDiagnostiX software (Institut Straumann AG, Basel, Switzerland). The implant positions were fixed by the prosthetic constraints imposed by the position of the future prosthesis (Fig 12).

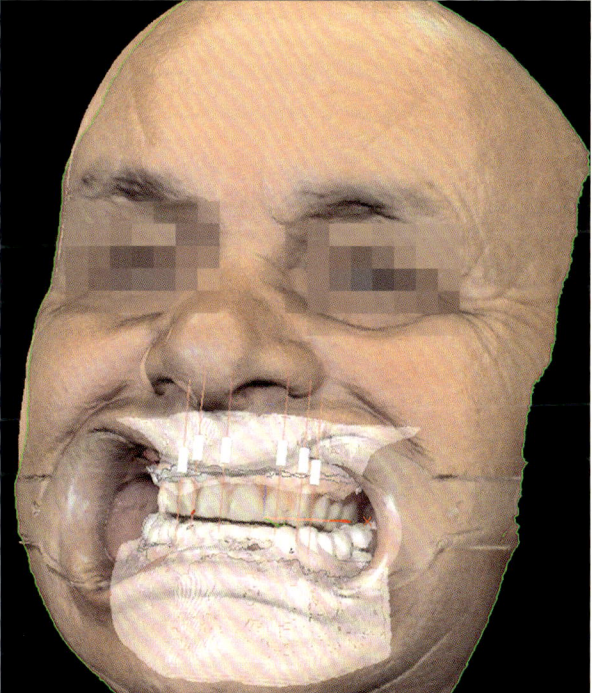

Fig 12   The final result of the merging procedure. The surgery was planned based on esthetic and prosthetic requirements.

3.5   Dynamic Facial Scanners

Dynamic facial scanning, meaning capturing facial movement and transferring the result to a realistic digital animation of the human face, is the next big step in creating the virtual patient. Such technology has been already introduced in the movie industry, where movies are made without having any actual actors involved. Its use in dentistry could have a significant impact on digital workflows and the creation of a virtual patient.

However, capturing detailed 3D facial animation is difficult because it requires the recording of complex facial movements at different scales. Mimicking the complex muscle motion and skin wrinkling and folding involved in human facial expressions is challenging, as detailed skin features are extremely difficult to capture.

There are multiple approaches to capturing 3D facial expressions, including 3D scanning, marker-based motion capture, structured-light systems, and image-based systems (Huang and coworkers 2011). Despite technological improvements, acquiring high-quality facial recordings remains a difficult task. Some devices can, for example, acquire high-resolution facial detail such as pores, wrinkles, and age lines, but typically only for static poses. Marker-based motion capture systems can record dynamic facial movements with very high temporal resolution (up to 2,000 Hz), but due to their low spatial resolution (usually 100 to 200 markers), they are not capable of capturing expressive facial details such as wrinkles (Huang and coworkers 2011). Recent progress in structured-light systems (Zhang and coworkers 2004; Li and coworkers 2009) and multi-view stereo reconstruction systems have made it possible to capture 3D dynamic faces with moderate fidelity, resolution, and consistency, but their results still cannot match the spatial resolution of static face scans or the acquisition speed of marker-based motion capture systems.

As this technology is developing rapidly in disciplines other than dentistry, its dental application will hopefully be available sooner that we currently imagine.

3.6 Shortcomings and Future Technical Improvements

Creating a virtual patient with all the necessary information in a single dataset is the ultimate goal of digital dentistry. Imagine if, at the patient's first appointment, all the necessary parameters could be recorded, including CBCT data, IOS data, and facial information, all in a single dataset with superimposed images of the patient, a dataset that is readily available on your computer screen.

Currently, technical difficulties remain and create inaccuracies during this process:

- Variation in image quality of the different datasets to be merged/superimposed
- Difficulties arising from such superimposition requiring the recognition of identical landmarks on two different images; this process is more complicated when, for example, a facial scanner image is

merged with an IOS image, because as IOS is performed intraorally and facial scanning extraorally, there are no matching landmarks to be used

Although teeth can be used as landmarks, there are limitations, as described earlier in this chapter. By exposing the teeth during the facial scanning procedures or using markers attached to teeth, the process may be simplified and improved, but this is not possible in edentulous cases. To try to address this, Tahmaseb and coworkers (2012) used pre-installed mini-implants mounted with scanbodies as landmark references.

More accurate devices and integrated systems, such as the one described in Chapter 10.3, are required to enable the predictable use of this technology in daily dental practice.

3.7 Conclusions

We are currently witnessing a paradigm shift in the clinical procedures and technical methods of dental rehabilitation. Currently available CAD/CAM technology for diagnosis and treatment planning, for guiding the surgical placement of implants, and for the design and fabrication of removable or fixed implant-supported prostheses, has the potential to revolutionize the field of dental implantology.

The soft-tissue profile information obtained through 3D facial scanning is undeniably an ideal supplement to these existing scanning technologies. Merging facial scan information with data obtained from CBCT and digital intraoral scanners allows prosthetic designs that fully accommodate the esthetic demands imposed by the external profile of the patient, while still adhering to surgical constraints. Improvements in combined surgical and prosthetic planning will be of benefit to patients and clinicians alike. There is currently no single dental software package that can be used for comprehensive diagnosis and surgical treatment planning, as well as digital prosthesis design.

With increasing interest from academia and industry, the number of commercially available single- and multiple-camera systems for prosthodontic applications can only be expected to grow. Recent initiatives undertaken by industry leaders to develop open software standards for dental applications will hopefully permit the seamless integration of 3D facial scan data with other 3D sources, including CBCT and digital intraoral scanning.

However, since the technology is still in its infancy, including its potential applications in prosthodontics, there is an urgent need for more scientific evidence to corroborate or refute the applicability of facial-scanning technology in dentistry. Indeed, this seems to be the greatest challenge to address in the coming years.

4 <u>Software Packages</u>

C. Evans

Software packages are critical to the successful implementation of digital workflows in implant dentistry. Software is available to cover all aspects of the digital workflow, which can be summarized in the following chart (Fig 1):

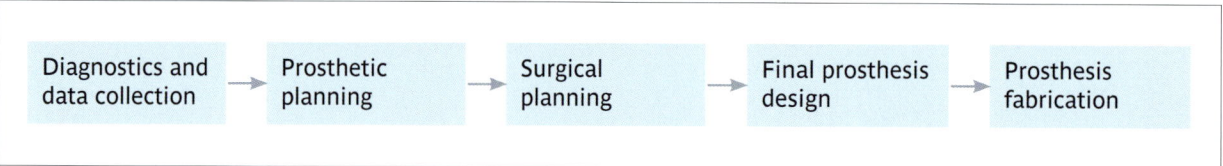

| Diagnostics and data collection | → | Prosthetic planning | → | Surgical planning | → | Final prosthesis design | → | Prosthesis fabrication |

Fig 1   The digital workflow.

Digital workflows and solutions allow team members to readily communicate and share information regarding treatment proposals, as long as all team members have access to the appropriate software. A comprehensive solution can integrate all aspects of the software into one seamless workflow.

The software architecture can be either open or closed. Open software provides the clinician with considerable freedom to work in the digital environment without being restricted to a single system. Information can be freely exchanged across different software platforms. A closed software system requires all team members to have access to a particular software package and may restrict the sharing of information or cause breaks in the digital workflow.

Open software also provides access to a comprehensive range of product files for different implant systems, including prosthetic components and anatomical crown forms, and the ability to produce a customized crown anatomy for the intended prosthetic design. Additionally,

the operator can control the prosthetic manufacturing process, selecting a centralized or localized production facility depending on requirements of the particular clinical case.

Most software packages offer solutions for a variety of user experience levels. Novice CAD/CAM users may require software with a "wizard" function so that they can produce restorations with minimal knowledge of the software package, while advanced users may prefer an advanced level of user control and the additional functions with the possibility for complete customization of different parameters.

Closed software can restrict the ability of the user to share and export different aspects of the digital process. Some companies offer further "add-ons" that may allow file formats to be exported to overcome these limitations. This limits users in their ability to create files that can be easily opened in different software packages, instead requiring the user to remain within the architecture of a single closed system.

4.1 Diagnostics and Data Collection

Treatment-planning software may enable the merging of facial scans, intraoral scans, clinical photographs, and radiographic data so that a "virtual" patient can be created. Digital Smile Design packages (Figs 2a-b) allow the clinician and the patient to preview treatment proposals for the replacement and restoration of the dentition prior to implementing active treatment. The clinician can then take note of, and potentially avoid, complications or areas of difficulty that might arise during treatment. Some planning software allows for a 2D reconstruction only, while others allow for 3D reconstruction (Coachman and coworkers 2016; Gimenez-Gonzalez and coworkers 2016). Importing color photographs of the existing clinical situation facilitates the graphical simulation of proposed changes, providing the patient with a clear idea of the final prosthetic plan. This can be a valuable communication tool for patients and clinicians.

Traditionally, a diagnostic wax-up of the prosthetic plan would be completed on a diagnostic stone cast. The diagnostic functionality within a software package allows for a "virtual wax-up" to be performed on a "virtual model" in the CAD software program. This information can then be merged with conventional photographs for a trial preview or linked to radiographic data for surgical planning.

One advantage of this digital procedure over conventional processes is that many different design proposals can be readily created by duplicating the design orders and that different treatment options can be previewed by both the patient and clinicians (Figs 2 to 6).

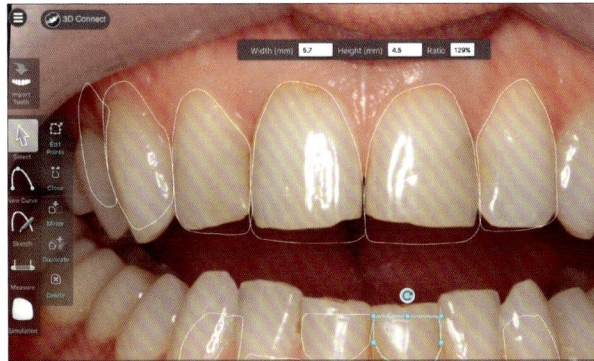

Fig 2a   Digital design.

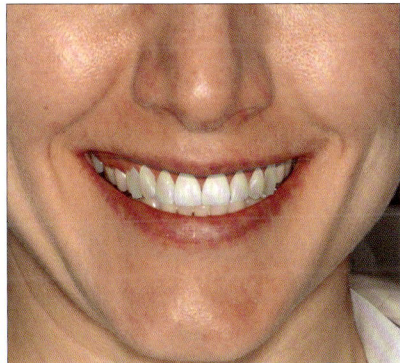

Fig 2b   Digital Smile design.

Figs 2a-b   Smile Designer Pro (Tasty Tech, Toronto/Ontario, Canada) tooth simulation.

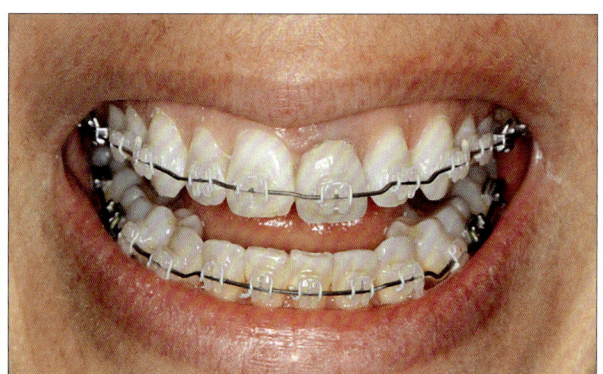

Fig 3   Failed tooth 21.

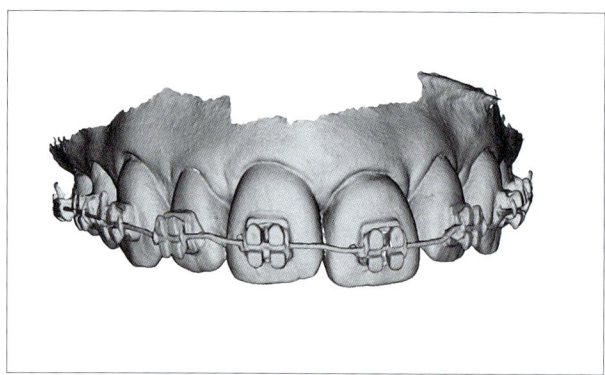

Fig 4   Surface scan.

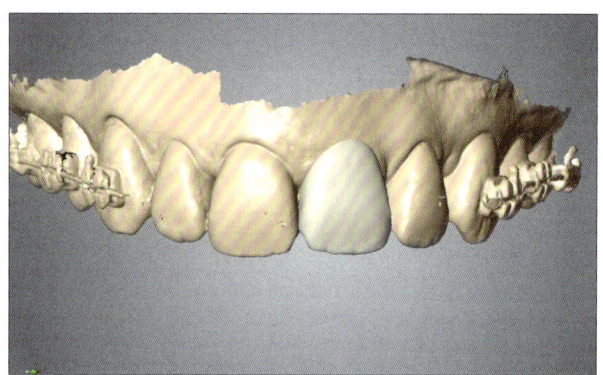

Fig 5   CAD design proposal after virtual extraction of tooth 21 and digital removal of the orthodontic archwire and brackets.

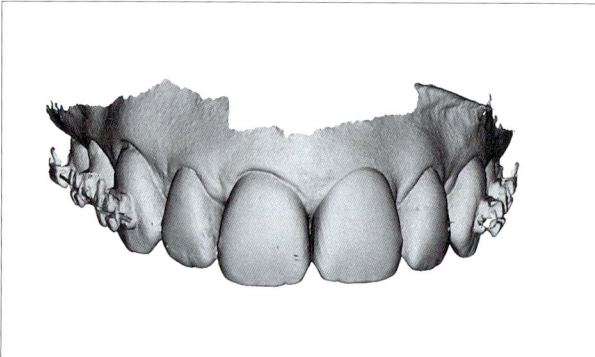

Fig 6   The exported STL can be used to produce a manual cast.

4.2 Prosthetic and Surgical Planning

Implant-planning software can merge radiographic data from a CT or cone-beam computed tomography (CBCT) scan with the surface scan of the intraoral situation. The standard radiographic data format is DICOM (Digital Imaging & Communications in Medicine). The standard surface-scan format is STL (originally an abbreviation for stereolithography, also known as Standard Tesselation Language).

The first step in this sequence is to correctly merge and align the two datasets within a software package to ensure optimal accuracy of the planning process (Figs 7a-b). The ability of the software to identify areas of similarity between the two datasets is critical in order to align and merge the CBCT scan data with the STL or surface scan data.

Artifacts, including motion artifacts and data loss from metallic restorations known as "beam hardening," may influence the quality of the CBCT scan. Such artifacts could prevent the identification of similar surfaces necessary for the accurate merging of the different file types. Appropriate segmentation of the CBCT scan is necessary for a clear identification of the areas of commonality. Segmentation is the formatting of the image to assign a "label" to every pixel in that image sharing a certain characteristic (such as grayscale value), thereby changing the image into something that is easier to analyze.

In cases of complete edentulism, radiographic (fiducial) markers such as prepared marker objects or radiopaque teeth located within a trial set-up are required, to serve as identifiable points on the acquired images so that the surface scan and CBCT data can be merged successfully. The extent of the field selected in the CBCT may also influence how successfully the data is merged.

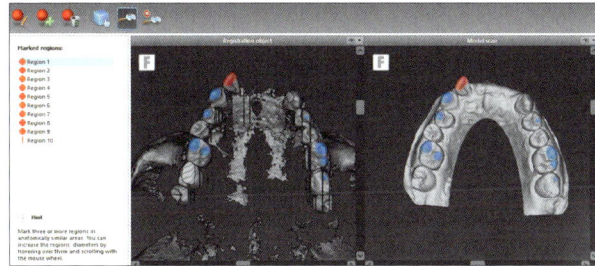

Fig 7a Selection and alignment of data points on the segmented CBCT with corresponding points on the surface scan in the coDiagnostiX software (Dental Wings, Montreal, Ottawa, Canada).

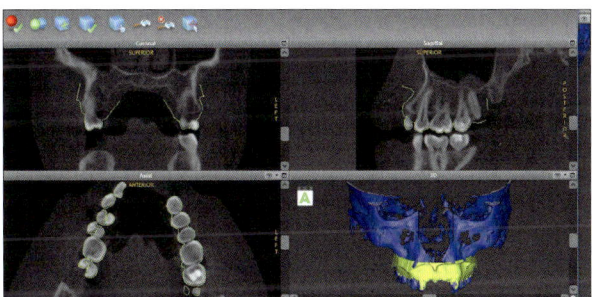

Fig 7b Alignment of the cast to the segmented DICOM from the CBCT in coDiagnostiX.

A limited field of view CBCT may provide insufficient data points for successful merging of the CBCT with the surface scan, particularly if there is an artefact on the CBCT from metallic objects. CBCT segmentation to separate the arches assists in correctly locating the images. The ability to fine-tune the alignment of datasets without relying solely on automatic registration points is a desirable feature of a software package.

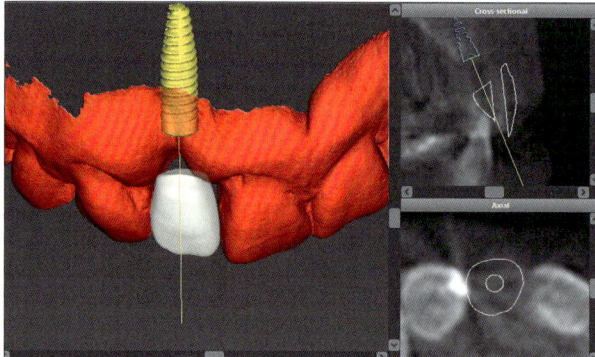

Figs 8 and 9   Stock tooth shapes in coDiagnostiX shown on the CBCT and surface scan.

As always in dental implant therapy, the treatment planning process is restorative-driven. The prime consideration is the correct positioning of the necessary replacement teeth.

Following successful alignment of the surface scan to the CBCT dataset, the software will need to allow the import the restorative plan including the replacement tooth and soft tissue form. There are three options for developing the restorative solution:

- Stock tooth form
- Custom CAD design
- Importing a clinical tooth position from a diagnostic set-up

4.2.1   Stock Tooth Shapes

Following successful alignment of the surface scan to the CBCT dataset, a stock tooth shape is imported from a library incorporated into the software (Figs 8 and 9). This option provides a simple and rapid solution for creating a basic prosthetic plan, which can then be used to produce the surgical plan. There are limited options for the development of customized gingival formers or healing abutments, and the prefabrication of abutments or provisional restorations for immediate loading is not possible.

4.2.2   Custom CAD

The clinician or dental technician will create a comprehensive virtual diagnostic tooth set-up using CAD software, having imported a surface scan and aligned this with the CBCT dataset of the clinical situation. A comprehensive prosthetic design proposal can be produced in the CAD software that accommodates the correct occlusal relationship and three-dimensional tooth positions, creating a dataset that is greater than the simple sum of its parts (Figs 10 to 13).

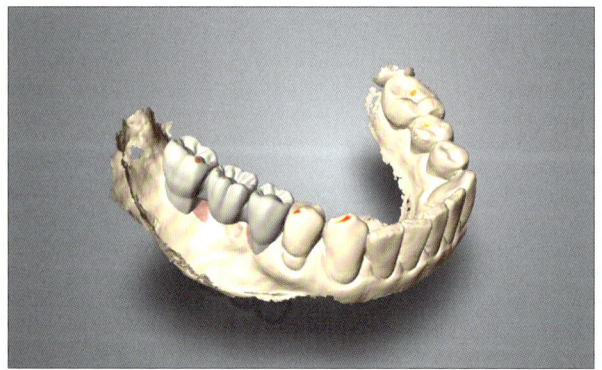

Fig 10   Surface scan with CAD.

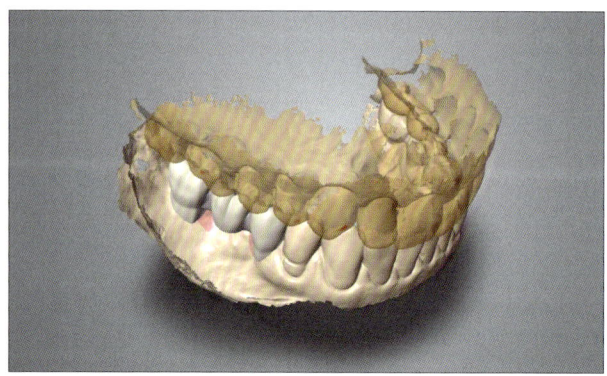

Fig 11   Occlusion verified.

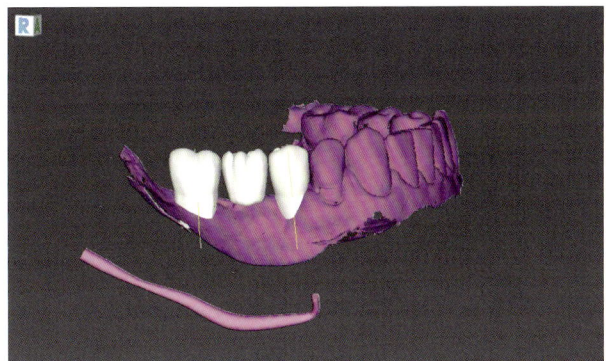

Fig 12   Synergistic transfer to CoDiagnostiX.

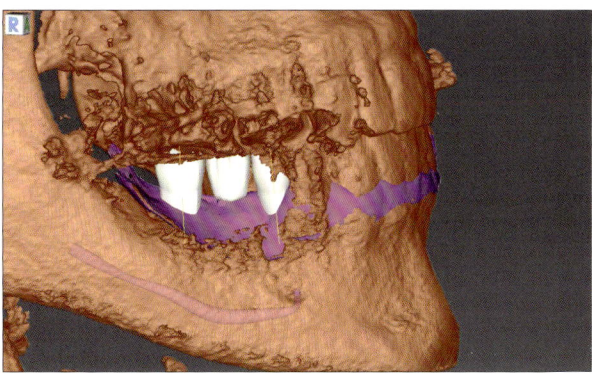

Fig 13   Final planning and the CBCT.

Using a synergistic function, the coDiagnostiX (Dental Wings, Montreal, Ottawa, Canada) software is able to merge the intended tooth and appropriate implant positions; once completed, it is also possible to design the development of the ideal implant position. If required, customized healing abutments or prosthetic components can then be manufactured from this design prior to implant surgery.

A final surgical plan can be developed and printed for reference by the surgical team (Fig 14).

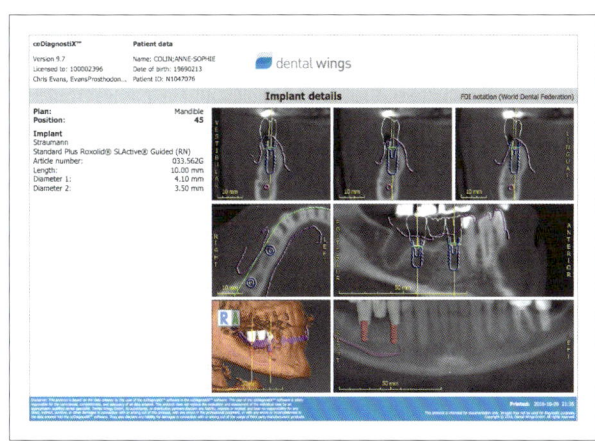

Fig 14   Final surgical plan.

4.2.3   Importing a Clinical Tooth Position from a Diagnostic Set-Up

This option uses a multi-point alignment function within the software successfully merge multiple datasets within one treatment plan. In this case, a surface scan of a physical diagnostic wax-up is imported and aligned using the same processes described above. Multiple layers representing multiple datasets are then created within the software to facilitate treatment planning.

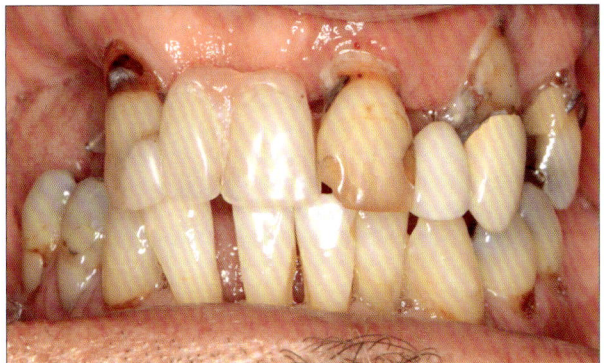

Fig 15   Failing dentition.

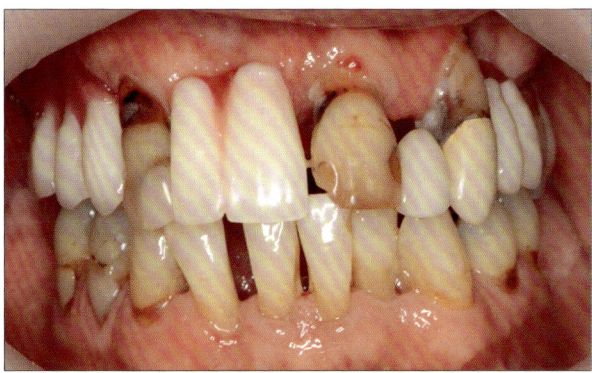

Fig 16   Diagnostic set-up try-in.

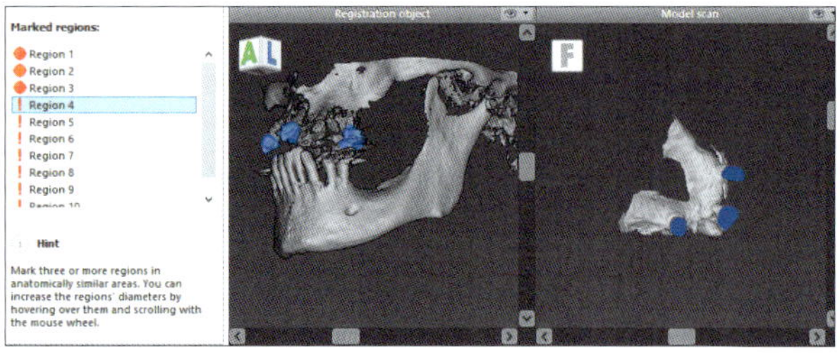

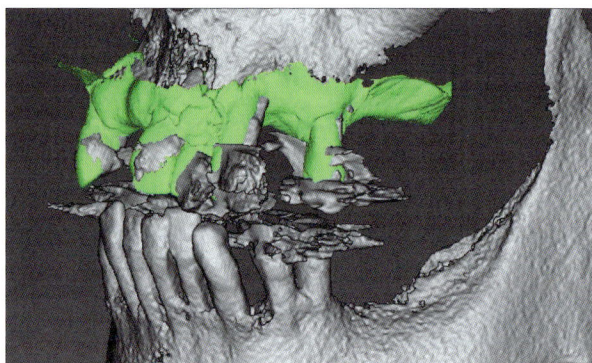

Fig 17   Merging data.

This planning process will allow all team members to view the treatment proposal in detail, even on mobile devices via cloud integration, so that the plan can be fully evaluated before treatment commences (Figs 15 to 20). On completion of the planning process, the surgical documentation can be printed for dissemination to the treatment team, as well as for ordering the required components.

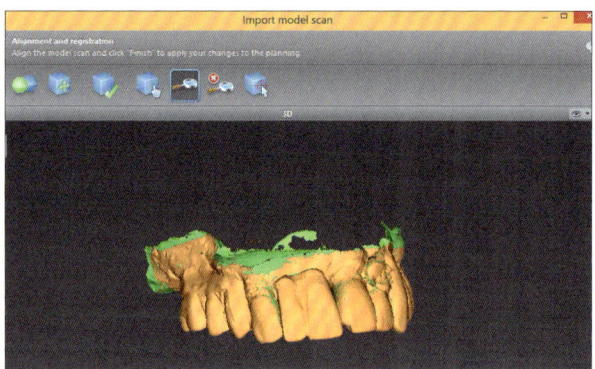

Fig 18   Alignment of surface scan.

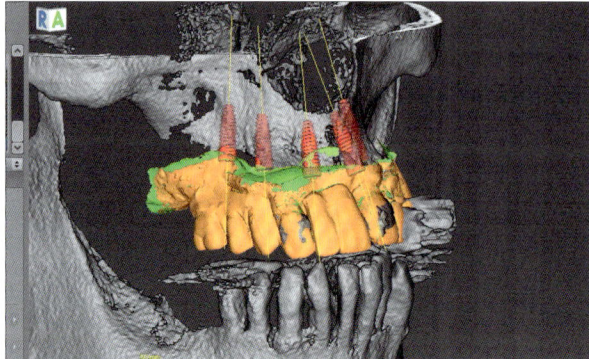

Fig 19   Alignment of wax-up with surface scan.

Fig 20   Implant planning according to the diagnostic set-up.

4.3 Computer-Assisted Design (CAD)

CAD software allows for the final prosthesis to be designed virtually. The entire process is covered, from the diagnostic set-up to the final design for simple or complex, fixed or removable prostheses. The software uses specific design parameters to control the manufacturing tolerance within the system. Angulations of implant positions, abutment shapes, and contours can be individually customized. A preloaded selection of stock tooth shapes is provided in the library; many of these shapes are based on existing denture-tooth morphologies available for commercial use. The software also facilitates the development of custom tooth shapes and anatomies that the dentist or dental technician may prefer.

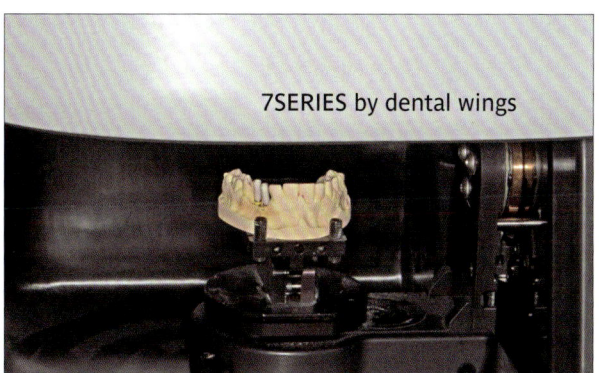

Fig 21   Working cast in a laboratory scanner.

4.3.1   Final Prosthetic Design

The function of the software is to take the reconstructed surface scan, which can be an intraoral scan or a scan of a physical model constructed from an analog impression, and accurately position the virtual dental implant within the dataset.

It is important that the correct scanbody library be referenced in the software set-up to ensure correct and accurate replication and meshing of the geometry. The design steps are similar, irrespective of whether an intraoral scan or a laboratory scan of a cast is used. The complete contour of the scanbody must be clearly shown in the surface scan for the software to accurately identify the scanbody location; missing data on the scanbody outline will limit the accuracy of the merging process. Deeply placed or extremely divergent implants can influence the ability of the software to correctly identify the scanbody and hence the true implant position or alignment (Flügge and coworkers 2016; Gimenez-Gonzalez and coworkers 2016). It is important to use scanbodies that are compatible with the software interface. Failure to do so may prevent the software from recognizing the scanbody geometry (Figs 21 to 25).

The design process should allow complete customization of the emergence contour from the implant shoulder. The material parameters encoded into the software will prevent inadvertent over-reduction of the material in the design process, which can create points of premature failure (Figs 26 and 27).

Abutment contours and parallelism can be carefully controlled, and it is easy to configure the addition or removal of the layers of information on the screen for a clear visualization of the design parameters (Figs 28 and 29). Cross-sectional views can be made to ensure material thickness requirements are satisfied (Fig 30).

One clear advantage of the digital workflow for restoring implants in the esthetic zone is the ability of the software to duplicate or match restoration contours simply, rapidly, and precisely. Subgingival contours established by provisional restorations can be readily duplicated and copied to the final restorative design, ensuring that the final restoration closely matches a provisional previously shown to provide adequate peri-implant mucosal support (Figs 31 to 37).

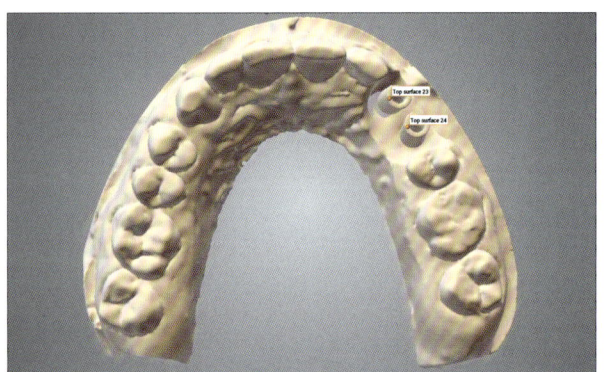

Fig 22   Scanned working cast with implants.

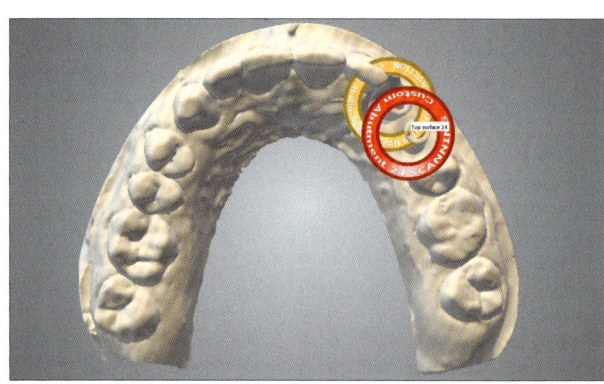

Fig 23   Implant positioning in the software.

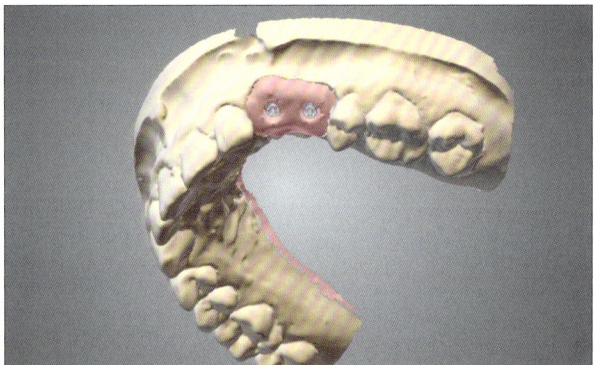

Fig 24   Scanned working cast.

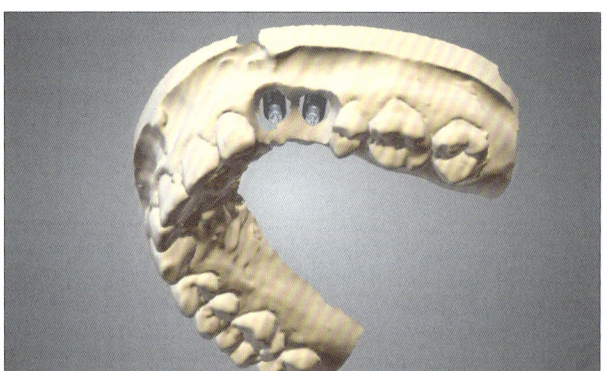

Fig 25   Soft-tissue layer removed from the scan.

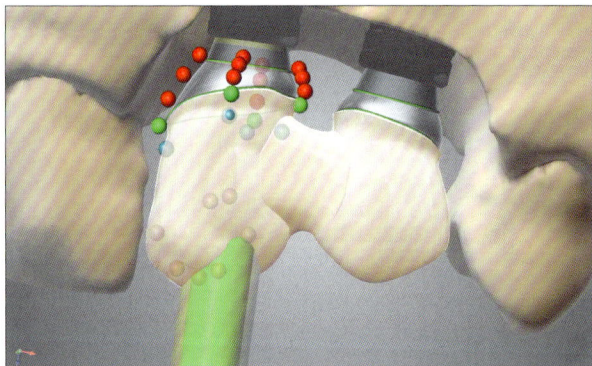

Figs 26 and 27   The contours of an abutment can be modified by moving the circular node. Different colors are used to represent different positions on the restoration.

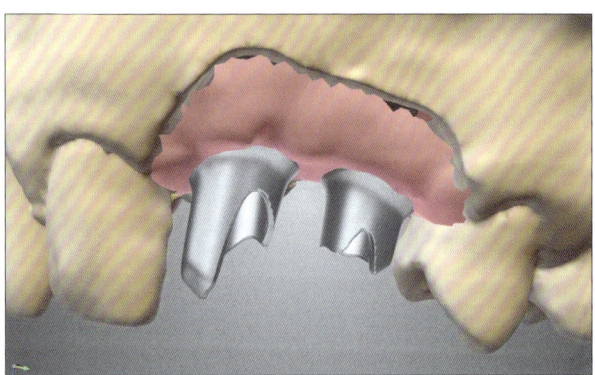

Fig 28   Abutment parallelism.

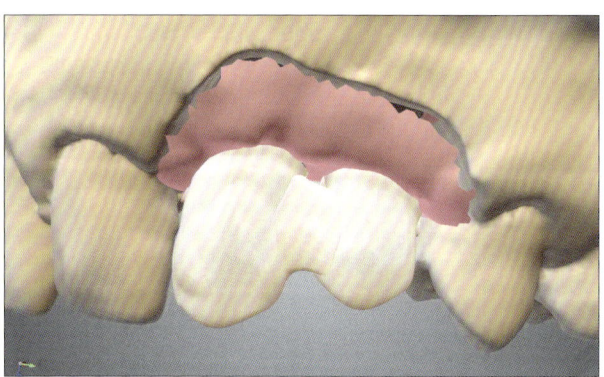

Fig 29   Framework layer added.

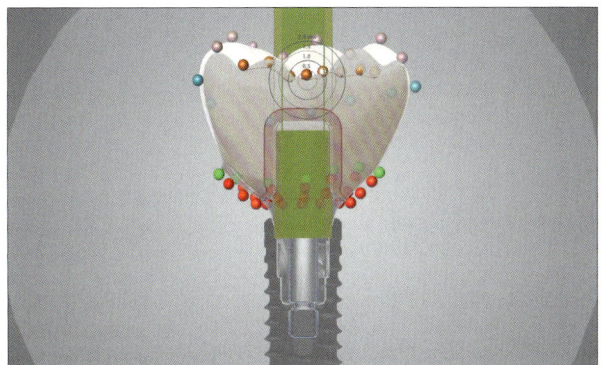

Fig 30   Implant cross-section.

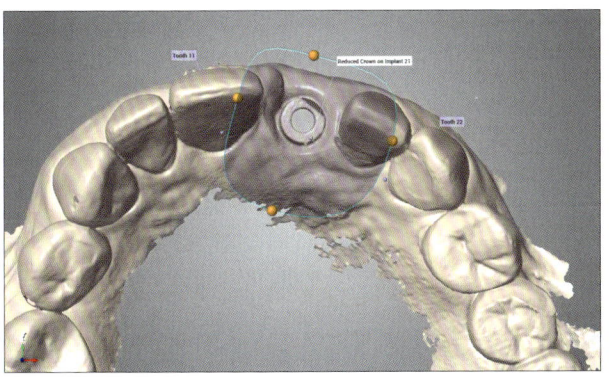

Fig 31   Intraoral scan.

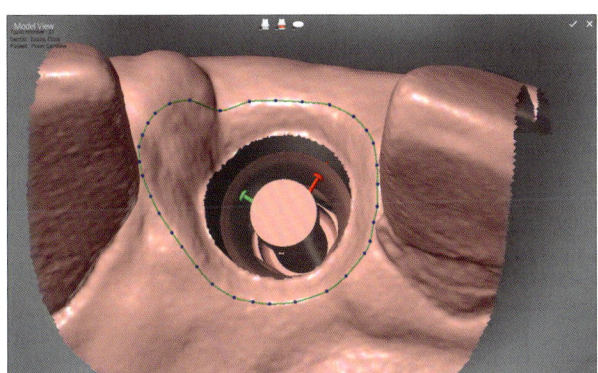

Fig 32   Specifying the mucosal contour of the restoration on the scan.

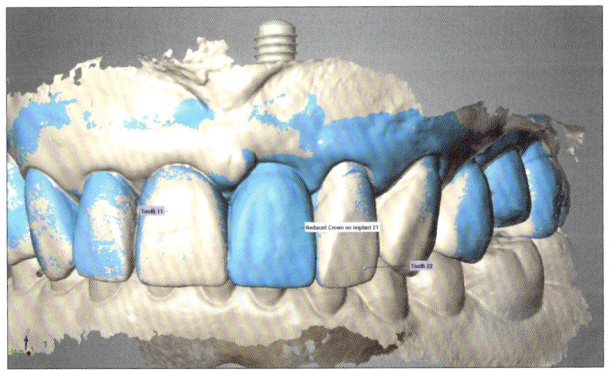

Fig 33   Superimposition of the diagnostic provisional restoration on the scan.

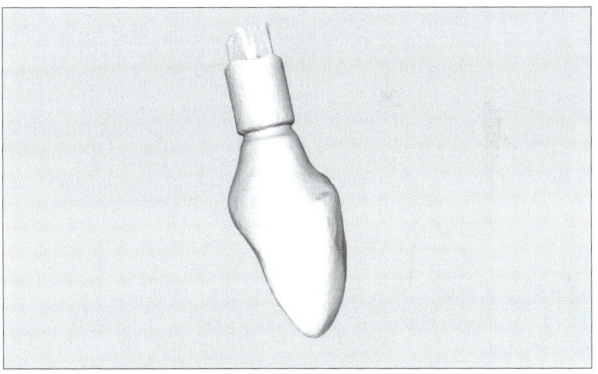

Fig 34   Scan of an implant-supported provisional.

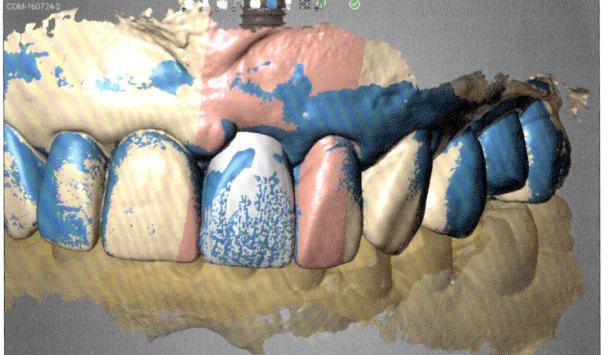

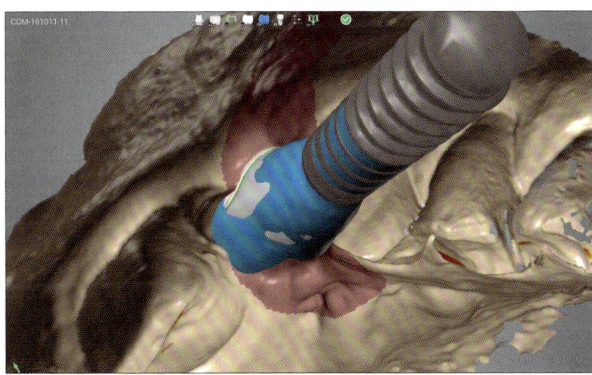

Figs 35 and 36   Adapting the restoration to the provisional restoration.

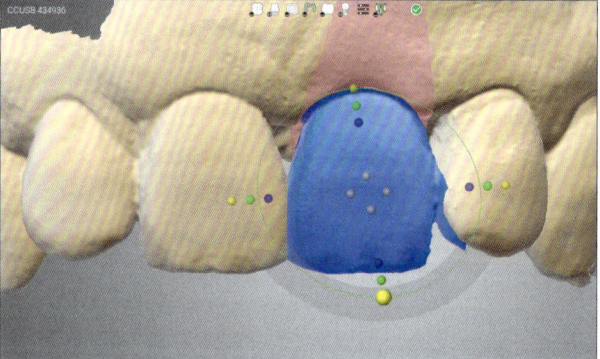

Fig 37   *Verification of the implant position and cross-section.*

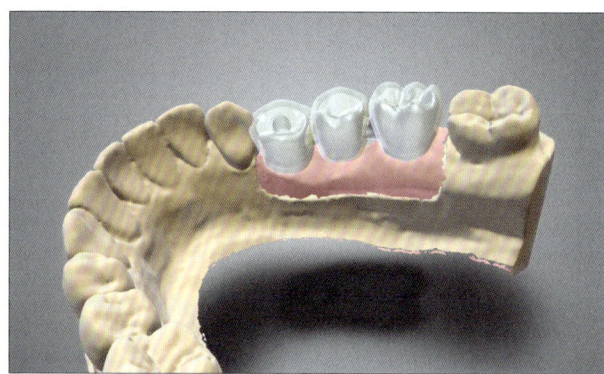

Fig 38   *Full-contour design.*

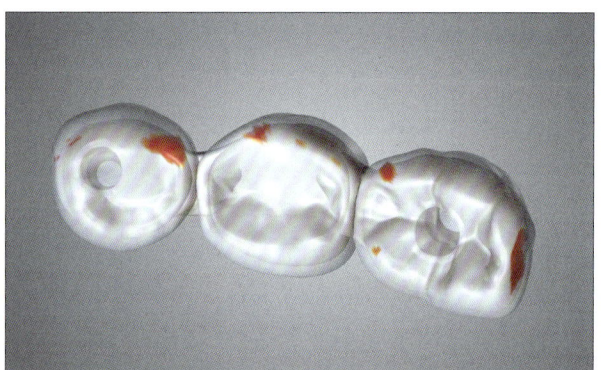

Fig 39   *Final design.*

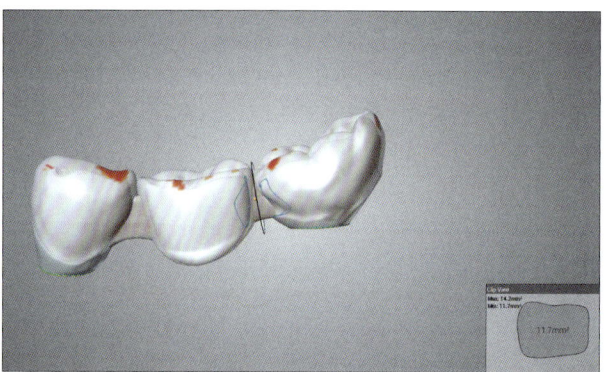

Fig 40   *Verifying the connector thickness.*

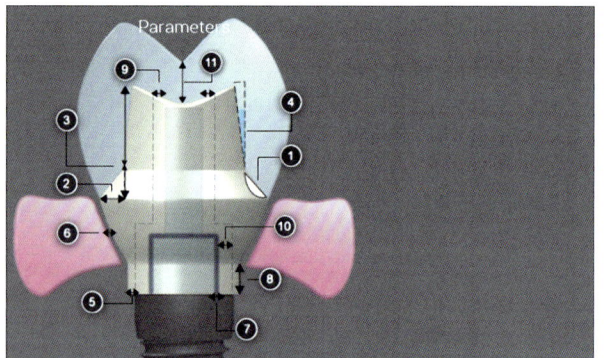

Fig 41   *Full range of possible abutment adaptations.*

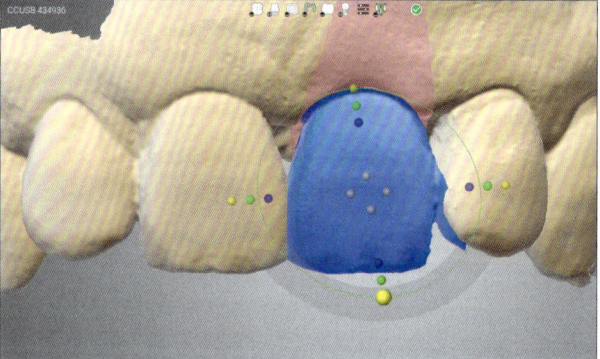

Fig 42   *Tooth 21 anatomy mirrored on tooth 11.*

A further advantage of CAD design software for the production of an implant-supported prosthesis is that the restoration is designed to full contour (Figs 38 and 39). If the design is cut back by the technician for application of veneering materials, this can be done to ensure an appropriate uniform thickness over the entire prosthesis, ensuring adequate support for veneering ceramic, for example. Furthermore, connector thicknesses can be calculated and confirmed as adequate for preventing material failure under functional load (Fig 40).

Abutment design parameters can be carefully controlled and customized to suit the clinical situation (Fig 41). The anatomy of the contralateral teeth can be copied and mirrored to produce symmetrical tooth forms (Fig 42).

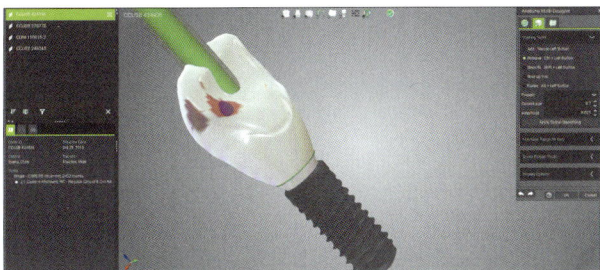

Fig 43 Opposing tooth indicated by red contact marks on the lingual aspect.

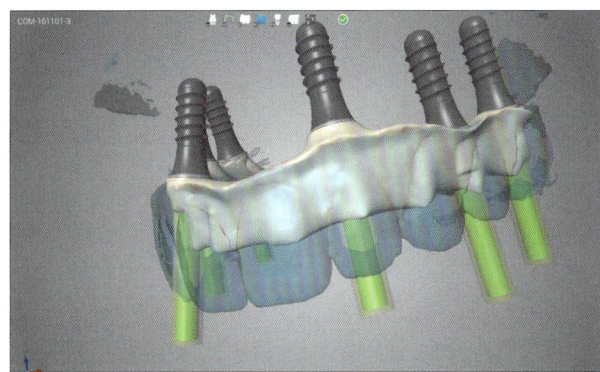

Fig 44 Full-arch reconstruction in CAD software with the final tooth position used to develop the framework design.

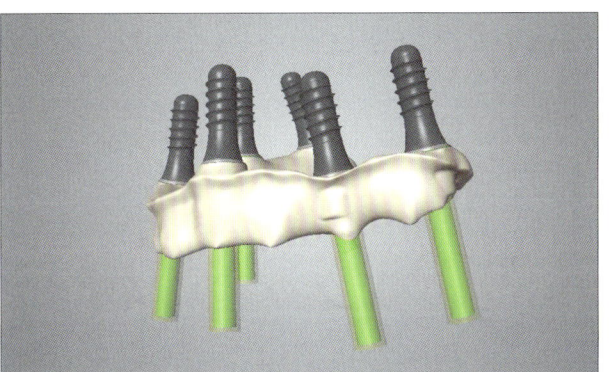

Fig 45 Framework contours.

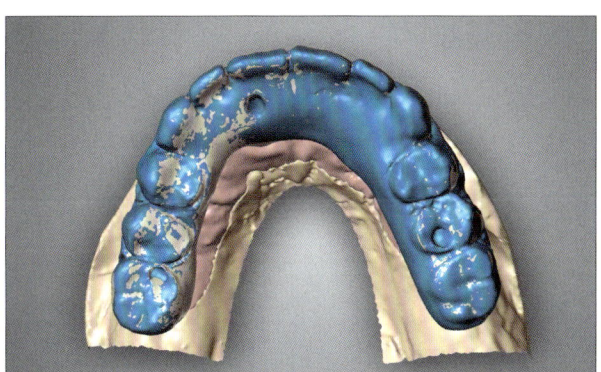

Fig 46 Final tooth position used to adapt the final contour of the restoration (occlusal view).

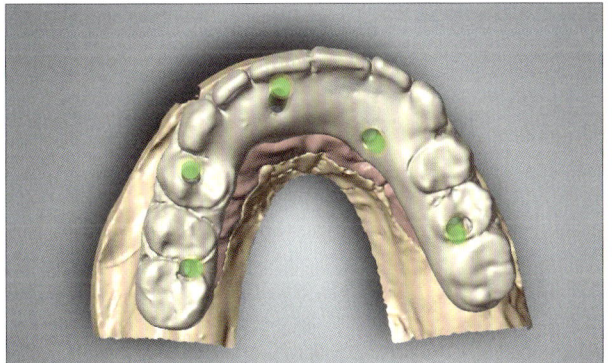

Fig 47 Final contour of the restoration form with the final tooth position layer removed (occlusal view).

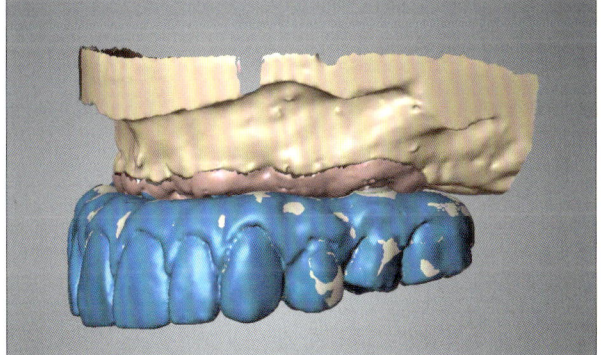

Fig 48 Final tooth position used to adapt the final contour of the restoration (lateral view).

Mirroring of adjacent tooth morphology or morphing the final contour to a diagnostic set-up as required allows complete customization of the final prosthesis (Fig 43). Adaptation of the final occlusal form can be viewed in animations of excursive jaw movements and the extent and degree of occlusal contact can be readily viewed.

Frameworks for full-arch restorations can be designed to completely support the overlying restorative material in a stock frame design or a fully customized design, based on the adaptation of the approved final tooth position (Figs 44 to 50).

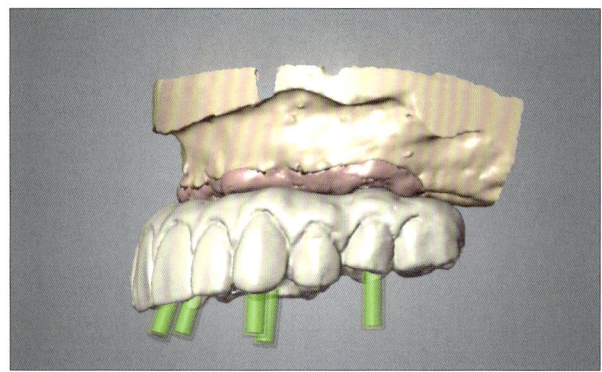

Fig 49   Final contour of the restoration form with the final tooth-position layer removed (lateral view).

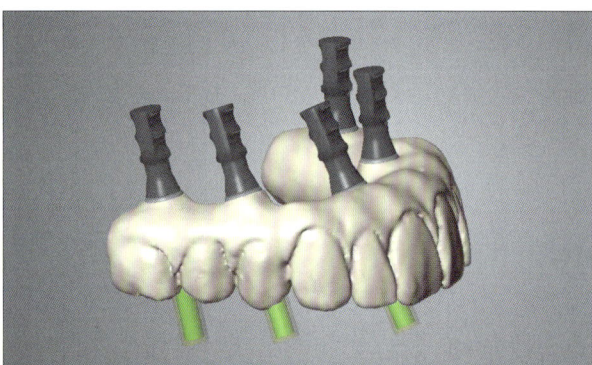

Fig 50   Final contour of the restoration form with the final tooth-position layer and virtual cast removed (lateral view).

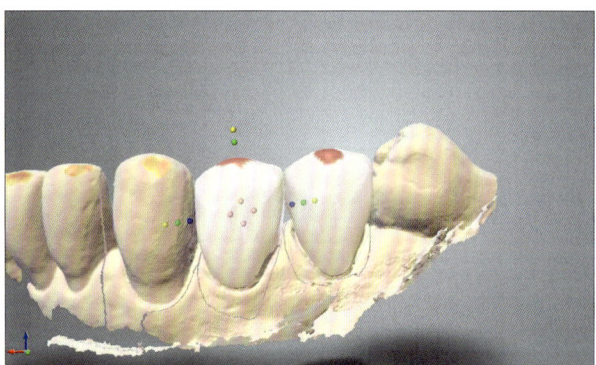

Fig 51   Occlusal contact intensity seen in yellow on the natural teeth and in red on the prosthesis indicating a restoration which is high in contact—the form should be adjusted until the contact color matches that on the natural teeth.

Occlusal and proximal surface contacts can be carefully adjusted using different tools within the software to smooth, add, or remove forms, similar to the way in which the dental technician manipulates dental wax in a manual wax-up (Fig 51).

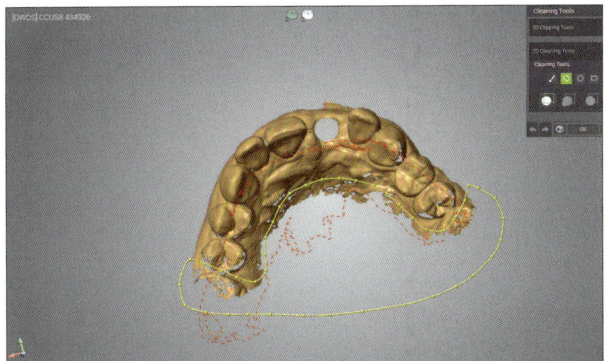

Fig 52   Surface scan area to be cleaned up using the selection tool.

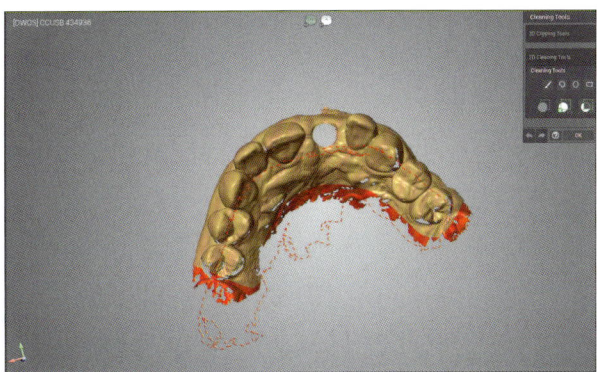

Fig 53   Area in red highlighted ready to be deleted.

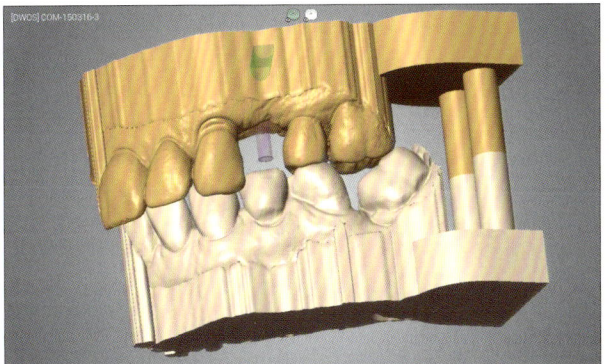

Fig 54   Articulator interface added to the virtual model.

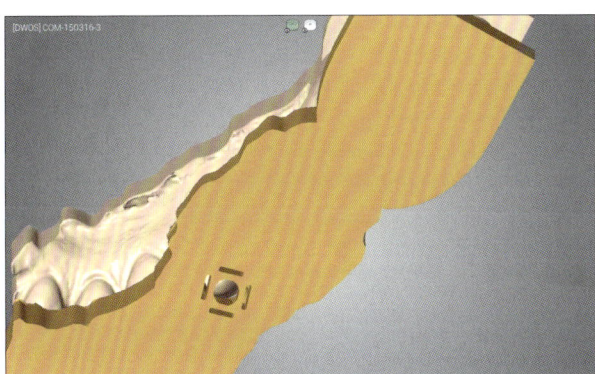

Fig 55   Repositionable analog pin hole inserted in the virtual model.

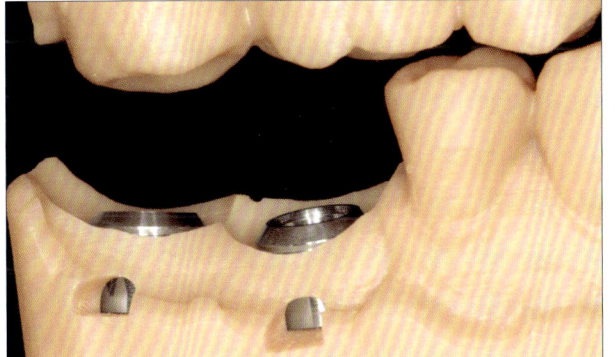

Fig 56   Reposition analogs inserted with viewing windows to confirm full seating within the model.

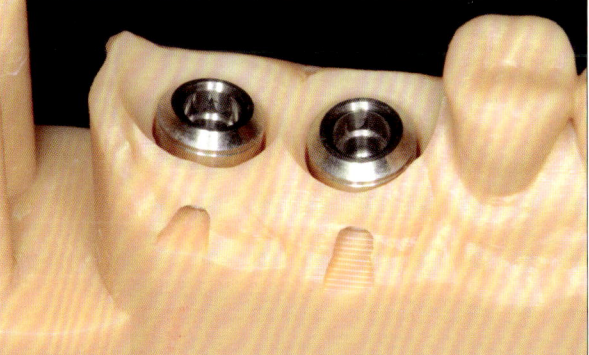

Fig 57   Contour of the model emerging from the implant shoulder matched to that of the restoration.

4.3.2   Model-Building

Model-building functions are used to design virtual models that can be printed or milled. The surface scan is cleaned to delete any unnecessary scan areas (Figs 52 and 53). A wide variety of articulator interfaces can be accommodated and the height and alignment of the model controlled to produce a replica similar to what the dental technician is used to working with (Fig 54). The software allows for a variety of implant analog replicas to be virtually positioned within the model. Unlike conventional implant replicas, which are immobile when poured in dental stone, these virtual analogs are repositionable. Viewing windows are created within the physical model to ensure that the analogs are fully seated (Figs 55 to 56).

Any emergence contour developed in the restoration during the CAD process will be automatically transferred to the model (Fig 57).

4.4 Computer-Assisted Manufacturing (CAM)

The last stage in the production of the final prosthesis is the milling process. Dental technicians can enlist the services of a centralized milling facility, using the export function of the software. Either a direct transfer or an "export and share" function can be set up such that data are seamlessly transferred directly to the milling facility. Specific milling tolerances are incorporated within the software packages, which need to be matched and calibrated with the selected milling machine to ensure the accuracy of the process.

4.5 Concluding Remarks

As with all computer systems, the software used in the digital workflow will need constant updates as further advances and changes are made by the developers. New functions may be added during each progressive update.

- Different software packages are often required to complete various stages of the digital workflow.
- These software packages need to be compatible so they can be used seamlessly throughout the entire digital workflow.

- Each software package should have the capacity to work on a variety of implant types, as well as the option to export digital information in the necessary file formats.
- Clinicians must be prepared to undergo continual training and learning, as the functionality of the software will likely change with every update.

5 Merging Digital Datasets

G.O. Gallucci, B. Friedland, A. Hamilton

This chapter reviews the merging of different digital files to reconstruct the orofacial anatomical structure in a virtual environment. The merging of files (digital data sets) is necessary because several digital files need to be compiled and accurately matched to create a virtual patient.

The accuracy of this matching process, which is explained in detail in this chapter, is of paramount importance to ensure that no accuracy is lost as the transition from virtual to analog is later performed to fabricate and deliver the prosthesis.

In the virtual environment, the operator will plan the implant position(s), design a surgical template for guided implant surgery, and design/manufacture the prosthetic elements for clinical delivery. All this digital work occurs on, and across, several matched files.

However, the digitally designed guides or prosthetic elements are based on digital files obtained from IOS (intraoral surface scanners) or EOS (extraoral surface scanners) as positional references. Thus, the clinical accuracy of the digitally fabricated elements will completely depend on the precision of the file-merging process in the digital environment.

5.1 Scanning Technologies and Related Datasets

Several techniques are used to scan different orofacial anatomical structures. This is in part due to the technology used for digitization, which results in a variety of file formats. Chapter 2 describes in detail the principle of intraoral and extraoral surface scanners (IOS and EOS) and how they produce a detailed rendering of the scanned object surface (Fig 1).

However, IOS/EOS scans do not provide volumetric information but only the surface characteristic of the scanned object; hence the name "surface scanner." For instance, when a surface scan is observed from its internal aspect, the reconstructed image appears hollow, or empty. The "external" view displays the full details of the scanned surface, whereas the "internal" aspect lacks definition (Figs 2a-b).

Consequently, a surface scan does not provide any information regarding the underlying anatomy that is required for planning implant placement. Thus, surface scanners need to be matched with DICOM files obtained from a CBCT.

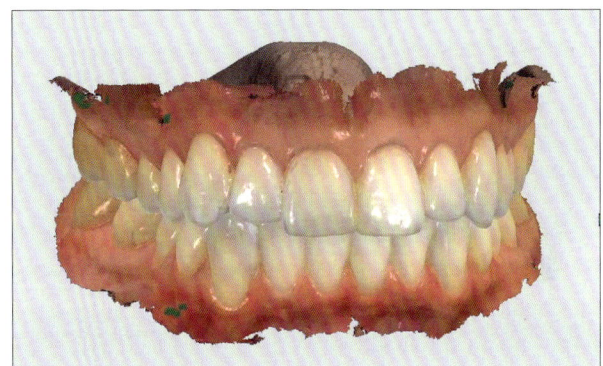

Fig 1   IOS scan with color rendering.

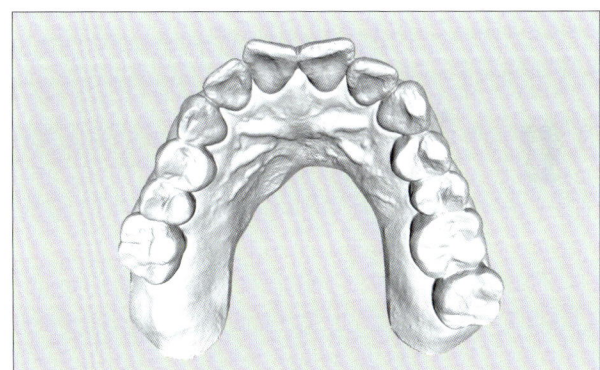

Fig 2a   "External" view of a maxillary surface scan.

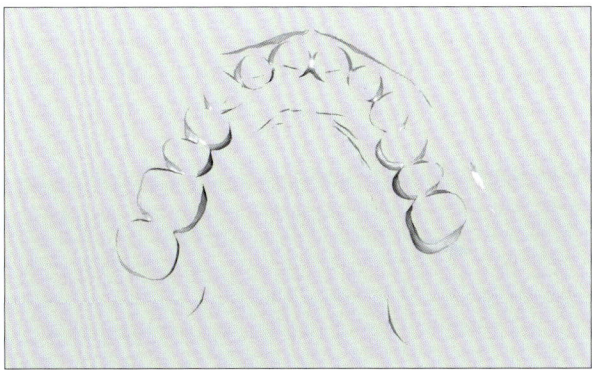

Fig 2b   "Internal" view of the same scan.

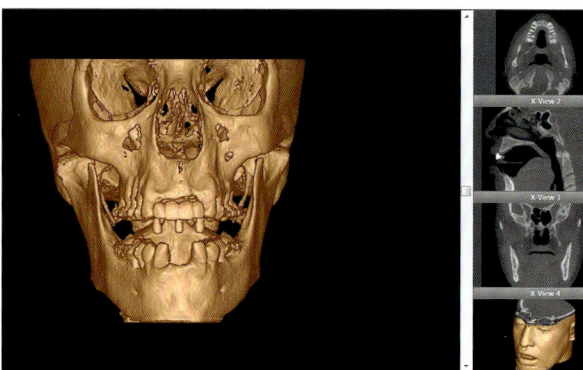

Fig 3   *CBCT 3D rendering with different view planes.*

Cone-beam computed tomography (CBCT) scans produce 2D image slices of the patient, which can then be displayed individually or as a stack to generate a 3D image. The surface definition of CBCT scans is not as precise as that obtained with a surface scanner, which is why CBCT DICOM files should be merged with files from surface scanners (Fig 3). CBCT scans produce volumetric data of the skeletal structure of the region of interest. CBCT data contain voxels (three-dimensional data bits), as opposed to the pixels (two-dimensional data bits) of the surface scan. Consequently, a digital image of the volume and the three-dimensional shape of the underlying bony structure is rendered and can be manipulated by the viewing software (Fig 3).

Unlike surface scans, CBCT uses ionizing radiation. Whereas the total radiation exposure during dental CBCT is generally lower that with other types of computed tomographic imaging, at least where limited fields of view are employed, dental CBCT examinations normally involve significantly higher radiation doses to patients than plain radiography. In this context, careful consideration should be given to avoiding repeated or unnecessary exposure by careful planning and by considering the risk and benefits of CBCT scans.

CBCT has displaced the use of medical CT in implant dentistry because CBCT units are less expensive, expose patients to less radiation, and are more compact, allowing for in-house use in a dental office. However, there are several factors to consider when a CBCT scan is to be used for planning as part of a digital implant workflow.

5.2 Accuracy of CBCT Scans

The accuracy of CBCT scans is important to clinicians in the diagnosis and preoperative planning for implant surgery. In the absence of confounding factors, the deviation of a CBCT scan is at least one voxel (0.3 mm³) according to the 5th ITI Consensus Conference (Focas 2018). It seems unlikely that this deviation would compromise the safety or efficacy of virtual implant planning or guided implant surgery. However, this known variation should be accounted for during the presurgical diagnostic planning. In this context, resolution is a key parameter for CBCT image quality.

Resolution refers to the ability of a CBCT scan to differentiate two objects and to reproduce fine details of the object being studied. The resolution of CBCT images is lower than that of intraoral radiographs. Several factors can affect the quality of a CBCT scan, such as changes in the angulation of the patient's head, movement artifacts, scatter, the reconstruction algorithm employed, voxel size, radiation exposure, and other factors.

5.3 Field of View (FoV)

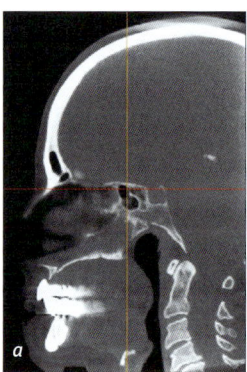

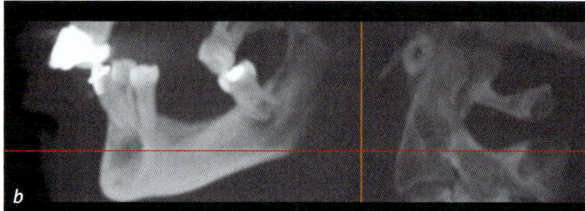

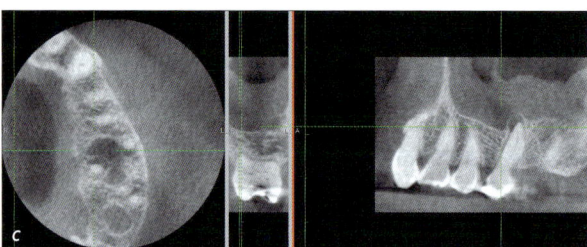

The radiological field of view is the volume of interest selected for imaging. A FoV can be set to different sizes to capture the desired anatomical structures. This can vary from the size of a single tooth to the size of the skull (Figs 4a-c). A larger FoV means a higher radiation exposure. While the use of CBCT is only lightly regulated in some countries, in others (including EU countries), the risks and benefits of the exposure are carefully assessed, and recommended practices include restricting FoV and voxel size to reduce the total radiation exposure of the patient. However, for dataset merging, a medium-size FoV (jaw-sized) is recommended. A smaller FoV (quadrant-sized) is not recommended due to the reduced surface area for dataset merging, which may lead to inaccuracies. When CBCT and surface scan data are merged, it is advisable to include the entire jaw in the CBCT scan to ensure sufficient data points can be matched and used to merge the images. Consequently, digital procedures may involve higher radiation doses than conventional procedures.

Figs 4a-c   Different FoV sizes. Large FoV—skull-sized. Significant radiation exposure of sensitive structures (a). Medium FoV—jaw-sized (b). Small FoV—quadrant-sized (c).

5.4 Beam Hardening and Scatter

Beam hardening and scatter (Fig 5) are mechanisms that both produce artifacts in the form of dark streaks between two high-attenuation objects, such as metal and bone. These mechanisms also result in bright streaks seen adjacent to the dark streaks (Boas and Fleischmann 2012). In the oral cavity, high-attenuation objects include metal (e.g. amalgam, crowns with metal, posts) and some non-metallic objects (such as gutta-percha or endodontic sealers). Scatter on a CBCT scan directly affects the trueness of the scanned object. When a CBCT scan is taken, it may be helpful to separate the maxilla from the mandible with a wax rim or other non-attenuating material to minimize or avoid scatter from the opposing arch. The reduction of imaging artifacts is a key factor in merging datasets, as the images of the teeth are normally used for merging proposes. The presence of scatter may cause inaccuracies within the file-merging process, jeopardizing the clinical outcome.

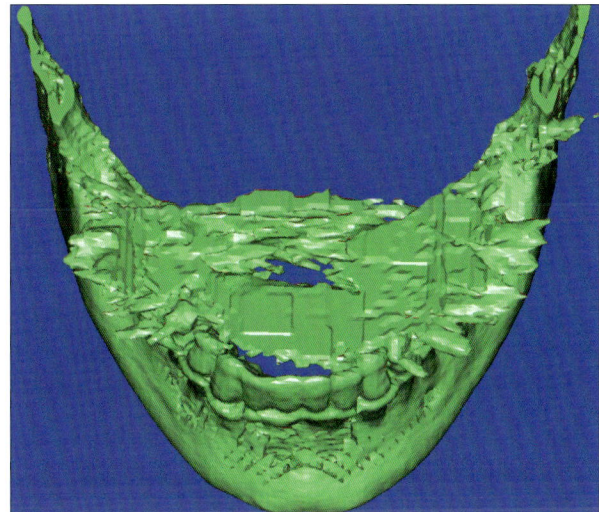

Fig 5   Mandibular CBCT with significant scatter on the occlusal surface.

5.5   Preparation a Patient for a CBCT Scan

It is recognized that errors can accumulate in the course of a digital workflow process, just as they may in conventional workflows. An effort should therefore be made to reduce errors at each step of the process—this is particularly important when taking a CBCT scan, since ionizing radiation is used.

The preparation of the patient for a CBCT scan should include the visualization of the prosthodontic planning. Radiographic templates or intraoral markers should be worn during the acquisition of the CBCT image. The separation of the upper and lower jaws should be ensured in order to minimize or avoid the "spreading" of imaging artifacts from one jaw to the other. A cotton roll placed in the vestibular area helps separate the lips and cheeks from the dentoalveolar complex, potentially improving the quality of the CBCT images.

5.6 Merging Files

When it comes to digital planning in implant prosthodontics, the image properties offered by surface scanners and CBCT are both necessary to provide complete information of the area of interest. However, these two types of 3D images result in different file formats. Thus, most implant-planning software allows for the merging of DICOM and STL files.

This process is very simple to achieve and provides a complete 3D rendering of the field of interest in terms of both surface and volume (Figs 6a-b).

5.6.1 Merging Datasets Using Common Anatomical Structures

DICOM and STL files are usually merged using implant-planning software, although some CAD/CAM software may also offer this feature. Specific details of the actual process may vary according to particular software used, but the general principles are similar.

First, the DICOM dataset is imported, segmented and aligned. Segmentation is the process of segmenting or partitioning a digital image for the purpose of identifying the boundaries of one type of tissue from that of another, for example, bone from gingiva (Mansoor and coworkers 2015).

Next, the STL file is imported into the same software. In the process shown in Fig 7, the operator uses the tooth morphology to identify and mark clearly identifiable regions in both files to guide the merging process. It is recommended to spread the distribution of merging points bilaterally over four areas. Some software packages offer an automatic recognition feature. The system then employs a "best match" algorithm to merge the DICOM and STL files into a new dataset.

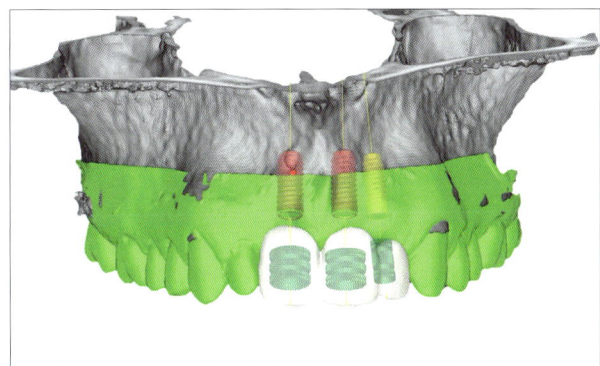

Fig 6a   3D Rendering of merged DICOM (gray) and STL (green) data.

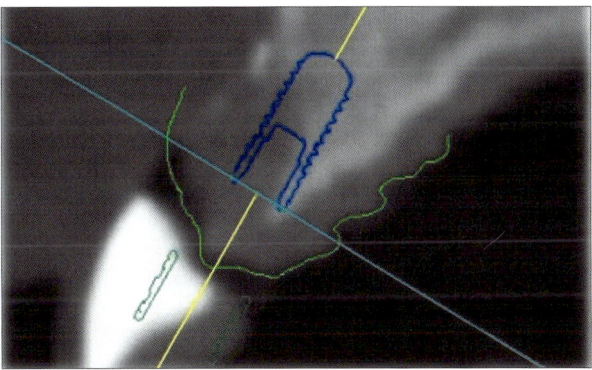

Fig 6b   Sagittal view of merged files.

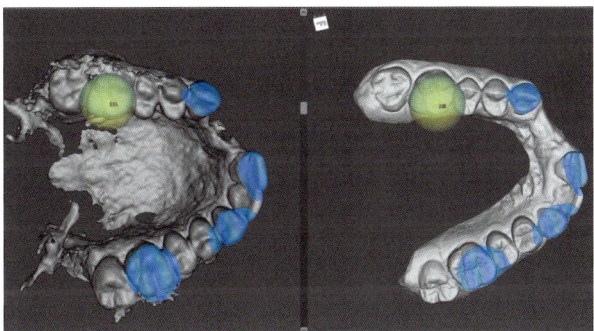

Fig 7   Merging process in the planning software displaying the DICOM (left) and the STL (right) files. Blue: Marked files. Green: Areas selected to indicate the matching areas for the software.

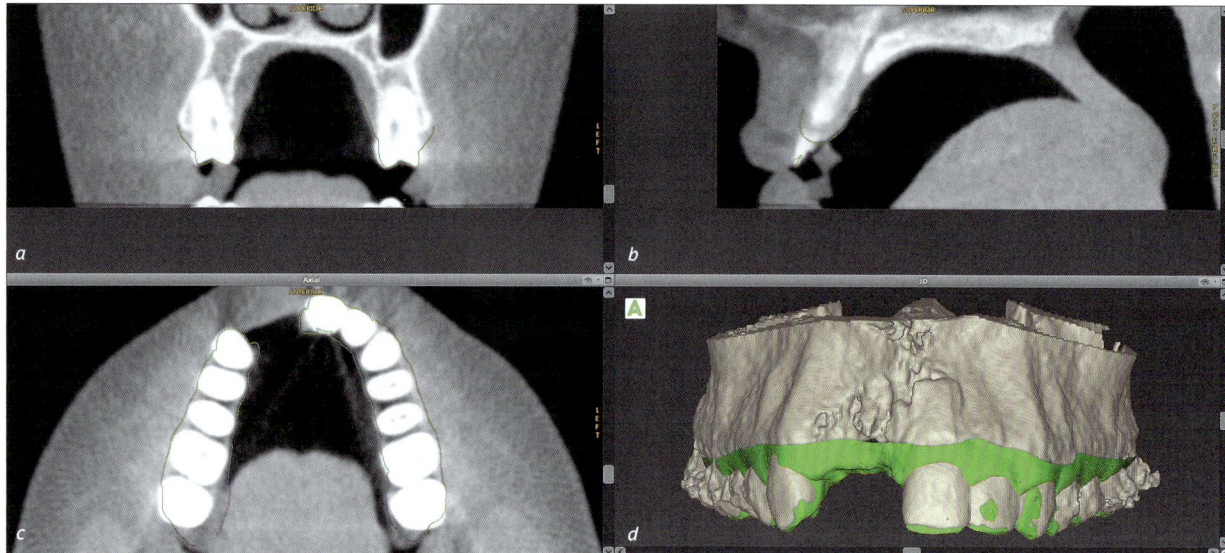

Figs 8a-d   Different views where the accuracy of the match can be verified in all planes.

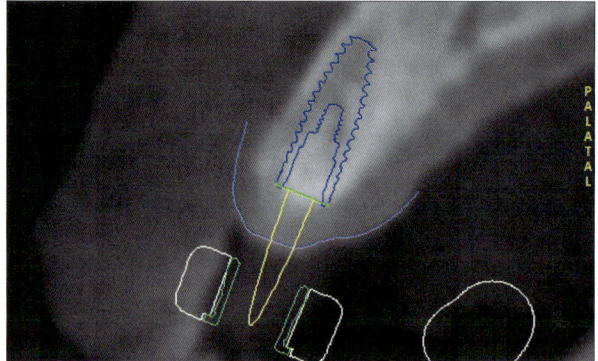

Fig 9   Sagittal view of the merged DICOM and STL files, virtual implant planning and the digital design of the surgical guide and sleeve in place. Gray: CBCT. Blue: Virtual implant. Light Blue: STL merged. Green: Guide sleeve. White: Surgical guide design.

Once the initial matching is completed, most software provides for user validation of the merging process and provides the opportunity for manual adjustments. In the validation window, the operator can scroll across the matched files to assess and validate the accuracy of merging (Figs 8a-d). At this point, manual adjustments can be made to ensure a precise match.

The accuracy of the match (alignment) between DICOM and STL files has direct clinical implications. During the implant planning, the implant position is based on the information obtained from the merged files (Fig 9). The operator will set the implant position based on the anatomical volume provided by the DICOM dataset and the tooth setup/soft tissue outline provided by the STL file.

Once the implant position is established, the next step is the fabrication of a surgical guide. Here, the planning software uses only the STL file for the design of the surgical guide. Since the planned position of the implant determines the position of the template guide sleeve, any inaccuracies in the merging process may cause serious complications at the time of implant placement. Consequently, careful verification of the accuracy of the merging process is recommended for the avoidance of intrasurgical complications or implant malpositioning.

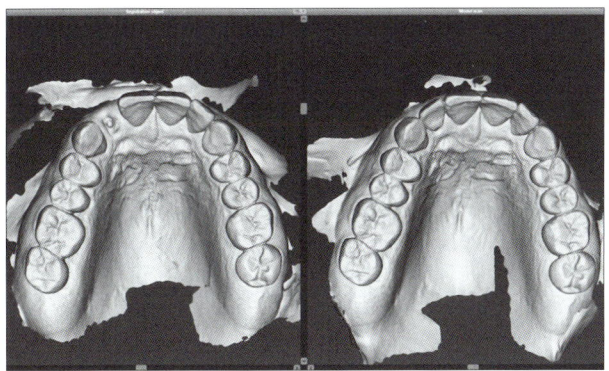

Fig 10   Merging steps for two STL files: Tooth 12 missing (left) and with failing crown in place (right).

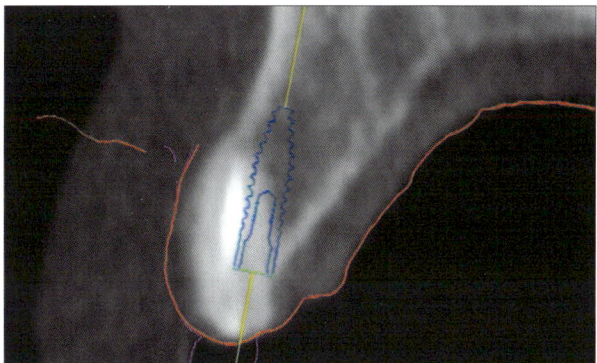

Fig 11   Planned implant position in the sagittal view. Gray: DICOM dataset. Blue: Planned implant. Orange: First STL file (without tooth). Purple: Additional STL file (with tooth).

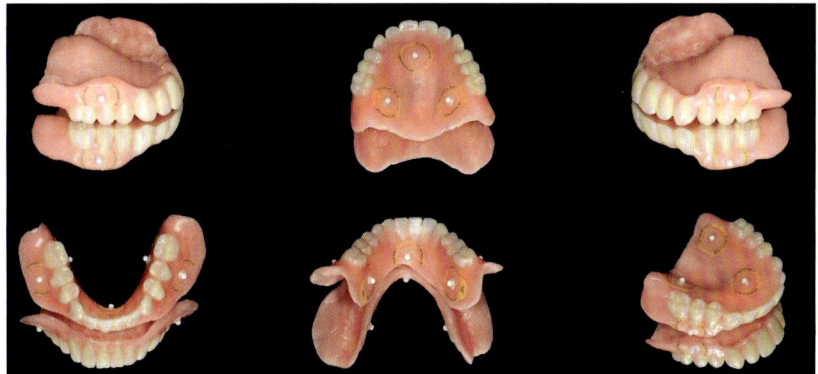

Fig 12   Adhesive radiographic markers are strategically positioned on the tooth setup in order to proceed with scanning.

5.6.2   Merging Additional STL Files

Once the first STL file has been merged with the DICOM dataset, additional STL files can be added using the first STL file as the merging reference. This technique allows for merging of STL files taken at different clinical time points, providing different outlines. For instance, an IOS/EOS scan of a missing tooth can be taken by reproducing the edentulous area; the area can then be re-scanned with a transitional prosthesis or a tooth set-up in place. Next, these two scans are merged in the planning software to provide a view of the edentulous mucosal surfaces and the tooth positions at the same time. Fig 10 shows the merging steps for two STL files, one with tooth 12 missing (left panel) and a second STL file with the failing crown in place (right panel). Once these files are aligned with each other, they can also be aligned with the DICOM dataset.

Fig 11 shows a sagittal view of the planned implant position where the multiple merging of files permits the visualization of the position of the gingiva (orange line of the first STL file) and the outline of the clinical crown (purple line of the second STL file) in relation to the planned implant position.

5.6.3   Merging Datasets Using Radiographic Markers

Adhesive radiographic markers (CTSpots, Beekley Medical, Bristol, CT, USA) (Fig 12) can assist in adding accuracy to digital implant workflows. The use of radiographic markers may provide greater precision in merging different datasets (files). This technique is commonly used when the patient is edentulous or when the 3D rendering of the CBCT scan is distorted by scatter. In these scenarios, the identification of anatomical structures common to both datasets may be impossible, and radiographic markers are used to guide the merging process. Radiographic markers are commercially available or can be custom-made from dental materials such as composite resin. Metallic markers are not recommended, as they will introduce scatter.

The principle of this technique is to acquire both the IOS/EOS and the CBCT scans with markers in place. When the files are imported into the planning software, the radiographic markers are clearly identifiable for the merging process, as shown in Fig 13.

Matching digital files to reproduce orofacial structures in a virtual environment is an essential phase of the digital workflow. The operator must ensure the accuracy of

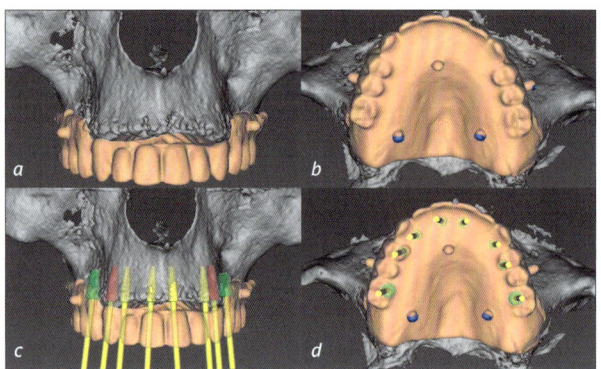

Fig 13   DICOM dataset of an edentulous patient merged with an STL file of the tooth setup. Frontal view of the merged DICOM and STL data (a). Occlusal view showing the result of merging the files using the radiographic markers (b). Frontal view of the implants planned for a fixed rehabilitation (c). Occlusal view of the planned implants (d).

the matched files, as a mismatched dataset may produce clinical inaccuracies. Although the technical aspects of the merging process are not complex, it is recommended to collaborate with a digital lab that is fully equipped to carry out this step or to have in-office trained staff perform a digital file match. Given the clinical relevance of this step in terms of treatment accuracy, the treating clinician must understand its clinical implication, verify the proposed matching and treatment plan, and ultimately approve the process.

6 Digital Workflows in Implant Prosthodontics

G. Gallucci

Conventional (analog) techniques are currently the predominant method used in implant prosthodontics. They have been in place since the early days of implant dentistry. However, the incorporation of digital dental technology (DDT) into modern oral implantology has given rise to new clinical workflows. For example, the digital design of a surgical guide to translate the planned implant position to the clinical environment will be performed almost entirely within a virtual environment. Or—in the case of fabrication of a zirconia abutment by the dental lab—digital technology will be employed for producing the abutment. In these circumstances, the use of digital technology is an enabling step.

But there are also other planning, surgical, and prosthodontic steps that may use either a digital or a conventional workflow. In this context, selecting the appropriate environment for the workflow (conventional, digital, or a combination of the two) should not be solely based on the technology itself, but also on the best approach to the treatment needs of that particular patient and site. This chapter will explore how DDT is applied to patient care.

The workflow for implant-prosthetic therapy comprises elements such as the environment, the different treatment phases, and the technology and techniques used by the operator and auxiliary staff. Table 1 shows examples of different environments (analog, digital, and clinical) and their outputs or clinical steps that achieve the final objective of restoring missing dentoalveolar structures with implant-supported prostheses. It is important to mention that digital and analog environments can be used alternately within the same workflow. For instance, a conventional diagnostic impression may be digitized by an extraoral scanner (EOS) to proceed in a digital environment. Conversely, a digital "impression" by an intraoral scanner (IOS) may be used to manufacture, by additive or subtractive techniques, a model on which implant prostheses can be fabricated using conventional techniques.

While purely conventional or exclusively digital workflows can be selected, both would need to translate into the clinical environment with the required precision needed to place a dental implant in the correct position or to deliver an implant crown with an acceptable clinical fit.

The incorporation of digital technology brings new techniques to the field of implant dentistry that are more related to computer sciences than to clinical dentistry in general. The management of digital datasets and the transfer and merging of digital files across different environments calls for additional training for all members of the dental team. For instance, the segmentation of a DICOM file (from CBCT radiography), the virtual planning of a dental implant, the integration of an STL file (from an IOS) into a CAD/CAM software package, or the feeding of a CAD to a manufacturing unit, all require new training and new skills.

We are therefore seeing the emergence of a new entity, the "digital lab," that supports the data management inherent in DDT. These digital labs may be associated with conventional dental laboratories or may be standalone entities providing an array of digital services, often via the internet.

Table 1 Overview of the different environments (analog, digital, and clinical) and their clinical outputs.

Environment	Planning	Implant placement	Prosthodontics
Analog techniques (conventional lab)	• Diagnostic stone casts • Diagnostic wax-ups • Radiographic stents	• Surgical stents • Transitional prostheses • Immediate provisional prostheses	• Stone casts • Fabrication of provisional prostheses • Abutment selection and manufacturing (casting) • Final implant prostheses
Clinical	• Patient evaluation • Risks assessment • Preliminary impressions • Try-in of functional wax-up • Treatment plan	• Conventional implant placement (freehand) • Guided implant surgery • GBR techniques	• Implant level impressions • Provisionals • Abutment selection • Abutment try-in • Framework try-in • Delivery of final prosthesis
Digital technology	• Digital health records • Digital radiology • CBCT • Planning software • Intraoral scanning (IOS) • Extraoral scanning (EOS)	• Intraoperative digital radiology • CBCT • Intraoral scanning at the time of implant placement	• Intraoral scanning • CAD/CAM
Digital techniques (digital lab)	• Management of digital files • Digital wax-up • Stereolithographic models (3D printing) • Milling of models • Digital design of surgical guide for guided implant placement	• Virtual implant planning • Proposed surgical protocols	• Dataset management • Scan data to CAD system • CAD • Milling of abutments (CAM) • Milling of implant restorations (CAM)

6.1   Digital Workflows Applied to Patient Care

A fully digital workflow, as represented in Fig 1, consists of diagnostics steps, planning steps, surgical steps, and prosthodontic steps. It begins with data files obtained with an intraoral scanner (STL) and CBCT (DICOM) being merged within the planning software. Within this software, the implant positions are planned virtually, guided by the desired prosthetic design. Next, a surgical guide is digitally designed and 3D-printed to assist implant placement. After the osseointegration period, a working IOS or "digital impression" is taken. The resulting STL file is manipulated in a CAD software package to fabricate the implant-borne prosthetic components.

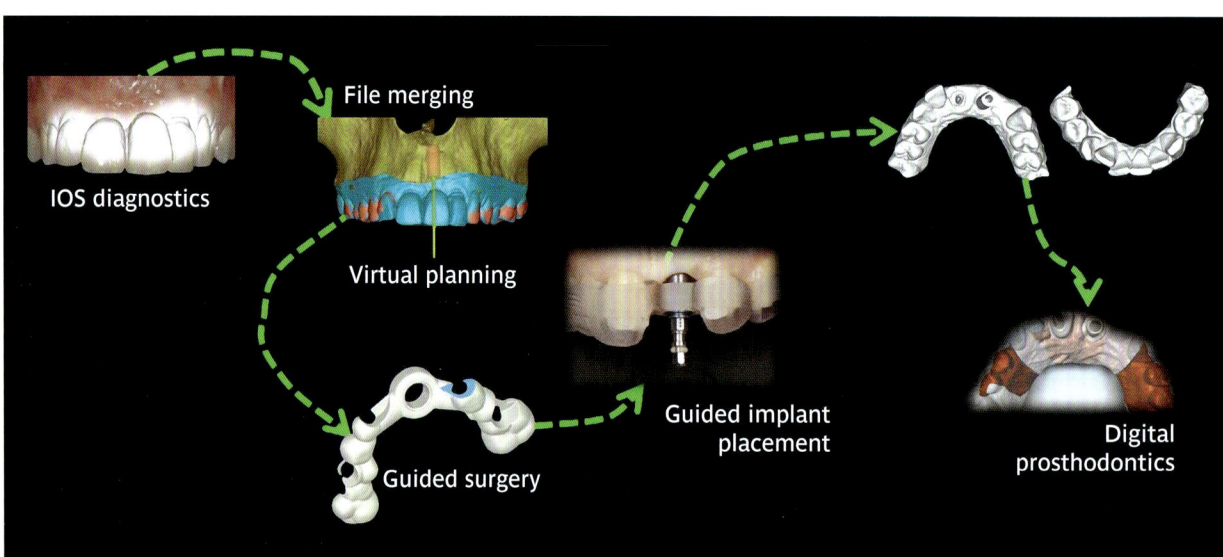

Fig 1   Digital workflow for implant prosthodontics. IOS: Intraoral scanner.

6.2 Diagnostic Steps of the Digital Workflow

The digital datasets normally obtained from the patient are either a digital diagnostic model obtained with an IOS or EOS scan of a physical (cast stone) diagnostic model.

These digital impressions (surface scans) are normally present in STL file format. Sometimes, depending of the scanner used, the output may be in a proprietary format that can only be read by the native system. STL files are relatively easy to handle and should be kept as a part of the patient's electronic health record. The diagnostic scans are imported into the implant planning (CAD) software either by directly reading the files from their location on the server, by way of a web transfer (ftp), or by direct transmission from the IOS unit to the digital lab. Fig 2 shows a representation of an STL file with diagnostic IOS data. (Chapter 4 addresses the topic of surface scanners in detail.)

Diagnostic IOS data can be imported into CAD software to perform a digital diagnostic tooth set-up. Fig 3 shows a representation of an STL diagnostic file imported into a CAD station on which a diagnostic tooth set-up for a missing lateral incisor is being modified.

The software can modify the original STL file to create a virtual representation of a conventional model, including the insertion of implant analogs and dies of tooth preparations.

Another method used to digitize the orofacial structures is digital 3D imaging. Here the patient is exposed to ionizing radiation to obtain a CBCT. Unlike surface scans (STL files), which produce a high-resolution 3D volume, DICOM files render a 3D volumetric representation of the scanned object with relatively poor surface definition. DICOM files can be relatively large, depending on the resolution used when scanning the patient. The DICOM files should also be considered as part of the patient's electronic health record. Various software packages exist for viewing or manipulating of DICOM files. In oral implantology, DICOM files are imported into a virtual implant planning software package (Fig 4).

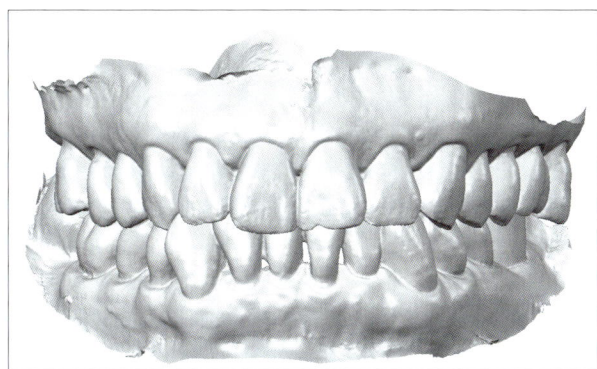

Fig 2 Frontal view representation of an STL file.

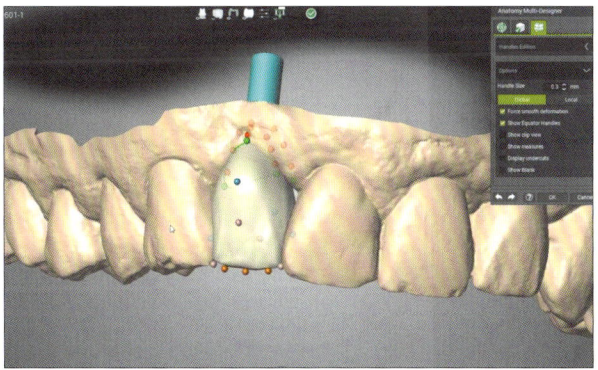

Fig 3 Representation of an STL diagnostic file imported into a CAD station with a digital set-up for tooth 12.

6.3 Planning Steps of the Digital Workflow

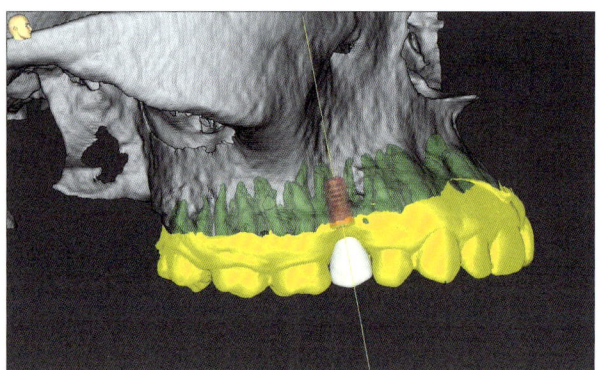

Fig 4   Virtual implant software. Gray 3D structure: Segmentation of DI-COM file showing only bone. Green 3D structure: Segmentation of DICOM file showing only teeth. Yellow 3D image: STL file obtained from an IOS unit showing teeth and soft tissue, merged with the DICOM file. Red: Virtual implant planning. White: Digital tooth set-up.

Once the DICOM files are imported into a virtual implant planning software package they can be "segmented", to reduce the 3D area, to refine the image by removing scatter or other artifacts, or to separate the different anatomical elements within the file (gray and green 3D structures in Fig 4). The DICOM files can be merged with the STL file (yellow image in Fig 4). The merging techniques and their clinical significance are described in more detail in Chapter 5.

The next step is to incorporate the desired prosthodontic outcome to virtually plan the appropriate restoration-driven implant position (red implant replica, Fig 4). This may be achieved either by importing additional STL files of an analog wax tooth setup, by using a digital tooth setup tool included in the software package, (white 3D tooth, Fig 4), or by a dual scanning technique in which the patient is scanned with a denture, then the denture is scanned by itself with radiographic markers, and these two scans are subsequently merged in the planning software. Following this step, the appropriate implants can be selected from a digital library and appropriately positioned relative to the adjacent anatomical structures and the prosthodontic planning, as shown by the red implant in Figure 4.

6.4 Surgical Steps of the Digital Workflow

Once the implant position has been defined, the same virtual implant planning software can be used for the digital design of a surgical guide. This design is then exported to an STL file for a 3D printer or milling unit for the manufacturing of the designed guide (Figs 5a-b).

Guided implant placement is discussed in detail in Chapter 7. Here, a surgical guide assists accurate implant placement by transferring the planned implant position to the surgical field. Using a digitally fabricated guide at the time of implant placement may often be the first step out of the digital environment into the clinical field, so it is of paramount importance to verify the clinical fit and stability of the guide. A common design feature of surgical guides is the inclusion of inspection windows that allow for visual verification of the accuracy of fit.

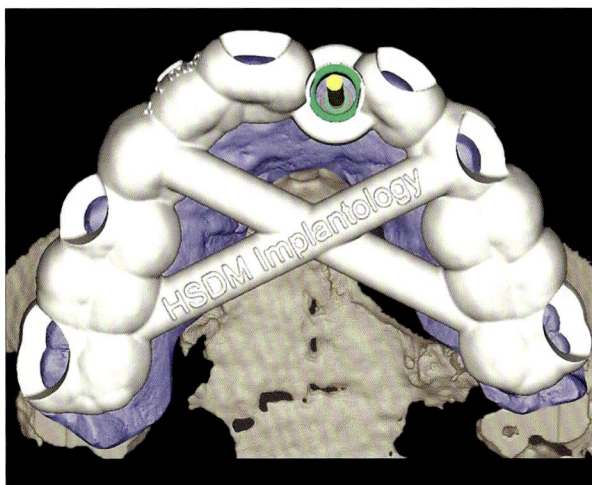

Fig 5a   Digital design of a surgical guide.

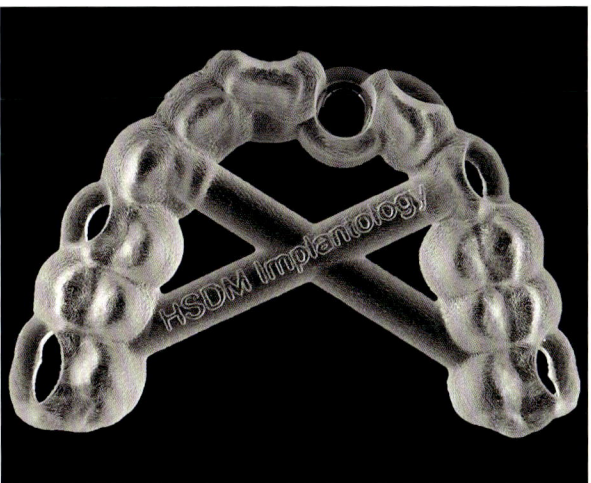

Fig 5b   3D-printed surgical guide.

6.5 Prosthodontic Steps of the Digital Workflow

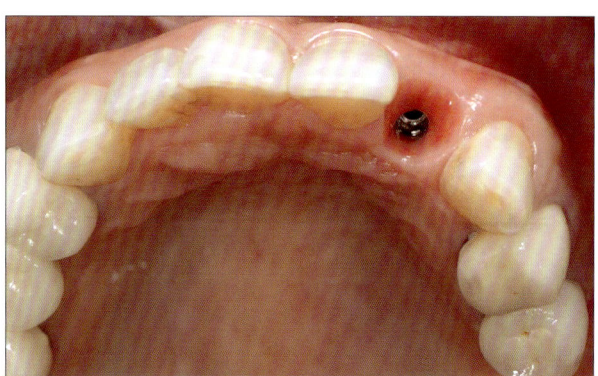

Fig 6a   Intraoral view of implant and peri-implant soft tissue condition before IOS scanning.

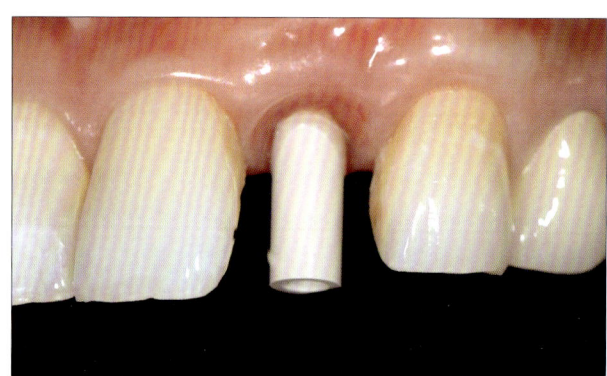

Fig 6b   Scanbody in place.

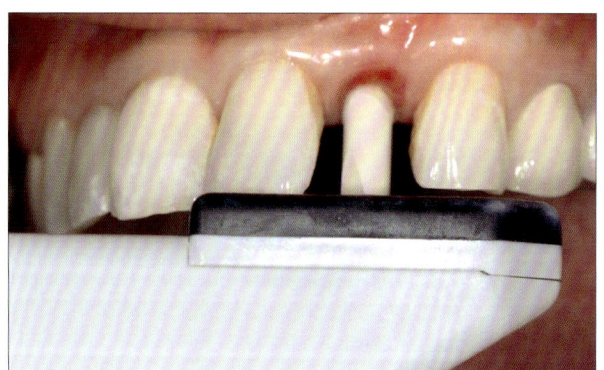

Fig 6c   IOS wand during used for intraoral digitization.

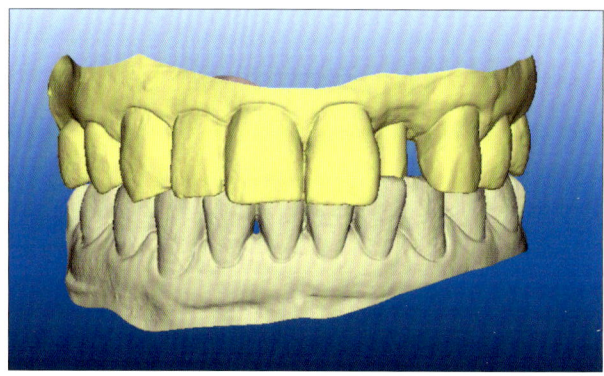

Fig 6d   IOS scan of the area of interest with scanbody replica.

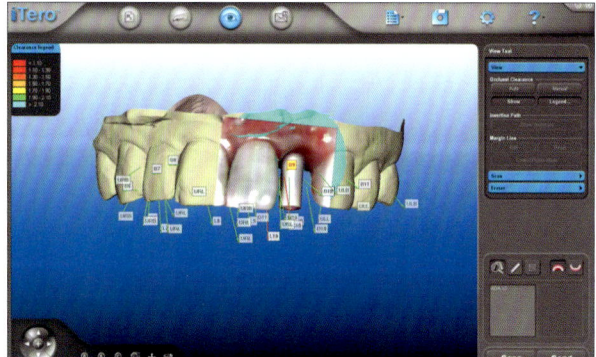

Fig 6e   IOS assessment window (shade).

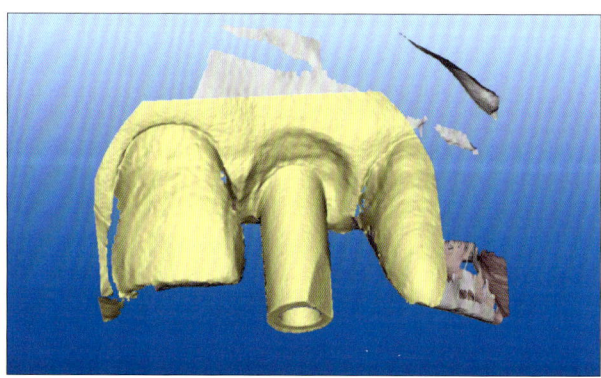

Fig 6f   STL with "socket" for repositionable analog.

Following successful osseointegration, IOS scans are made to transfer the implant position from the oral cavity to the digital lab. Figs 6a-f illustrate the clinical sequence of a digital implant "impression" with a digital scanbody in place and the resulting STL file.

There are several possible variations in workflow at this stage. Figs 6a-f show a complete IOS scanning sequence with a new scan being taken after soft tissue maturation. Alternatively, there exists the possibility of modifying the original diagnostic IOS scan into a working/final virtual model containing the reproduction of the implant position after placement. To achieve this, the operator can simply erase the area of interest clinically modified by the implant placement and amend the existing diagnostic IOS scan by re-scanning only the area of interest with the scanbody in place. This file is then merged with the original, minimizing the duplication of steps and renders the process more time efficient.

This STL file is now imported into the CAD station to begin the prosthetic fabrication via CAD/CAM processes. Fig 7 shows CAD views of a digital fabrication for an implant-supported prosthetic framework. The precise implant position and orientation is recognized by the orientation of the scanbody captured in the STL file, allowing the digital lab to proceed with the digital selection of prosthetic components for the fabrication of the final implant restoration. CAD software provides sophisticated tools that permit virtual modifications of the contour and dimensions of the CAD/CAM implant-supported prosthesis.

Once the CAD design is completed, the output file—in STL or a proprietary format—is usually sent to a milling station or, in some cases, to a 3D printer (Fig 8).

The CAM phase of the workflow is normally handled by the dental laboratory. Once manufactured, the prosthesis is sent to the clinician for a clinical try-in or for delivery. This step also represents a transition from the digital to the clinical environment; again, the verification of clinically accepted fit must be ensured.

Further verification may be achieved by using the model builder to manufacture a physical replica of the working IOS scan. These models can incorporate implant analogs on which implant prostheses can be placed for checking the fit, or for adjustment before clinical delivery (Figs 9a-e).

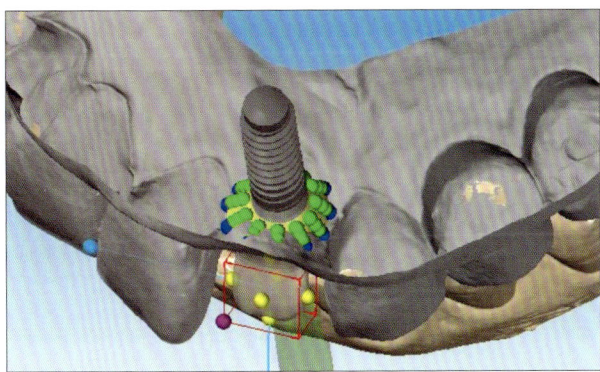

Fig 7 CAD station screenshot showing a single implant crown framework being designed. Green dots: Modification tool for the transmucosal area of the framework. Yellow dots: Modification tool for the coronal area of the framework.

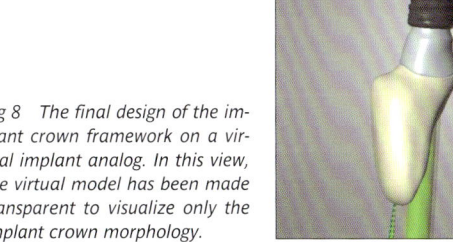

Fig 8 The final design of the implant crown framework on a virtual implant analog. In this view, the virtual model has been made transparent to visualize only the implant crown morphology.

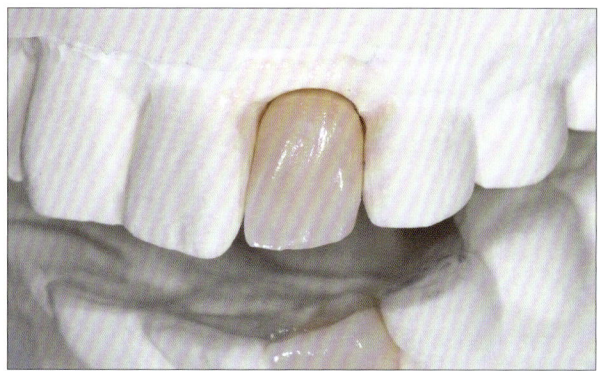

Fig 9a   CAD/CAM implant crown adapted on milled model.

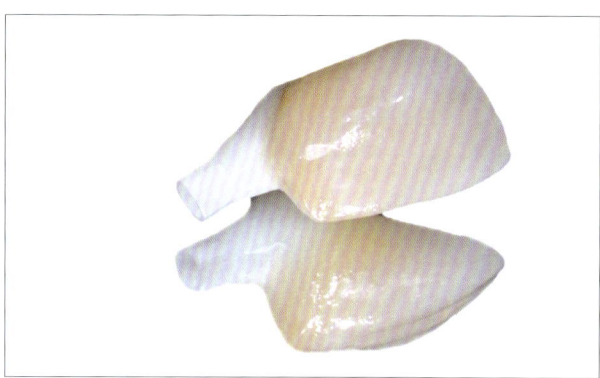

Fig 9b   CAD/CAM implant crown.

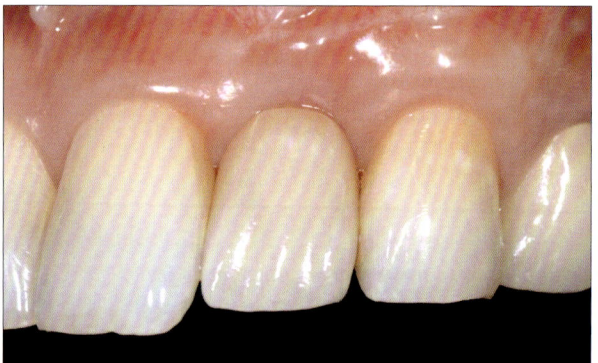

Fig 9c   Close-up view of intraoral fitting of CAD/CAM implant crown.

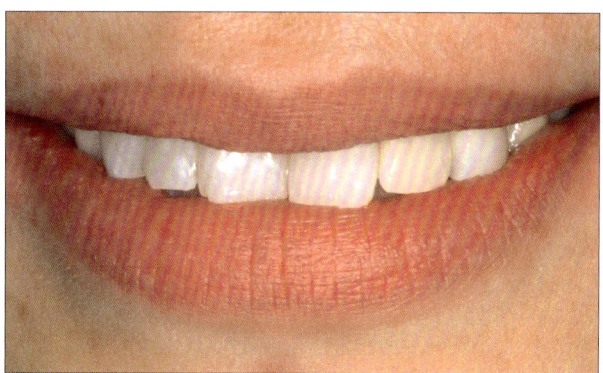

Fig 9d   Extraoral view of CAD/CAM implant crown.

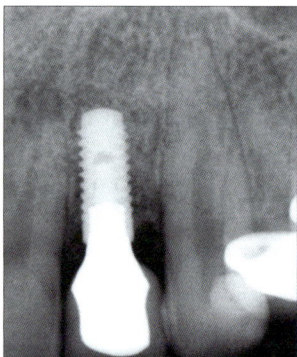

Fig 9e   Radiographic evaluation of the fit of a CAD/CAM implant crown.

6.6 Alternative Steps in Digital Workflows

The processes described above represent a simplified version of the full digital workflow. While these steps describe the common navigation throughout the process, there are several possible workflow variations at both the digital and the clinical levels. For example, a hybrid implant-prosthodontic workflow includes some steps that are performed using conventional methods and other steps that are performed digitally. Other examples include the taking of an IOS for the final prosthesis at the time of implant placement or the fabrication of all-digitally designed and manufactured implant-supported crowns without ever creating any physical model.

Another variation is the capability of cross-communication between different software packages. The preoperative planning of a case can thus take place on a CAD/CAM station and the resulting planning information can be shared with other team members, either in the same location or remotely, by linking the CAD/CAM software in real time with a virtual implant-planning system. In this way, modifications can be made on either software package to optimize the prosthetic design and implant position (Fig 10).

This feature is clinically significant, as it creates a virtual environment for the synergistic planning of cases that is accessible by all team members.

As the field of DDT develops, other variations of the digital workflow may evolve. However, it is of paramount importance that team members understand the basic elements described in Table 1 as key components of a digital implant workflow. Diagnostic, planning, surgical, and prosthodontic steps will commonly need to be adapted to the specific characteristics of a specific case, creating a customized workflow with a digital, conventional, or combined environment for each patient.

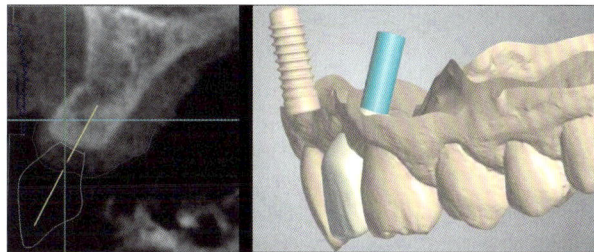

Fig 10   The CAD software (right) is used to determine the tooth set-up. This information is then retrieved by the surgical planning software (left). Once the two software packages are linked, changes can be seen simultaneously in real time on each station.

7 Computer-Guided Surgery

A. Tahmaseb

Prosthetically driven implant placement, considering the surrounding anatomical structures, has been a subject of interest to dental clinicians for several years now. Correct implant positioning is paramount to achieve favorable esthetic and prosthetic outcomes and to provide adequate access for maintenance to help prevent future complications. Extensive and meticulous planning is a prerequisite of successful dental treatment in general and implant treatment in particular. Dental professionals have been using various planning tools for decades, including study casts mounted in articulators, diagnostic wax-ups, and markers on radiographs.

But the introduction of cone-beam computed tomography (CBCT) in implant dentistry was a true breakthrough, particularly as these devices resulted in lower radiation exposure than conventional computed tomography (CT) scanners (Loubele and coworkers 2009; Guerrero and coworkers 2006; Harris and coworkers 2012).

Combined with implant-planning software, CBCT imaging makes it possible to plan the best restoration-driven implant position within the surrounding vital anatomical structures in a "virtual" computer environment. The resulting digital data are then used to fabricate computer-generated surgical guides (drilling templates) via CAD/CAM. This process ultimately results in the transfer of the planned implant position from the computer to the patient, with the surgical guide directing the implant osteotomy and the insertion according to plan. The goal is to achieve the predicted ideal implant position surgically without damaging the surrounding anatomical structures (Widmann and coworkers 2010).

7.1 Terminology

Guided implant surgery systems use a combination of hardware and software to facilitate the planning of implant positions. The resulting positions are then converted into surgical guides or loaded into positioning software using a variety of methods.

Jung and coworkers (2009) have categorized these methods as either dynamic and static systems:

- **Dynamic systems** communicate the selected implant positions to the operator using visual cues displayed in real time on a computer monitor rather than using rigid intraoral guides.

- **Static systems** (or computer-aided implant surgery, CAIS) use prefabricated surgical guides for implant placement. The original plan cannot be modified, since prefabricated surgical guides do not allow for intrasurgical changes in implant positions.

For this reason, a clear description of these systems, their modes of application, and their precision can be of assistance to clinicians interested in these techniques.

7.2　Systems Used in Guided Surgery

7.2.1　Dynamic Systems: Navigated Surgery

In dynamic guided-surgery protocols, planning software into which CBCT data have been imported is used to plan implant positions. Surgical navigation devices with an optical tracking system are then used to facilitate insertion of the implants at the preplanned positions. For example, the MicronTracker (ClaroNav, Toronto, Canada) (Fig 1) uses stereoscopic vision in real time to detect and track specially marked objects. These marked objects, known as optical tracking targets, are connected to the surgical handpiece and to the patient's jaw (Fig 2). The optical tracker then tracks these markers and displays on a screen the real-time location of the instrument tip via 2D images of the sagittal, axial, and coronal views of the patient scan (Fig 3). The surgeon can follow the surgery on the screen in real time and modify the procedure if necessary, for example if an anatomical obstacle such as a nerve has to be avoided (Fig 4).

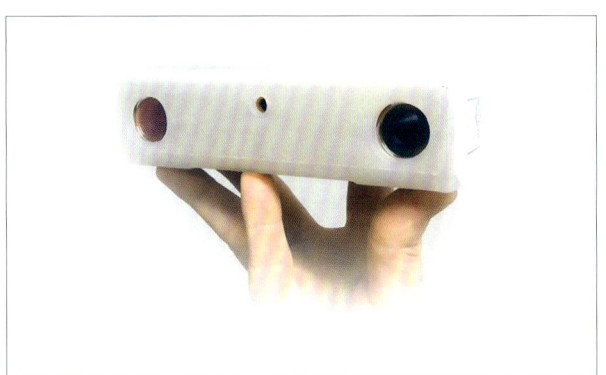

Fig 1　MicronTracker (ClaroNav).

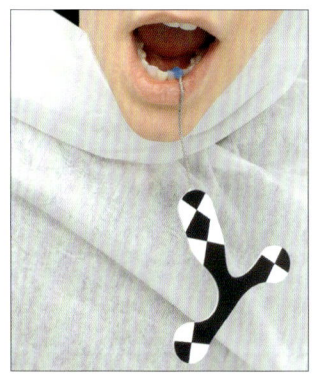

Fig 2　The marked objects are connected to the surgical handpiece and to the patient's jaw.

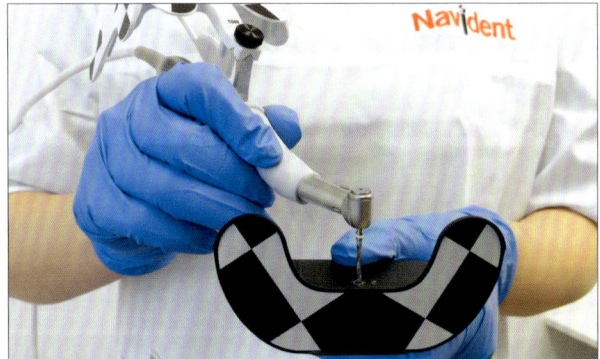

Fig 3　The optical tracker tracks these markers and displays the real-time location of the instrument tip on 2D images.

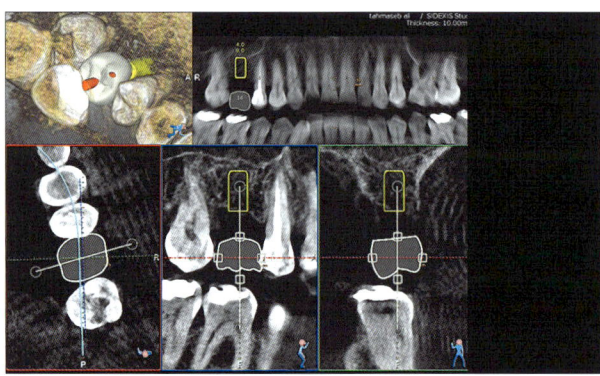

Fig 4　Planning software for a navigation system: Virtual implant insertion prior to the actual surgery.

Surgical navigation systems are often referred to as dynamic systems because it is possible for the surgeon to modify the surgical procedure and the implant position in real time, deviating from the initial plan if necessary. Since the surgeon can visualize an avatar of the drill in 3D, relative to the patient's previously scanned anatomy and to the presurgical treatment plan, modifications can be made during surgery based on significantly more information.

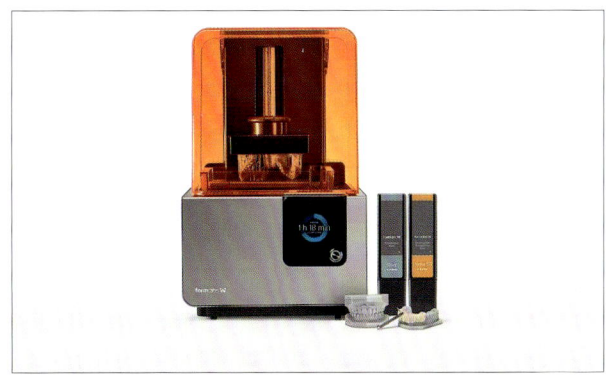

Fig 5   3D printer (Formlabs, Somerville, MA, USA) to print surgical guides.

7.2.2   Static Systems: Guided Surgery

Computer-guided (static) surgery systems use different methods for the fabrication of surgical guides, such as stereolithography (rapid prototyping), three-dimensional (3D) printing (Fig 5), or mechanical positioning devices (Fig 6) that convert the radiographic template to a surgical equivalent on a computer through transformation algorithms (Jung and coworkers 2009) (Figs 6 to 15). Stereolithography is a technique for creating solid three-dimensional plastic objects from computer-aided design (CAD) data by selectively solidifying an ultraviolet-sensitive liquid resin (photopolymer) using a laser beam (Laney 2007). This process is also known as 3D layering or 3D printing. In implant dentistry, these physical models can reproduce the true maxillary and mandibular dimensions.

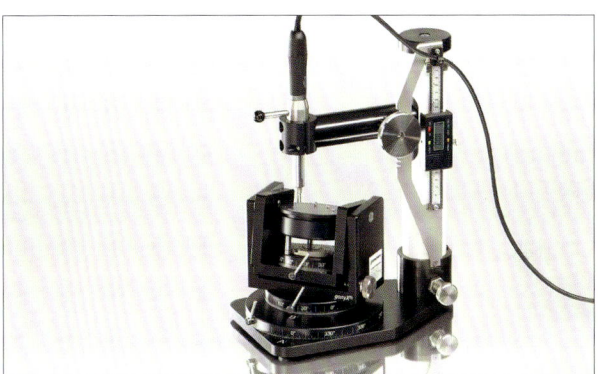

Fig 6   GonyX (Straumann) device for the fabrication of surgical guides.

In both stereolithography and 3D printing, the implant position coordinates (the geometrical 3D positioning data) are used to design a surgical guide. Often, as demonstrated in Fig 6, the design software is integrated into the planning software (coDiagnostiX). This software creates a file in a format that can be exported to a 3D printing device.

If the surgical guide is produced mechanically, devices such as the GonyX instrument (Institut Straumann AG, Basel, Switzerland) require the implant coordinates to be entered manually. A master model forms the basis for the scanning template and the surgical template. The scanning template contains information about the desired prosthetic outcome in the form of radiopaque teeth and is visible on CBCT images.

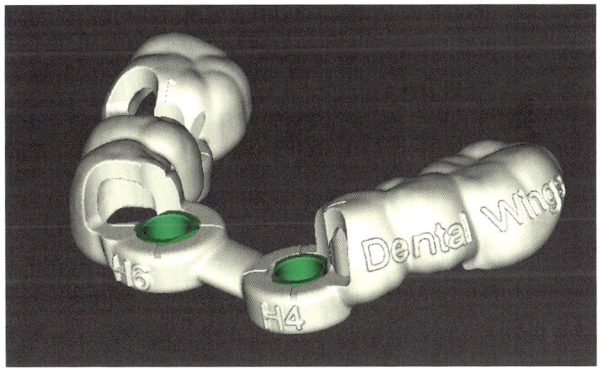

Fig 7   Dentalwings/Straumann coDiagnostiX: Integrated software to design a surgical guide to be 3D-printed as a surgical guide.

The scanning template is connected to a Templix plate with three reference pins. These are indexed using the GonyX instrument to confirm the accurate transfer from the digital implant plan to the fabricated surgical guide (Fig 8). The clinician can import the 3D data set (DICOM) directly into the planning software.

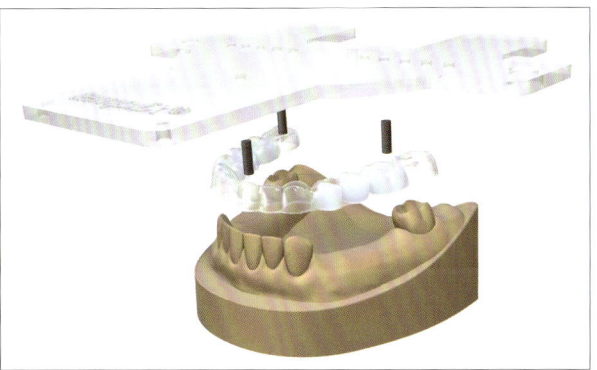

Fig 8   Templix – the link between digital implant planning and surgical guide fabrication.

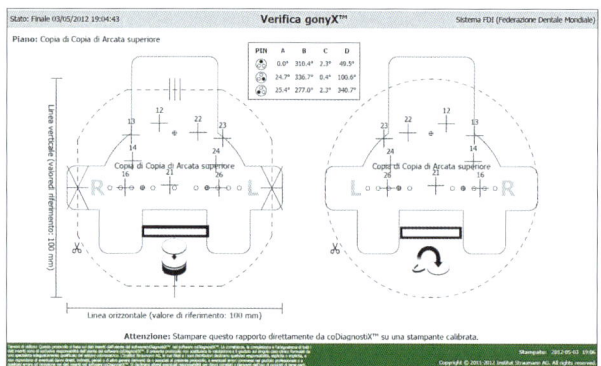

Fig 9   GonyX verification template.

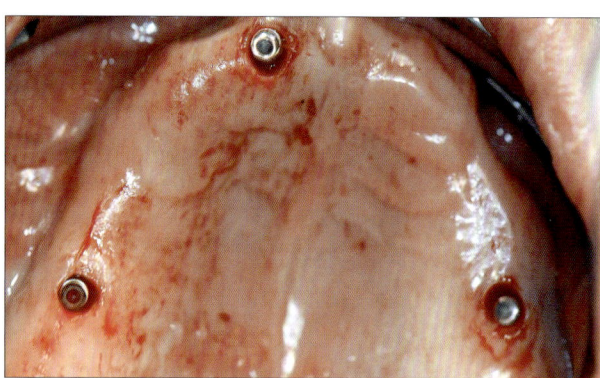

Fig 10   The reference mini-implants in an edentulous maxilla.

Once implant planning has been completed, the software delivers a plan for producing the surgical guide using the GonyX instrument. The plaster cast and scanning template are positioned in the GonyX instrument using a verification template produced from the software and printed on paper (Fig 9). Each implant position is generated by the planning software and imported into the GonyX device, using four dials to set the spatial coordinates (A, B, C, and D) for each implant position. The GonyX device is then used to drill appropriate holes in the template for the drill sleeves.

Obviously, there are still many analog steps in this process, making it susceptible to human error, which may have a significant detrimental impact on the surgical outcome.

Static (guided) systems are classified according to the type of drilling guidance within the surgical guide. For example, some systems use multiple surgical guides, each with sleeves of a specific diameter, while others have one guide into which to fit sleeves of progressively increasing diameter to match the drill in use. Some

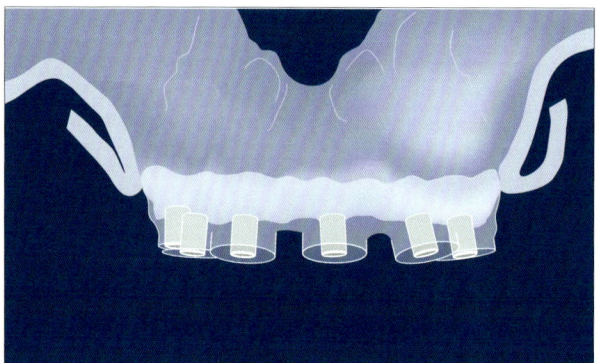

Fig 11   Bone-supported surgical guide.

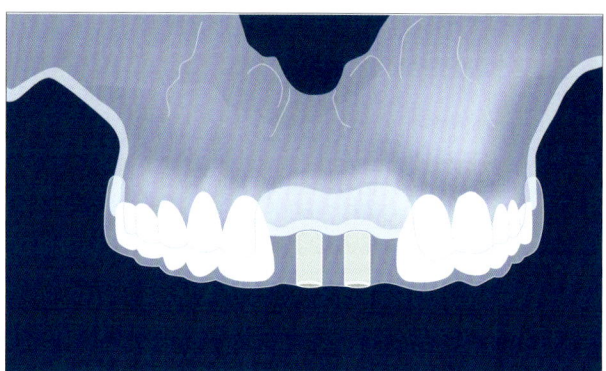

Fig 12   Tooth-supported surgical guide.

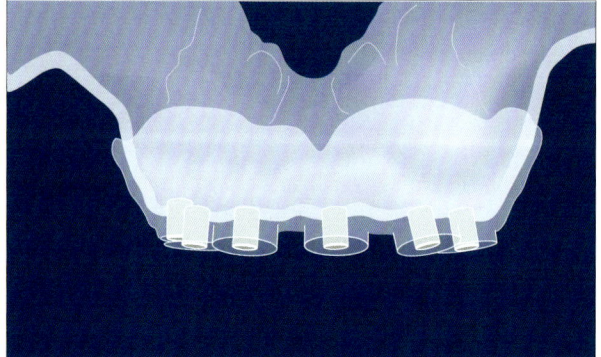

Fig 13   Mucosa-supported surgical guide.

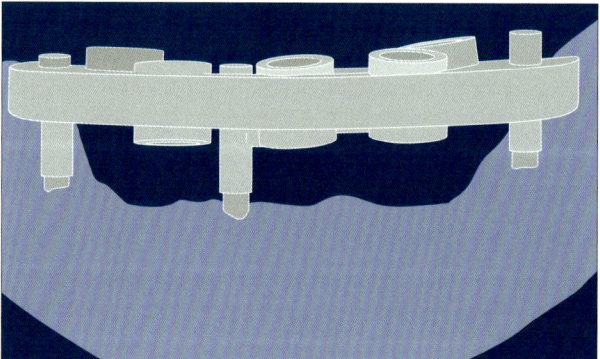

Fig 14   Fixture-supported surgical guide.

systems have drills with vertical "stops" to achieve depth control, while others use visual markers to aid control of the osteotomy depth.

Some static (guided) systems allow guided placement of the implant itself; so-called "fully guided systems" (Pettersson and coworkers 2010a, Tahmaseb and coworkers 2010; Tahmaseb and coworkers 2011). In some systems, the implants are placed manually after a template has been used to prepare the osteotomy, and in others only the initial osteotomy is prepared using a computer-aided surgical guide. (Ersoy and coworkers 2008; DiGiacomo and coworkers 2012; DiGiacomo and coworkers 2005). These are known as "partially guided systems."

Some systems use preinstalled mini-implants as reference points for computer-aided surgery (Cassetta and coworkers 2013; Tahmaseb and coworkers 2012). These mini-implants are used to stabilize the surgical guide, but also to calibrate images by connecting scanbodies to them. Different radiopaque reference markers (e.g., gutta-percha, radiopaque denture teeth, composite resin) may be placed in radiographic templates worn during the scanning process, either using a distinct scanning template or by adding the appropriate materials to the patient's existing dentures.

7.2.3 System Precision

Computer-guided and computer-navigated implant procedures are often recommended where bone quantity is limited, or for critical anatomical situations such as the placement of an implant adjacent to the mandibular nerve. Therefore, knowing the maximum implant deviations these systems allow is highly relevant to daily clinical practice.

It is important to distinguish between *accuracy* and *precision*, as these two terms are frequently used together. *Accuracy* refers to the closeness of a measured value to a standard or known value. *Precision* refers to the closeness of two or more measurements to each other. The analysis of the accuracy achieved using this technology has commonly been conducted by measuring the difference between the planned implant position and the actual implant position after insertion, at various levels. Some authors use criteria such as entry point, apical position, or angular deviation, while others work with 3D coordinates (such as X, Y, and Z axes), making it difficult to meaningfully compare different systems.

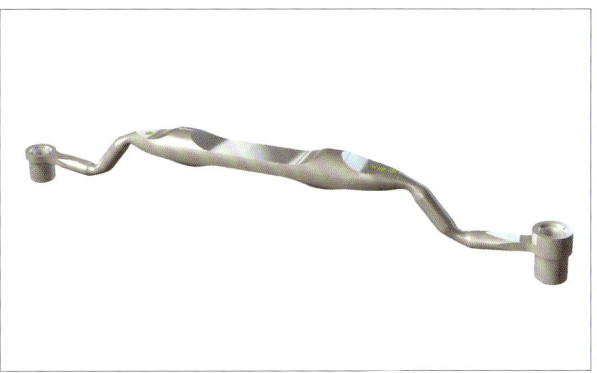

Fig 15   Drill handle (Straumann) to adjust the surgical guide to the drills with increasing diameter.

In their systematic review, Tahmaseb and coworkers (2014, 2018) demonstrated that different levels of qualitative and quantitative evidence were available for computer-aided implant surgery (CAIS), with high implant survival rates (admittedly after only 12 months of observation), achieving a variable level of accuracy. They demonstrated that, although the average accuracy remained within the clinically acceptable range, the maximal deviations were unacceptable. The data analyzed in this study showed inaccuracies at the implant entry point of 1.12 mm, with a maximum of 4.5 mm, and inaccuracies of 1.39 mm at the implant apex, with a maximum of 7.1 mm.

In another systematic review, Jung and coworkers (2009) stated that static systems tend to be more accurate than dynamic ones. However, most of the publications on navigated surgery have been clinical studies, whereas most articles on static protocols have been laboratory-based (on models, cadavers, etc.), where more accurate measurements are possible. This greater accuracy can be explained by better access, greater visual control of the axis of the osteotomy, the absence of movement in the cadaver or model, and the absence of saliva or blood. However, in a recent clinical trial, Block and coworkers (2016) stated that dynamic navigation can achieve a level of implant placement accuracy that is similar to static guidance—and that, at any rate, is a clear improvement over freehand implant placement.

It is important to note the use of navigation technology is associated with a considerable learning curve, as clinicians are generally not used to performing surgery using indirect line of sight. Jung and coworkers (2009) claimed that with more experience of the system, surgeons will gain proficiency and may use the technique with less trepidation.

7.3 Positioning the Surgical Guide

Static surgical guides can be categorized as follows:

- Bone-supported surgical guides
- Tooth-supported surgical guides
- Mucosa-supported surgical guides
- Fixture-supported surgical guides
  (on mini-implants or secured by osseous pins)

7.3.1 Bone-Supported Surgical Guides

Bone-supported surgical guides are designed such that the guide rests directly on bone. Thus, when these surgical guides are used, a large mucoperiosteal flap must be elevated to expose the bony structure in order to place the surgical guide.

Tahmaseb and coworkers (2014) concluded that a statistically significant lower accuracy of placement was observed with the use of bone-supported surgical guides in comparison to the other types of surgical guide mentioned here. This might be caused by bone-supported surgical guides being manufactured based on 3D-scan data only. Liang and coworkers (2010a, 2010b) showed that image quality can vary between devices with different resolutions. 3D imaging is also subject to distortion artifacts similar to those in conventional radiography due to factors such as patient movement and positioning, anatomical phenotypes, etc., which can affect the accuracy of the images and therefore the data used to create a surgical guide.

7.3.2 Tooth-Supported Surgical Guides

Tooth-supported surgical guides are supported by remaining natural teeth or fixed restorations. Such guides may be produced in the laboratory based on an analog cast, or via a digital workflow.

The emerging technology of intraoral scanning has significantly influenced digital dentistry in general and computer-guided surgery in particular. Intraoral scanners (IOS) can digitally capture the teeth and the surface structures of the oral cavity and add considerable value to these digital workflows (Joda and Brägger 2013). By superimposing CBCT and IOS images via surface-to-surface matching ("best-fit" method) using anatomical landmarks such as teeth, a realistic digital view of the patient's hard and soft tissues can be created. A digital set-up of the planned prosthetic restoration can then be added to this dataset, allowing prosthetically-driven implant planning to be completed taking all hard and soft tissues and all prosthetic requirements into consideration.

It has been suggested that merging CBCT and IOS images can improve the fit and accuracy of static surgery guides (Nkenke and coworkers 2004; Rangel and coworkers 2013). However, surface-to-surface superimposition can be negatively influenced by many factors; the registration accuracy inherent in commercial virtual implant-planning software is significantly influenced by the processing of data imported by the user and by other factors, potentially resulting in clinically unacceptable deviations being encoded in surgical guides.

For example, discrepancies between CBCT and surface-scan modeling resulting from inaccurate registration can be transferred to the surgical field and may result in deviation between the planned and achieved implant positions (Flügge and coworkers 2016). Also, Pettersson and coworkers (2012) showed in a clinical study that the greatest deviations were found in the scans of patients who had moved rather than remaining still during scanning.

7.3.3 Mucosa-Supported Surgical Guides

Mucosa-supported surgical guides are usually based on the double-scan technique. Here, the first dataset is a CBCT scan of the patient wearing the original radiographic template or existing denture with the addition of spherical radiopaque markers (Fig 16). To adjust the resulting DICOM (Digital Imaging and Communications in Medicine) dataset, an additional scan of either an existing or newly developed radiographic template, or a new denture with radiopaque markers (e.g., gutta-percha), is taken (Fig 17). The spherical markers on both images are used to superimpose the images to create a digital model of the anatomical structures and the relevant restorative information retrieved from the scanned diagnostic prosthesis. In this way, these images are calibrated.

This dataset is then converted into a 3D image viewed in implant planning software that provides different imaging sections/planes: panoramic, sagittal, axial, etc. In this way, the planned implant positioning can be evaluated in different planes, assessing any anatomical limitations as well as the prosthetic needs of the patient.

It is generally recommended to start planning the implant in the *sagittal* view, where there is a clear image of the orofacial plane of the surgical site and associated anatomical structures (mental nerve, sinus, etc.) so the implant can be planned according to the anatomical situation. Moreover, as the outlines of the planned prosthetic device are also visible in this view, the prosthetic requirements can also be considered. The *occlusal* view is used to refine the position such that the screw access of the prosthetic device is ideally positioned. The *panoramic* view is mostly used to refine the implant position mesiodistally and in respect to adjacent teeth

or implants. Also, when planning multiple adjacent implants, the panoramic view is used to check the parallelism of the implants used in the prosthesis (e.g., implant-supported bridges).

However, when fully edentulous patients are treated, one cannot be certain that the scanned prosthesis or existing denture is always positioned in precisely the same reproducible intraoral position; nor that, once the surgical guide has been manufactured, it in turn is always placed in exactly the same position (Tahmaseb and coworkers 2014). Some systems attempt to use bite registration to achieve the right position, but even with this technique, the thickness and resilience of the mucosa, as well as the bite forces, can substantially affect the position. This could be one of the reasons for the inaccuracy of these techniques. Clinicians must be aware that errors might occur with these approaches.

7.3.4 Fixture-Supported Surgical Guides

Surgical guides can be supported by additional components. These can be preinstalled like reference (mini-) implants (Tahmaseb and coworkers 2012) or intrasurgically, e.g., transmucosal pins.

Tahmaseb and coworkers (2014) concluded that guides supported by mini-implants achieved a high level of accuracy where the final restoration could be prefabricated and successfully inserted based on data retrieved from the computerized planning. Also, in a clinical study, Gallucci and coworkers (2015) showed that transitional implants can, besides holding the surgical guide, also support the provisional restoration during postoperative healing, which can help prevent unintentional loading of the implants resulting in non-integration.

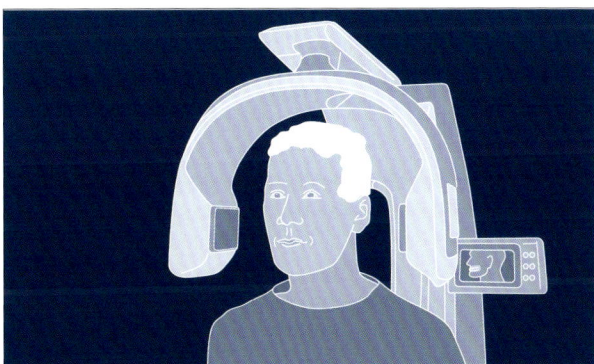

Fig 16   Double-scan technique: CBCT imaging of the patient wearing a radiographic template together with radiopaque markers.

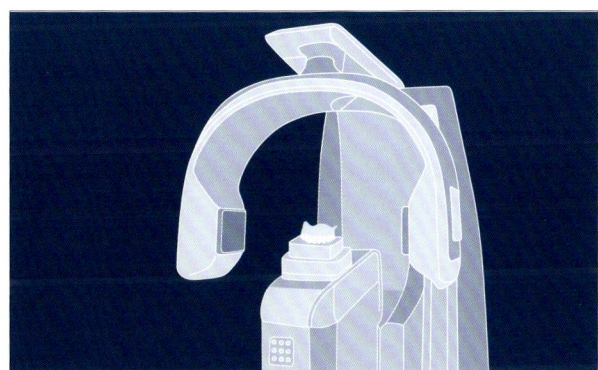

Fig 17   Double-scan technique: CBCT imaging of the CBCT template with radiopaque markers.

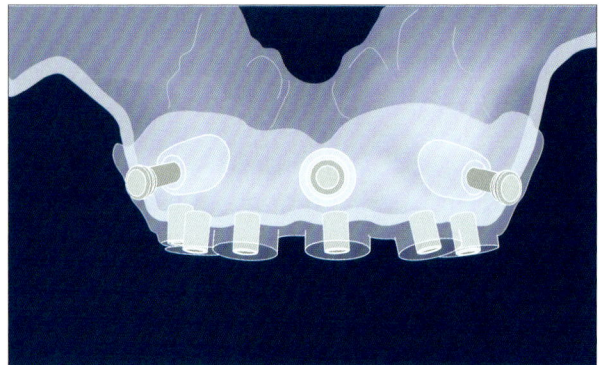

Fig 18   Mucosa-supported surgical guide with fixation pins.

Transmucosal osseous pins can also stabilize mucosa-supported surgical guides intrasurgically (Fig 18). They are inserted at the time of surgery and position the guide accurately and in line with the preoperative planning. The position of these pins can be planned with the relevant software; however, there is no conclusive assurance that the surgical guide is placed in the exact preplanned position.

How the surgical guide is supported during the procedure has a significant impact on accuracy. It has been reported that bone-supported surgical guides performed significantly less well compared to tooth- and mucosa-supported guides (Tahmaseb and coworkers, 2014).

7.4 Prefabrication of Prostheses and Immediate Loading

One of the advantages of guided surgery could be the possibility of prefabricating the restoration prior to implant placement to enable immediate implant loading. Theoretically, the final implant positions will already have been determined by computerized planning. The resultant geometrical positions of the future dental implants might therefore be used to create a virtual model of the postoperative situation. This information can then be used to design and fabricate the prosthetic superstructure.

Tahmaseb and coworkers (2011) showed in a clinical trial in fully edentulous patients that when transitional mini-implants were used prior to the actual planning and eventual implant insertion, the accuracy and precision of a prefabricated superstructure was comparable to the classic approach where the superstructure is fabricated from an impression of the inserted implants after implant insertion. They showed that when appropriate precautions were taken to avoid errors at different stages of the treatment, these preinstalled transitional mini-implants could improve the outcome when prefabricated prosthetic devices are used.

7.5 Limitations

Although guided implant surgery was originally hailed as a promising technique, various factors can make the treatment outcomes rather disappointing. Although to date there has been no evidence of possible shortfalls of individual steps of the digital workflow and their interactions, it is possible to highlight some factors that might explain the frequency of unacceptable clinical results.

One of the main causes of implant inaccuracy, as stated earlier in this chapter, is the variability in the precision and accuracy of CBCT data. Factors such as patient movement, positioning, and the way that the data has been processed may combine with variations introduced by the technical specification of different CBCT devices. Field of view (FoV) selection, the number of projections, acquisition and exposure factors (kVp, mA, scan time), and image-reconstruction algorithms can all influence the clinical outcome (Loubele and coworkers 2009).

Another contributory factor is the variable accuracy of the IOS. As with different CBCT devices, commercially available IOS all have their own specifications and levels of precision. Among the parameters that might affect the result are the deviations presented by each device, the practitioner's level of experience with that device, their individual ability or dexterity, and the scanning protocol used.

Variations in surgical guide accuracy can also result in unexpected outcomes. In addition to the factors already mentioned, drill and sleeve tolerances can affect the accuracy of the prepared implant bed. Koop and coworkers (2012) showed that, to achieve minimal deviations during surgery, it is essential to use the drill in a centric position, parallel to the cylinder. The use of longer sleeves and inserts may assist in this regard.

Recently, in another systematic review, Tahmaseb (2018) concluded that current guided surgery systems are less accurate in fully edentulous jaws than in partially edentulous jaws. This can be explained by a lack of reference points for both CBCT and IOS in fully edentulous patients as well as the technical shortcomings of these devices.

These and other issues can individually and cumulatively affect the result of guided implant surgery. Tahmaseb and coworkers (2010, 2011, 2012) showed in clinical and in in-vitro studies that excessive transitional steps (data conversions) between digital and analog processes could also introduce minor errors. Many small errors may cumulatively result in greater inaccuracies, which can significantly affect the outcome.

For these reasons, caution is advised when using guided-surgery techniques.

A certain level of experience in conventional surgical and prosthetic procedures is essential when using these guided techniques.

7.6 Future Developments

Following rather disappointing preliminary outcomes of early studies of guided surgery, many clinicians and researchers, together with industry representatives, have examined ways to improve the accuracy and precision of the technology. To overcome the imprecision of guided surgery, it is important to recognize each evolving factor individually and in combination.

Some novel CBCT devices deliver higher-quality images with lower radiation doses than earlier versions (Jacobs and coworkers 2018).

In the future, MRI technology will most likely take over from classic radiology in dentistry as well as general medicine, reducing the need for exposure to ionizing radiation. In dentistry, MRI techniques are currently used for the diagnosis of various diseases, including temporomandibular joint disorders and tumors (Shah and coworkers 2014). MRI has another application in implant dentistry in that it provides more precise data on bone height, density, and contour (Adeyemo and Akadiri 2011).

Ultrasonography has already been investigated as a possible alternative to radiology within dentistry (Wakasugi-Sato and coworkers 2010) and is currently used to detect maxillofacial fractures, exhibiting high sensitivity. In an in-vitro cadaver study, Chan and coworkers (2017) recently showed that ultrasound was as accurate in determining the height and thickness of the alveolar bone as either CBCT or direct measurements. Of course, further investigation is required to confirm the level of accuracy and define the indications in which these novel approaches could be applied.

Another rapidly developing technology is intraoral scanning. Although studies are not yet available to confirm required improvements, there is a trend for these devices to get faster, easier to use, and potentially more accurate.

However, conventional impressions, stone casts, and optional digitization with desktop scanners remains the recommended workflow, especially for fully edentulous jaws and longer edentulous spans (Wesemann and coworkers 2017).

8 <u>CAD/CAM Technology and Custom Bone Grafts</u>

A. Tahmaseb, G. Ragoebar, N. Al-Harbi

Tooth loss due to extraction, trauma, or disease is followed by varying degrees of resorption of the alveolar ridge. In such cases, the bone defect needs to be augmented to provide sufficient bone volume for the correct three-dimensional positioning of an appropriate implant and also to ensure overlying soft tissue support for good aesthetic and functional outcomes.

Several treatment strategies have been proposed, using natural or synthetic, particulate or block materials to augment bone defects in both the vertical and the horizontal planes (Esposito and coworkers 2009). Treatment selection is mainly based on the size of the defect. In the case of self-contained defects, the use of guided bone regeneration (GBR) is well documented (Chiapasco and Zaniboni 2009; Buser and coworkers 2013a, 2013b). It involves barrier membranes in conjunction with allografts, xenografts, or autologous particulate-bone augmentation materials. However, a rigid block graft may be recommended in larger defects.

Autologous bone block grafts can be harvested from intraoral or extraoral sites, depending on the size of the defect and the ability of donor sites. Disadvantages inherent in autologous bone harvesting include the risk of infection, donor-site morbidity, and graft resorption (De Santis and coworkers 2015). Allografts are also used to augment critical defects, but with varying outcomes.

Current advancements in computer-aided design and computer-aided manufacturing (CAD/CAM) technology and computerized planning based on cone-beam computed tomography (CBCT) help plan and treat augmentation cases. Digital radiographic images can be converted into virtual three-dimensional (3D) models that offers the surgeon a realistic impression of the patient's bone morphology. A three-dimensional defect can be augmented using virtual three-dimensional bone grafts, which can then be manufactured using additive CAD/CAM manufacturing techniques. Although it is possible to manufacture a custom biomedical scaffold for bone tissue engineering, the materials available for CAM techniques are not always suitable for direct bone augmentation in humans (Lehman and Casap 2014; Pruksakorn and coworkers 2015; Lee JS and coworkers 2014; Lee M and coworkers 2012; Klammert and coworkers 2010; Mangano and coworkers 2013).

Customised site-specific grafts could be a treatment option for bone augmentation in dentoalveolar indications. Although several reports have described the integration of the digital approach into bone augmentation procedures, little is known about the current applications, the fit of the custom grafts, or limitations of their use in maxillofacial bone augmentation.

The aim of this chapter is to provide an overview of the current clinical applications and the accuracy of custom patient-specific grafts for maxillofacial bone augmentation.

8.1 Milled Bone-Graft Materials

Currently, custom augmentation scaffolds are mainly made from allograft materials. The use of allografts to augment mandibular and maxillary defects has regained interest in recent years; however, the safety record of allografts has historically been a concern both of clinicians and of their patients. The clinical advantages—reduced donor-site morbidity, shorter intervention times, and the available amount of graft material—make allografts an attractive alternative for autologous onlay bone grafts. However, the health regulations of several European countries oppose the use of allografts for dental use.

Recently published reviews have addressed the origin, preparation, and processing of allografts to guide the clinician toward using safe and reliable graft products. A systematic review by Waasdorp and Reynolds (2010) recognized the potential of allogeneic onlay bone grafts but was unable draw any conclusions regarding the efficacy of allogeneic bone blocks due to the limited data available. Despite this, several companies offer patient specific allografts in many countries.

Bone augmentation workflows begin with three-dimensional imaging of the patient's bone defect using CBCT. Custom bone blocks are designed using specialized CAD software (Fig 1). Once the final design is approved by the surgeon, a block can be produced to allow a simplified surgical procedure with a prefabricated and accurately fitting graft. Venet and coworkers (2017) suggested that custom bone allografts can be successfully used for horizontal ridge reconstruction in the anterior maxilla, with demonstrated reduced morbidity and shorter total intervention time compared to conventional surgical procedures.

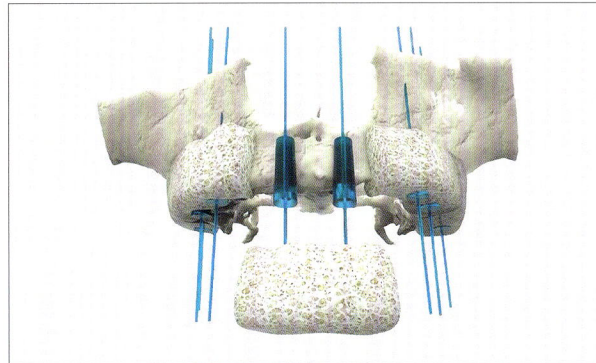

Fig 1 Design of an individual bone graft with future dental implants shown.

Defect-specific graft templates

Another option that facilitates the use of autologous material is to create a defect-specific graft template. CAD/CAM techniques can be used to prepare a graft-cutting guide as well as a surgical placement guide, for example in mandibular reconstruction using vascularized free bone flaps such as fibula, tibia, or iliac-crest bone (Ciocca and coworkers 2011).

Schepers and coworkers (2016) presented a clinical study based on CBCT images of a craniomandibular defect and high-resolution CT angiography of the lower-leg donor site, imported into CAD software. A planned reconstruction of the jaw defect was performed in a virtual environment. 3D models of the jaw defect and of the fibula were created, and the fibula donor flap was virtually cut and placed into the defect by computer simulation. By scanning the antagonist jaw, a diagnostic wax-up could also be incorporated with the planned occlusion, such that the implants could be planned and the fibula could be appropriately positioned to receive the implants at the same surgery.

Based on this information, it was possible to design and fabricate a surgical template for cutting the donor bone flap and an implant surgical guide.

Several reports have described the creation of physical surgical models onto which traditional titanium plates can be adapted extraorally. Ciocca and coworkers (2011) used a custom titanium mesh that served as a tray to hold particulate autologous bone and Bio-Oss granules (Geistlich, Wolhusen, Switzerland) in a case of an atrophic maxilla. After eight months, the regenerated bone was sufficiently strong to receive implants. The mesh was removed, and the implants were placed. No clinical problems or complications were detected during the twenty-month follow-up period.

8.2 Printed Bone-Graft Materials

Biomaterials in either particulated or block form have increasingly been used in attempts to reconstruct the alveolar ridge in an attempt to avoid the use of autologous bone and thereby minimize patient morbidity. However, when three-dimensional critical bone defects are to be treated, different approaches are available. These may be bone-block grafts (Lee HG and Kim 2015), guided bone regeneration (GBR) techniques (Jung and coworkers 2013; Simion and Fontana 2004) and augmentation with titanium mesh (Rasia-dal Polo and coworkers 2014; Beretta and coworkers 2015).

Although the use of autologous bone blocks is still considered the gold standard, donor site morbidity and possible complications such as soft-tissue dehiscence and failure because of graft instability are frequent major setbacks with these procedures. The use of allograft blocks was described as an alternative in some studies (Ahmadi and coworkers 2017). Unfortunately, the clinical outcomes when allografts are used may not be as predictable (Aghaloo and Moy 2008). The successful integration of bone grafts depends mainly on their adaptation, vascularization, and a stable fixation to the recipient sites (De Marco and coworkers 2005).

In recent years, 3D printing technology has undergone significant technical development. 3D printers are frequently standard equipment in dental laboratories, used in the fabrication of prosthetic devices. 3D printers are also often used in other medical fields. The three-dimensional shape of a bone defect can be retrieved from the CBCT dataset and a matching bone-block graft can be designed and fabricated using CAD/CAM technology. The technical advantage of 3D printing is that different biomaterials or even proteins and cells can be used in different layers during the production process, creating structures based on, and similar to, the natural biological condition.

In the current literature, the use of digital technology in the production of custom bone grafts using different approaches has been presented. The placement of direct custom bone grafts has been reported only in a limited number of publications (Mangano and coworkers 2013; Figliuzzi and coworkers 2013; Li and coworkers 2011; Schlee and Rothamel 2013; Mertens and coworkers 2013). Similarly, the number of publications reporting indirect customization, by manufacturing surgical guides and surgical models that help the surgeon visualize, plan, and prefabricate the custom graft are also limited.

Using CAD/CAM to customize bone grafts has several advantages. Some reports showed shortened overall intervention times, implying financial benefits (Figliuzzi and coworkers 2013; Li and coworkers 2011; Mertens and coworkers 2013; Zhou and coworkers 2010; Ciocca and coworkers 2001). Others rated the esthetics as good (Li and coworkers 2011; Mertens and coworkers 2013; Ciocca and coworkers 2011; Zhou and coworkers 2010; Modabber and coworkers 2012; de Farias and coworkers 2014; Stieglitz and coworkers 2014). Only a few studies mentioned complications (Mertens and coworkers 2013; Bellanova and coworkers 2013; Zhou and coworkers 2010; Lazarides and coworkers 2014; Stieglitz and coworkers 2014), which included wound infection, dehiscence, and the need for further surgical intervention.

8.3   Full 3D Planning of Free Vascularized Fibula Flaps for Maxillofacial Defects

A method for the prefabrication of a free vascularized fibula flap using dental implants and split skin grafts for complex rehabilitations has been described by Rohner and coworkers (2003). Schepers and coworkers confirmed the reliability of this technique in 2016, designing an individual bone block in the fibula of the patient. Virtual reconstruction of the bone defect is performed in a segmented fibula. The image of the fibula is derived from a CT scan of the lower leg and, after virtual segmentation, is positioned in a CBCT-based 3D model of the bone defect. Next, the implants are virtually planned in the segmented fibula in the position needed for maximal support of the planned prosthetic reconstruction.

Based on the virtual planning, a 3D printed surgical guide is produced that is placed on the ventral rim of the fibula and secured on the bone with miniscrews. Then the implant beds are drilled and the implants are inserted through the surgical guide. The fibula in which the implants are inserted is covered with a split-thickness skin graft. Five weeks after placement, the implants in the fibula are exposed. The virtually planned surgical guide for the fibular osseous flap is secured to the implants in the fibula, following which the osteotomies can be performed with a reciprocating saw. After removing the

surgical guide, a titanium bar is secured on the implants in the osteotomized fibula, and the denture is attached to the bar with clips.

At this time, the blood circulation within the graft is still intact to minimize ischemia. As soon as the defect in the maxilla is exposed, the fibula is raised as a free graft. The graft with the positioning splint is placed in occlusion intraorally. The graft is secured with osteosynthesis plates and monocortical screws. The fibular artery and veins are connected to the blood vessels in the neck. (The entire process is described in more detail in Chapter 13.13)

Schepers and coworkers (2016) showed in their clinical study that digital planning and 3D printing to virtually plan and execute reconstruction of maxillofacial defects with prefabricated fibula grafts pre-installed with dental implants is an accurate procedure. Their study included eleven patients, all of whom were treated for a malignant or benign tumor or for osteoradionecrosis. Five patients had received radiotherapy.

This approach seems to be a reliable technique that benefits from new digital technology and can be utilized when extreme augmentation is needed.

9 Digital Articulators

C. Evans

9.1   Introduction

When manufacturing restorations to replace teeth, the occlusal anatomy of the teeth should harmonize with the mandibular movements. Many occlusal concepts have been proposed over the years for the re-establishment of the occlusal anatomy. The common theory behind these concepts is that the occlusal anatomy is defined both by the temporomandibular joints and by the incisal guidance (Carlsson 2009; Gross 2008).

Dental articulators are used in treatment planning to analyze how teeth move relative to each other during the functional movements of the jaw and during prosthesis fabrication to aid the dental technician in producing an anatomical shape that closely resembles that of the natural teeth. A facebow is a tool that is used to transfer the terminal hinge axis to the articulator, allowing a more accurate alignment of the casts (Shillingburg and coworkers 1981).

The correct use of the articulator and facebow should enable the technician to develop anatomical restoration shapes that require minimal adjustment on delivery.

9.2 Mechanical Articulators

As defined by the Glossary of Prosthodontic Terms Ninth Edition (GPT9), an articulator is a mechanical instrument that represents the temporomandibular joints and the jaws and to which maxillary and mandibular casts may be attached to simulate some or all mandibular movements (Academy of Prosthodontics 2017).

GPT9 defines four classes of mechanical articulators:

- *Class I articulator (non-adjustable articulator)*
  A simple holding instrument capable of accepting a single static registration; vertical motion is possible.
- *Class II articulator*
  An instrument that permits horizontal as well as vertical motion but does not orient the motion to the temporomandibular joints.
- *Class III articulator (semi-adjustable articulator)*
  An instrument that simulates condylar pathways by using averages or mechanical equivalents for all or part of the motion; these instruments can align of the casts relative to the joints.
- *Class IV articulator (fully adjustable articulator)*
  An instrument that will accept 3D dynamic registrations. These instruments can align the casts to the temporomandibular joints and simulate mandibular movements.

Semi-adjustable articulators offer endpoint data input but no intermediate tracking of jaw movements. Fully adjustable articulators offer a high degree of adjustment by representing the jaw movements more closely. Adjustments can be input via conventional occlusal registration techniques or by a computed-aided analysis of the jaw movement using electronic feedback or ultrasound (Kordaß and coworkers 2002; Gärtner and Kordaß 2003)

The mechanical articulator is different from the true anatomical situation in that the movements reproduced by the mechanical articulator follow the structures of the mechanical joint compartment on that specific articulator. Because these structures are fixed and invariable over time, they cannot simulate the real masticatory movements, which are dependent upon such factors as muscle patterns, the resilience of the soft tissues, and the articular disc of the temporomandibular joint (Maestre-Ferrín and coworkers 2012).

Mounting stone casts on a mechanical articulator can introduce errors that may result in a final restoration that is too high in occlusal contact or that exhibits balancing-side or working-side interferences. These positive errors in occlusal registration often occur because a registration medium is placed between the tooth surfaces to make the clinical occlusal registration. Additionally, the presence of small positive surface bubbles on stone casts can further separate the occlusal surfaces from correct and true intercuspation. The laboratory technician will need to carefully assess all casts and check the accuracy of the occlusal registration provided to reduce errors.

Failure to accurately transfer the patient's true terminal hinge axis to the dental articulator via a facebow transfer can result in an occlusal morphology of the final restoration that does not balance with the true jaw movements. This may introduce balancing-side and working-side contacts which the patient will experience as occlusal interferences (Shillingburg and coworkers 1981; Maveli and coworkers 2015).

Digital registration of the occlusal contacts between teeth using intraoral scanning techniques has the advantage of not requiring a registration medium to be placed between the occlusal surfaces, enabling a more precise registration.

9.3 Digital Articulators

The types of articulator available for use within the digital environment has evolved and expanded as CAD software packages have been developed. Early CAD options allowed static evaluation of the occlusal contact positions at only maximum intercuspation. Newer software provides semi-adjustable and fully adjustable articulators, including facebow transfers, to be used within the digital design software.

Simple hinge-axis class I or class II 2 articulators may be appropriate for simple anterior or posterior single-tooth replacements with adjacent teeth that provide sound intercuspation with the opposing arch. Clinical cases with strong canine guidance, where the selection of a flat occlusal shape will require minimal adjustment, may also be suitable for use with a simplified articulator. In complex reconstructions with extensive implant restorations and complex occlusal anatomy, a precise occlusal design is necessary that reproduces the clinical jaw movements, reducing the need for chairside occlusal adjustments and aiding prosthesis delivery.

If a monolithic material is selected for the final restoration, there is limited opportunity for the clinician to adjust the occlusal morphology at chairside at the time of delivery. In these situations, a CAD/CAM articulation must be selected to develop an occlusal morphology that harmonizes with the patient's jaw movements. The final anatomic shape will need to be verified in the CAD process prior to milling. If an error is made, the restoration may need remaking, as occlusal adjustment to monolithic materials after fabrication may weaken the material.

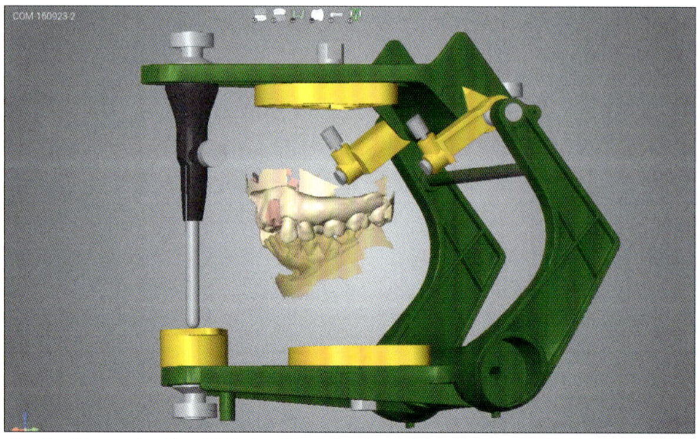

Veneered restorations will require a dental technician to manually adapt or build up material on a CAD/CAM framework. This route is chosen in clinical situations where esthetics plays a prominent role. In these cases, the use of a mechanical articulator will help dental technicians to evaluate their manual processes. CAD software that supports the integration of a class III or class IV adjustable articulator is indicated in these situations.

Three types of digital articulation exist within the digital workflow:

- Mechanical articulation with a digital interface
- Simple digital articulation
- Virtual digital articulation

9.3.1 Mechanical Articulation with a Digital Interface

The articulators used are class III or class IV articulators. Following a facebow transfer of the maxillary cast to the articulator, the plaster casts are mounted on removable plates on the actual mechanical articulator, which permits the scanning of the casts by a desktop scanner to locate them in the CAD software's "virtual" articulator exactly as on the mechanical articulator (Fig 1). This technique facilitates a facebow transfer to mount the casts, which assists the replication of the correct intermaxillary relationship with the terminal hinge axis. Software functions are available to simulate the complex movements of the mandible by conducting a review of the movements in protrusion, retrusion, immediate

Fig 1   Example of a digital articulator in CAD software, programmed after mounting models on a mechanical version of the same articulator.

lateral mandibular translation, and lateral excursions, using specified parameters for the set-up of the condylar slope, Bennett angle, immediate side shift, and incisal slope and height at the pin (Fig 2).

The occlusion can then be evaluated within the CAD software to investigate the areas of occlusal contact. The ability to visualize dynamic occlusion can also be used to check the design of the occlusal anatomy and allows any occlusal interferences to be resolved automatically (Solaberrieta and coworkers 2010) (Fig 3).

9.3.2   Simple Digital Articulation

There are two possible methods for simple digital articulation:

IOS scanning. The occlusal surfaces are scanned with an intraoral scanner (IOS) and imported into the CAD software. Using the occlusal scan function, the maxillary and mandibular scans are related to one another to provide a static maximal intercuspation position. Using the virtual articulation set-up function of the CAD software, these "virtual arches" are then positioned within the digital articulator using an arbitrary position and average preset values. This method is often used when sectional scans of the arch are made rather than full-arch scans. The virtual dynamic articulation function of the CAD software will indicate arbitrary contact positions within the limited range of movements that the system can simulate. This limited functional relationship may be adequate for single-unit cases in the anterior region; for posterior restorations, however, the lack of detail may produce occlusal interferences.

Model scanning with an occlusion medium. Physical casts are scanned, after which the software provides an option to scan an occlusal registration medium to provide the antagonist position rather than making a complete scan of the opposing cast. This technique facilitates an occlusal analysis, but one of limited accuracy. Its clinical use would be restricted to restorations where the final anatomy is copied from an accurate diagnostic wax-up or pre-existing occlusal morphology, or where the final restoration is a veneered ceramic restoration and the CAD procedure is used to develop a coping that will be manually veneered with a suitable material.

9.3.3   Virtual Articulators

Virtual articulators facilitate the evaluation of the static and dynamic jaw movements using virtual-reality technology (Maestre-Ferrín and coworkers 2011). They seek to improve the occlusal aspects of the restorative design by allowing analysis in occlusal contact positions as part of in the design process. Additionally, they can quantify the effects of resilience of the soft tissues on a time-dependent basis during chewing or eating and correct the digitally designed occlusal surface accordingly (Koralakunte and Alajanakh 2014; Solaberrieta and coworkers 2009).

The individual settings required for correct articulation within the virtual articulator are derived from an electronic trace or jaw-movement analysis used to program the virtual articulator (Fig 4). Three broad categories of jaw-movement recording systems are available:

- Ultrasound-based: JMAnalayser+ (Zebris Medical, Isny, Germany), ARCUSdigma (KaVo, Biberach, Germany)
- Voltage division methods: CADIAX (Gamma Dental, Klosterneuberg, Austria)
- Optoelectronic systems: CondyloComp LR3 (Dentron, Höchberg, Germany), Freecorder BlueFox (DDI-Group, Dortmund, Germany)

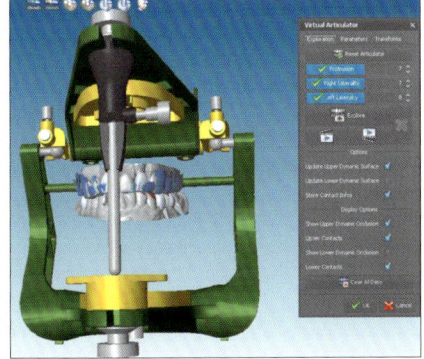

Fig 2   Articulation angles and adjustments can be virtually programmed in the CAD software.

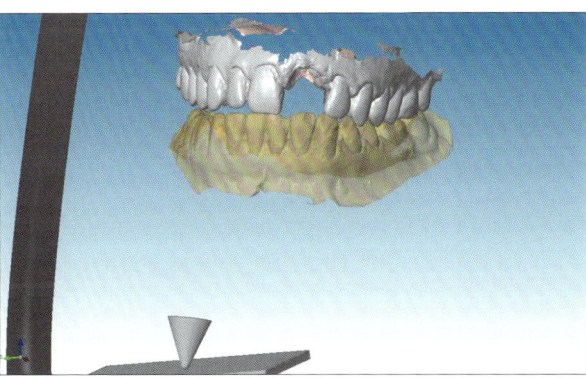

Fig 3   Left lateral excursive movements investigated in the CAD software.

As well as providing their own software for jaw-movement evaluation, most of these systems can provide values for setting up mechanical fully adjustable articulators, as well as export data for the CAD software to program the setting of the virtual articulator (Ahlers and coworkers 2015). While these systems can transfer condylar data, some do not support a true hinge-axis transfer with a digital facebow (Solaberrieta and coworkers 2013; Lam and coworkers 2016).

Recent advancements integrate jaw-movement tracking information with cone-beam computed tomography (CBCT) data to determine the anatomical position of the terminal hinge axis and to facilitate a more accurate evaluation of the occlusion. The CAD software then highlights the occlusal contact zones and automatically proposes the required modifications to the restorative design. It employs a collision-detection algorithm to dynamically calculate the occlusal surfaces.

The accuracy of virtual articulations has been reviewed and found to be as good as that of traditional mechanical articulators in terms of comparing the number of occlusal contacts found in both articulation types (Maestre-Ferrín and coworkers 2012).

9.4 Possible Future Developments

The next step in the development of virtual articulation systems is the integration of facial scanning data to produce a complete, functioning, "virtual patient" (Joda and Gallucci 2015b; Harris and coworkers 2016). This may provide an accurate location for the occlusal plane, which if incorrectly transferred can result in esthetic complications.

10 Fabrication Techniques and Materials

C. Evans

Recent developments in CAD/CAM technology and the increasingly industrialized manufacture of dental prostheses have provided a growing range of new materials with potential advantages (Le and coworkers 2015; Hebel and Gajjar 1997; Karl and Holst 2012):

- Monolithic restorative materials, reducing the possibility of veneering material fracture or chipping
- Biocompatible materials
- Metal-free restorations
- Reduced incidence of a lack of prosthesis passivity
- Improved fit of restorations
- Improved workflow efficiency
- Reduced production costs

10.1 Fabrication Techniques and Restorative Materials

Initial developments in CAD/CAM technologies for implant-supported restorations focused on reducing the incidence of framework misfit often found in prostheses made using the traditional lost-wax casting technique. This has always been a problem, especially with screw-retained prostheses to replace multiple missing teeth. Such casting misfits can be due to the differential volumetric shrinkage of the metals used in their fabrication. Various techniques have been used to overcome this problem, including sectioning and soldering gold alloy frameworks, laser-welding frameworks, Cresco Ti Precision (Dentsply Sirona, York, PA, USA), or fabricating implant-retained bridgework in smaller sections.

Modern dental CAD/CAM techniques can be used to mill the framework from a single block of material (a subtractive process) (Torabo and coworkers 2015; Dawood and coworkers 2015; Joda and coworkers 2017) (Table 1). This process uses a multi-axis milling unit with small tools to allow the intricate features of the definitive restoration, such as its occlusal anatomy, to be replicated from the digital design. Drawbacks include the wastage of a significant portion of the material during the process and tool wear, which may influence the final accuracy of the restoration (Kirsch and coworkers 2016). Furthermore, the accuracy of the restorative fit is limited by the size of the burs and the ability of the machine to manipulate the burs to match the requirements of the occlusal morphology. More recently, one company has sought to address this tooling limitation by developing of a compact laser-milling unit that allows the production of accurate surface details; however, at the time of this writing, this has not reached commercial maturity.

Table 1: CAD/CAM materials matched to milling techniques and tools used for processing (disc sizes are dependent on the milling unit)

Millable materials	Presentation	Wet/dry milling	Tools
Titanium	Discs	Wet	Diamond/carbide
Cobalt-chromium	Discs	Wet	Diamond/carbide
PMMA	Blocks or discs	Wet or dry	Carbide
Wax	Blocks or discs	Wet or dry	Carbide
Zirconia (presintered)	Blocks or discs Pin-supported	Wet or dry	Carbide
Zirconia (hot isostatically pressed, HIP)*	Blocks or discs	Wet	Diamond
Lithium disilicate	Blocks Pin-supported	Wet	Diamond
Resin-impregnated ceramics	Blocks Pin-supported	Wet or dry	Carbide

Other developments include additive rapid-prototyping techniques such as 3D printing, which can be used with a variety of materials. 3D printing can be classified based on the material used (Torabo and coworkers 2015; Dawood and coworkers 2015; Muyanaji and coworkers 2016):

1 Resin-based:

- **Stereolithography (SLA).** A photosensitive liquid resin polymer bath is activated selectively by laser curing to produce a solid object.
- **Photopolymer jetting.** A light sensitive polymer is injected onto a build tray by a printing nozzle.
- **Digital light processing.** Liquid resin is cured layer by layer from a projected light source.

2 Powder-based:

- **Binder jetting.** A powdered material is set by droplets of colored liquid, often water, sprayed from injector heads. The object is built up incrementally, layer by layer. The object will require post-production processing to strengthen or set the material.
- **Selective laser sintering (SLS).** Layers of particular powder material are fused into a model by a focused laser beam; the structure is self-supporting

3 Liquid-based:

- **Fused deposition.** A thermoplastic material is extruded onto a build tray to form a model.

Several factors have to be considered when choosing a material for implant-supported restorations (Joda and coworkers 2017). The extent to which the restoration can be produced entirely within a digital process will depend on many different factors, including:

- Esthetic expectations
- The planned retention mechanism (screw-retained vs. cemented)
- The size of the restoration
- Occlusal factors such as parafunction
- Anticipated ongoing maintenance requirements

Monolithic materials are attractive alternatives to layered ceramic build-ups in that they address the frequently reported technical complication of veneering material fracture (Pjetursson and coworkers 2014). While a monolithic material can be used for implant-supported restorations (Joda and Brägger 2014), highly esthetic restorations in the anterior region still require a certain degree of traditional manual intervention to produce a natural-looking restoration. Until further advances in esthetic materials for rapid prototyping are realized, a mixed digital/analog workflow will be required to produce restorations with complex natural characterizations.

Materials can be selected at one of three levels:

- Abutment level
- Framework level
- Integrated abutment/framework complex

10.2 Metal Alloys

Metal alloys have long been the standard material for abutments or frameworks used for implant-supported restorations. However, traditional cast gold alloys are increasingly being replaced by milled solid materials in an effort to reduce production cost and use more biocompatible materials.

10.2.1 Material Selection at the Abutment Level

The use of cast gold abutments has been proposed to reduce the "component stack" needed for implant-supported restorations by allowing direct screw retention of the abutment, eliminating the need for transmucosal abutment cylinders (Lewis and coworkers 1992) (Figs 1 and 2). While concerns about the tissue response to gold-alloy abutments have been voiced, the clinical significance of relevant histological observations has yet to be established (Vigolo and coworkers 2006; Linkevicius and Aspe 2008).

Titanium as an abutment material has sometimes been preferred to cast gold alloys, as an apical shift of the barrier epithelium within the connective-tissue attachment has been reported for gold-alloy abutments (Welander and coworkers 2008; Abrahamson and coworkers 1998; Abrahamsson and Cardaropoli 2007; Rompen and coworkers 2006).

CAD/CAM-milled titanium abutments can be used to support single-tooth restorations or bridgework if the thickness of the surrounding tissue adequately masks the abutment color (Leticia and coworkers 2016; Lops and coworkers 2016; Linkevicius and Vaitelis 2015). A significant advantage of CAD/CAM titanium abutments is that the precision of fit of the abutment interface is preserved; there is no risk of damage from laboratory workflow processes as there may be for gold abutments, such as investment-related damage to wax patterns or oxidation at the gold/abutment interface resulting in slight rotational inaccuracies.

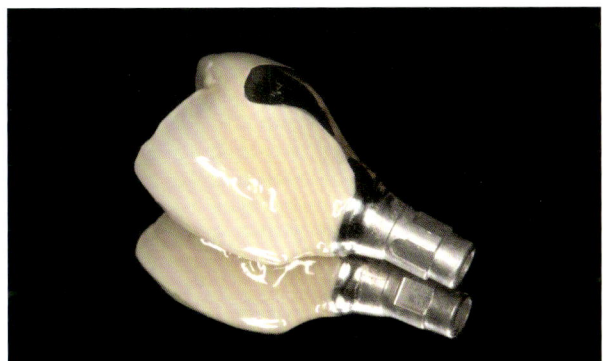

Fig 1 Metal-ceramic single crown made with a non-oxidizing gold-alloy abutment, with bonding alloy cast to the substrate, allowing the ceramic material to be directly built onto the complex. Mild oxidation of the abutment interface.

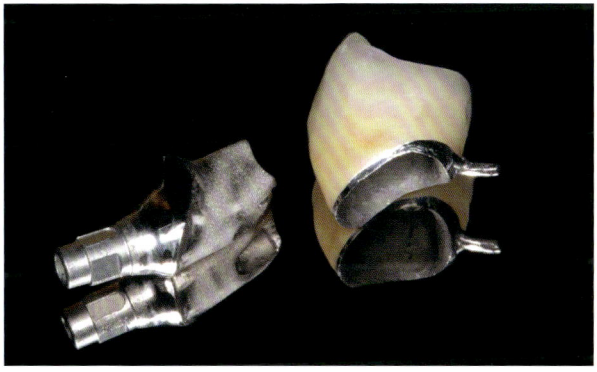

Fig 2 Two-piece custom gold abutment and separate metal-ceramic crown.

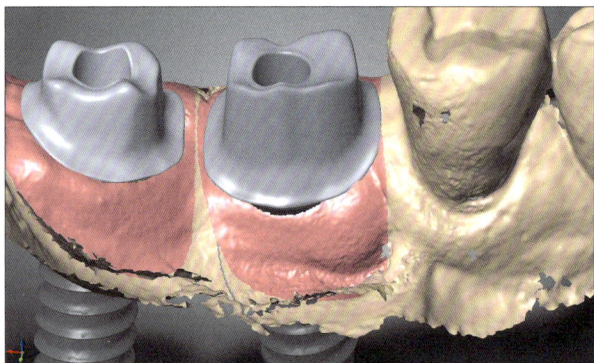 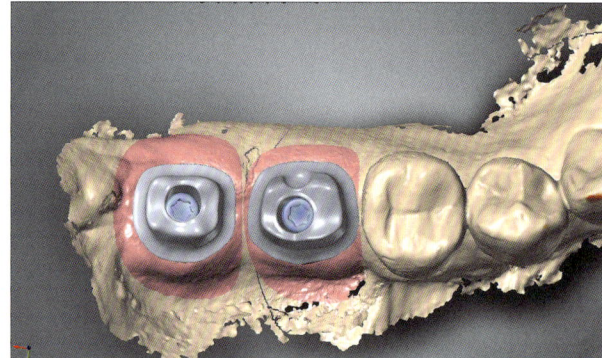

Figs 3a-b   CAD/CAM customized titanium abutments in design software (occlusal view).

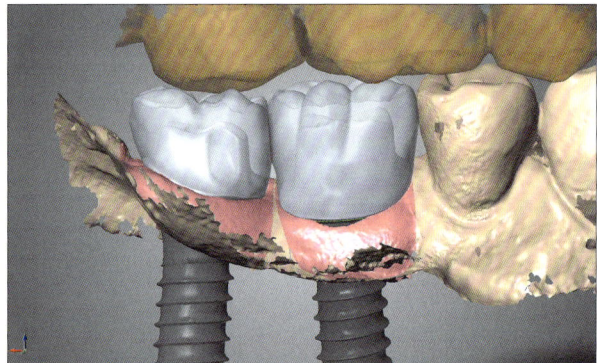 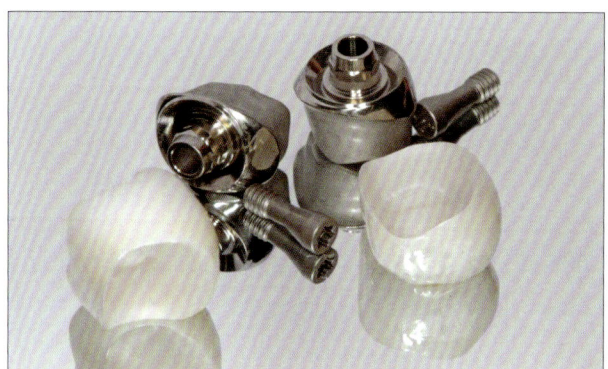

Fig 4   CAD/CAM-customized titanium abutments with prosthetic overlay.

Fig 5   Definitive CAD/CAM titanium abutments with monolithic zirconia crowns.

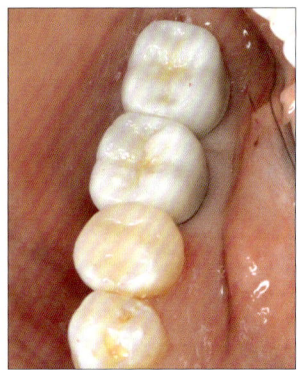

Fig 6   Definitive CAD/CAM prostheses in situ (occlusal view).

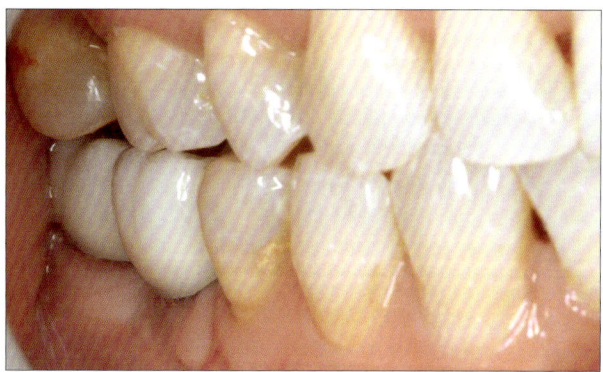

Fig 7   Definitive CAD/CAM prostheses in situ (buccal view).

Case 1 (Figs 3a-b to 7) illustrates the design of two custom CAD/CAM titanium abutments for cement-retained monolithic zirconia crowns.

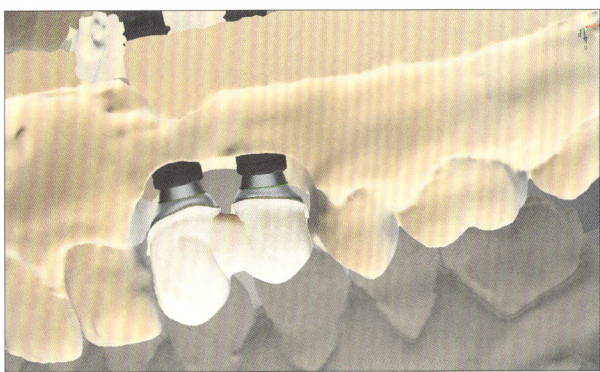 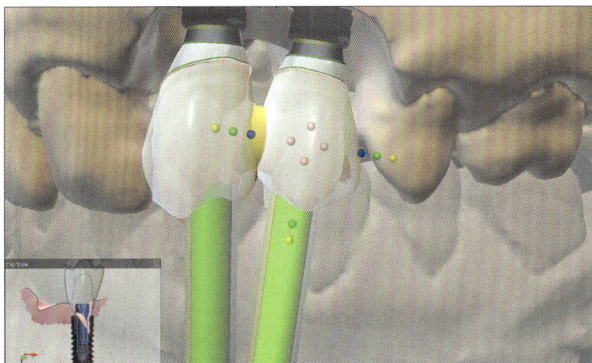

Figs 8a-b   Implant-supported replacement for teeth 23 and 24. CAD/CAM abutment and prosthesis in the design software.

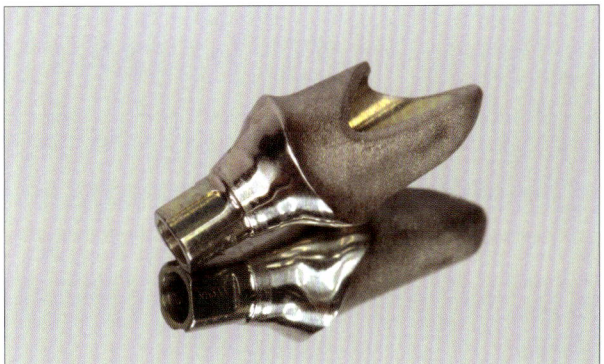 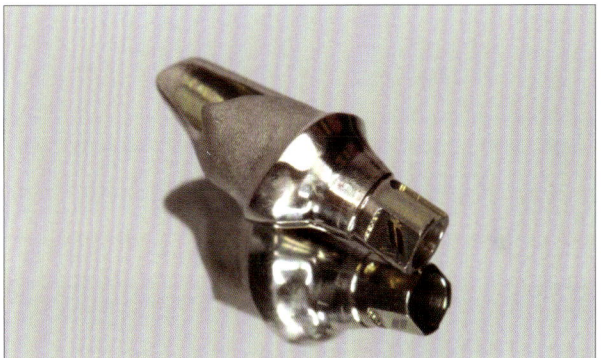

Figs 9a-b   Custom CAD/CAM titanium abutment. No oxide formation at the abutment interface.

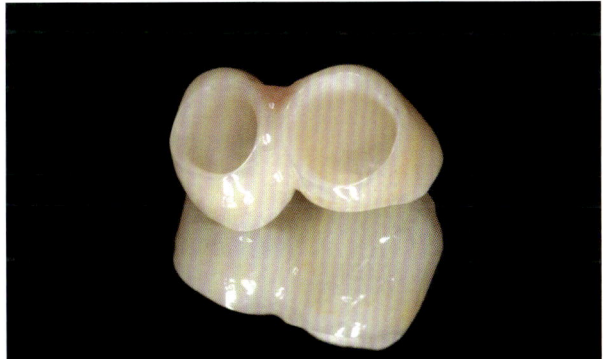 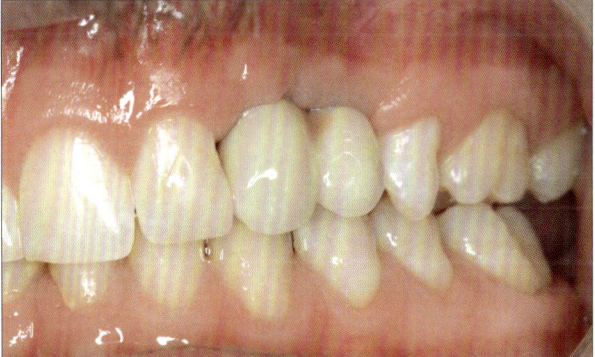

Fig 10   Cement-retained zirconia prosthesis ready for insertion.

Fig 11   Definitive cement-retained prosthesis with custom CAD/CAM titanium abutments.

Case 2 (Figs 8a-b to 11) illustrates the design of custom CAD/CAM titanium abutments to support a monolithic zirconia prosthesis designed as a splinted superstructure.

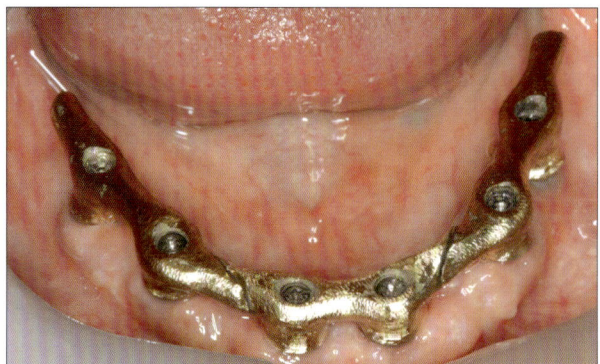

Fig 12a   A cast gold bar framework to reinforce a complete acrylic wrapping design.

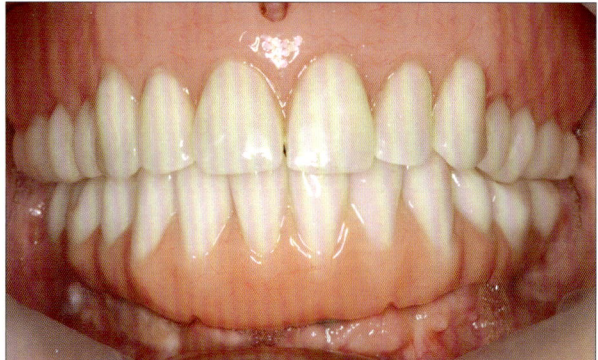

Fig 12b   Definitive fixed implant-supported prosthesis in situ.

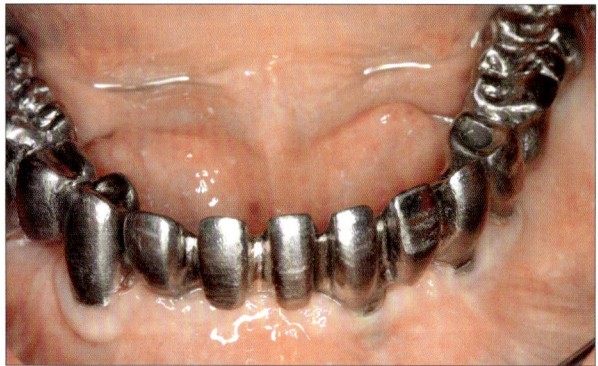

Fig 13a   Cast gold-alloy framework for an implant-supported metal-ceramic bridge.

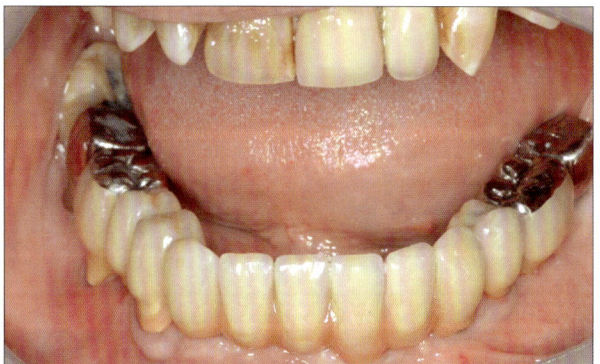

Fig 13b   Completed implant-supported metal-ceramic bridge.

10.2.2 Material Selection at the Framework Level

The fabrication of extensive metal frameworks to restore extended edentulous regions is technique-sensitive (Painz and coworkers 2013). Cast gold alloys have traditionally been used as the substrate material for the fabrication of complex complete implant supported prostheses (Figs 12a-b and 13a-b). However, widespread use of cast gold frameworks is declining due to the technical challenges associated with achieving precise and passive fit using lost wax casting processes, declining cost-effectiveness due to the increasing price of gold, and increased preference for more biocompatible materials (Abduo and Lyons 2013; Almasri and coworkers 2011; Ortorp and Jemt 2000; Jemt and coworkers 1999; Jemt 1995) (Fig 14).

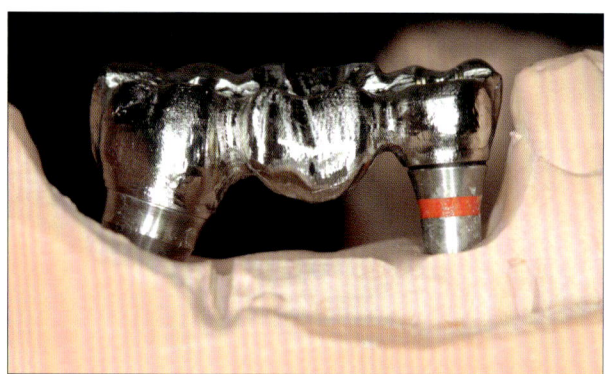

Fig 14   Ill-fitting cast framework requiring a remake, thus increasing cost.

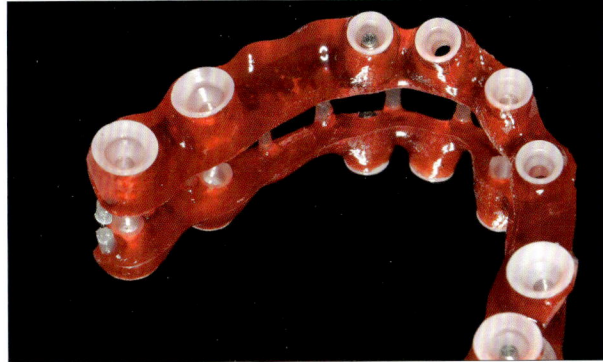
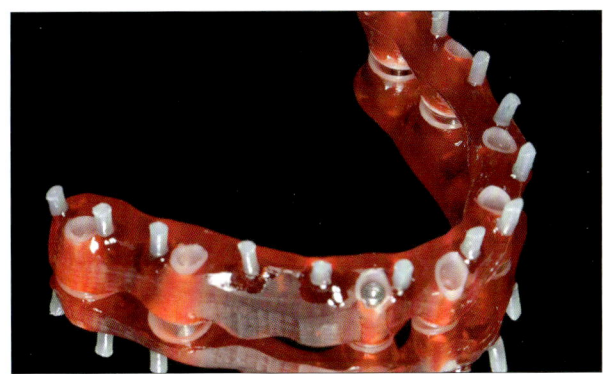

Figs 15a-b   A manual framework wax-up ready for copy-milling.

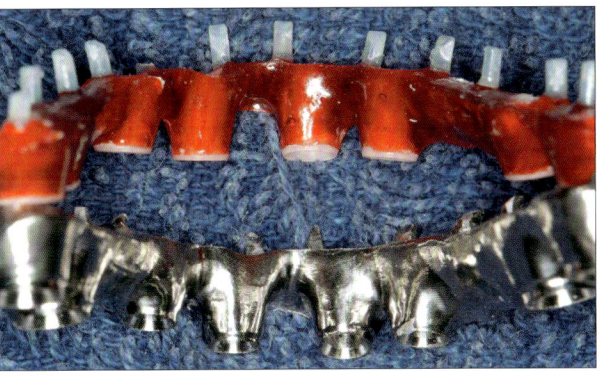

Fig 16a   Copy-milled titanium framework next to the original wax-up.

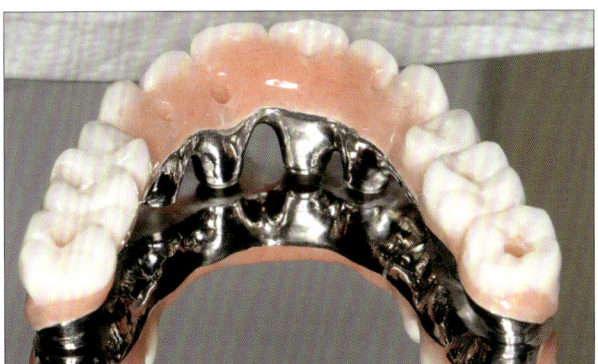

Fig 16b   Definitive full-arch fixed implant-supported prosthesis with acrylic resin teeth connected to the copy-milled titanium framework.

Prostheses for edentulous jaws are often designed to replace not only teeth, but also missing soft and hard tissues. The underlying frameworks can be used to support resin-layered replacement teeth, acrylic-resin teeth, ceramic veneers applied to replace both the teeth and gingival/mucosal structures, or a combination of a pink layer with individually cemented crowns.

Titanium was the first material used in the production of CAD/CAM frameworks and has been recommended as the first choice for superstructures in fully edentulous patients (Ortorp and Jemt 2012). It is covered by the greatest amount of clinical research to support its use, and generally the literature suggests that a subtractive manufacturing process (milling) can achieve an acceptable degree of fit, within the recommended clinical tolerance of 50 μm or less (Eliasson and coworkers 2010; Abduo 2014).

Early titanium frameworks relied on scans of manual wax-ups that were copy-milled using CAM software (Figs 15a-b and 16a-b).

Recent software advances provide CAD/CAM design options for metal frameworks, which support a fully digital workflow, allowing the final tooth position to be scanned and a complete digital design of the framework to be made without a manual framework-design process. The digital framework design has a known cut-back dimension applied relative to the designed final tooth position to create the appropriate space for veneering material.

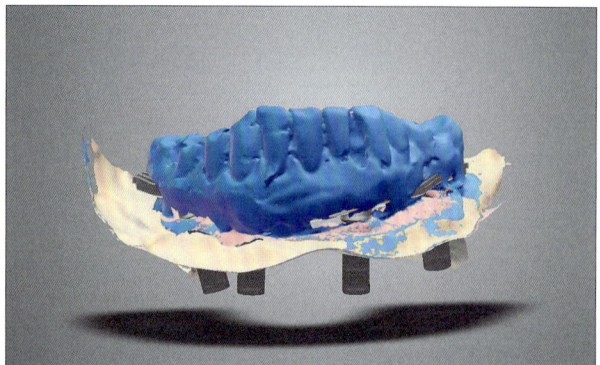

Fig 17   Final tooth position in the CAD software for the framework design.

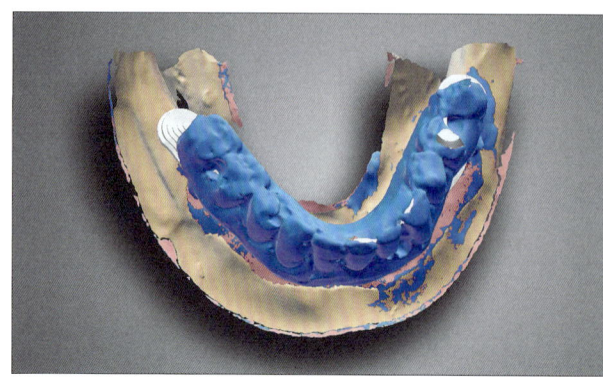

Fig 18   Final tooth position superimposed on the framework in the CAD software.

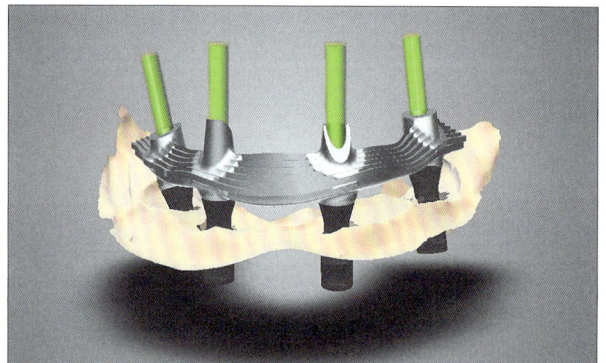

Fig 19   Framework with the final tooth-position layer removed.

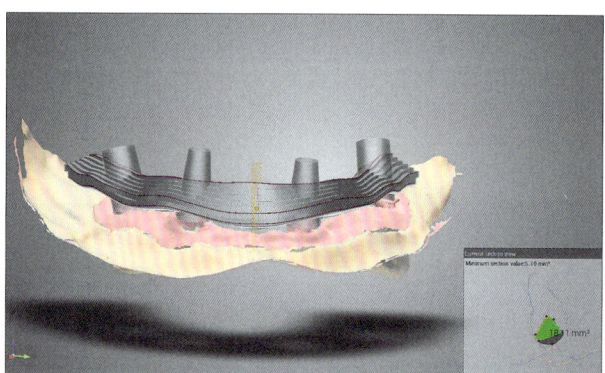

Fig 20   Verification of the cross-sectional area for adequate thickness.

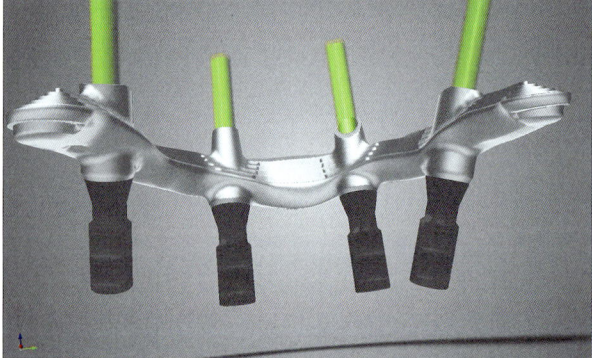

Fig 21   Verification of the position of the screw access channel in the framework.

Case 3 (Figs 17 to 24) demonstrates the complete CAD/ CAM design and production of a titanium framework supported by four implants. Technical complications with CAD/CAM frameworks such as fractures are comparable to those reported for conventional cast frameworks (Kapos and Evans 2014).

When a ceramic veneer is applied directly onto a metal framework, it is necessary to select an appropriate alloy that can develop an oxide layer capable of bonding to dental ceramics. Milled titanium frameworks for subsequent direct ceramic veneering are not widely recommended; the veneering material may often delaminate due to an insufficient oxide layer. To render the titanium surface suitable for reliable ceramic bonding, the surface must be modified, e.g., by air abrasion (Antanasova and Jevnikar 2016).

Alternative non-precious materials are also available for milled frameworks such as cobalt-chromium, which is rigid but less biocompatible (Svanborg and coworkers 2015) (Figs 25 to 30). Cobalt-chromium alloys are considered a better alternative to titanium, with a more predictable degree of ceramic bonding (Antanasova and Jevnikar 2016). These alloys are considered viable alternatives to metal-ceramic reconstructions because of their favorable mechanical properties and low cost (Svanborg and coworkers 2015).

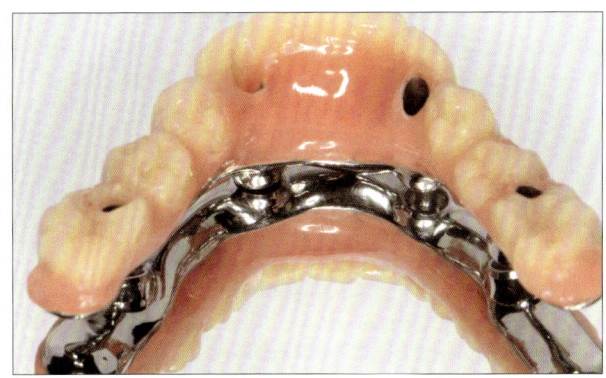

Fig 22a Case 3 Definitive titanium framework with acrylic resin veneer (occlusal view).

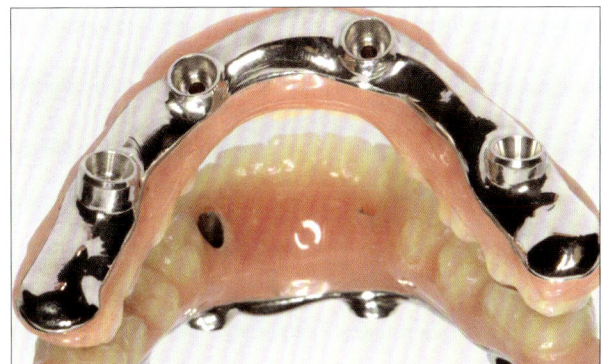

Fig 22b Case 3 Definitive titanium framework with acrylic resin veneer (intaglio surface).

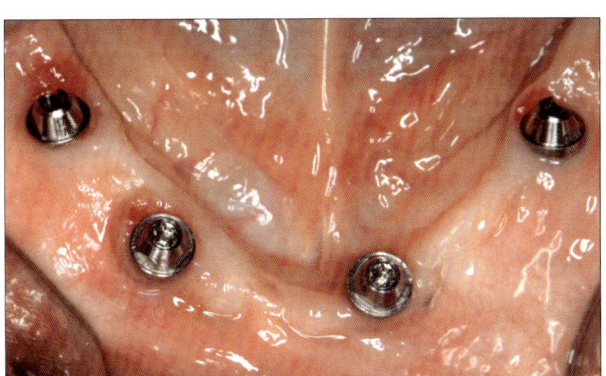

Fig 23 Definitive abutments, ready for insertion of the prosthesis.

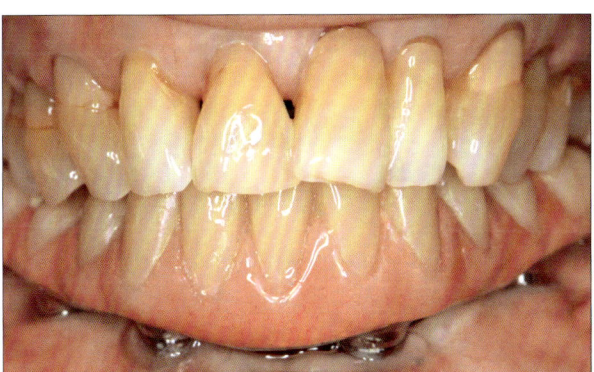

Fig 24 Definitive prosthesis in situ.

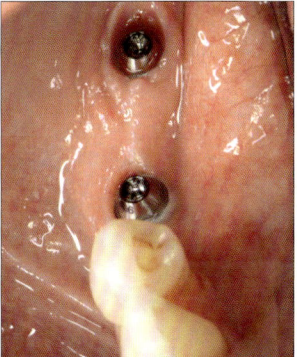

Fig 25 Abutment level choice of non-precious framework material.

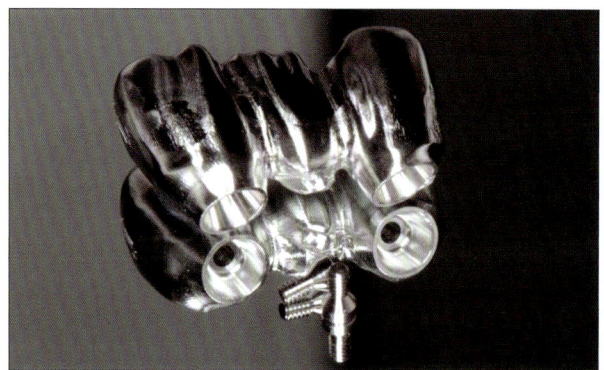

Fig 26   *Milled non-precious Coron framework to be ceramically veneered.*

In situations where the clinician may wish to use a traditional gold alloy, it is also possible to mill the digital design in wax to allow subsequent casting in gold (Figs 31 and 32).

Titanium frameworks are often lighter than cobalt-chromium frameworks; both are usually significantly lighter than cast gold frameworks (Paniz and coworkers 2013).

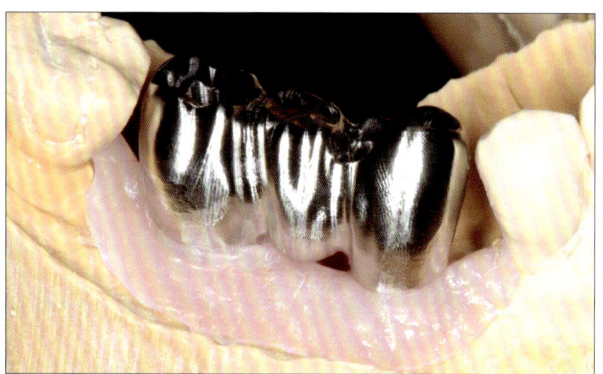

Fig 27   *CAD/CAM framework design. Precision of fit verified on the working cast.*

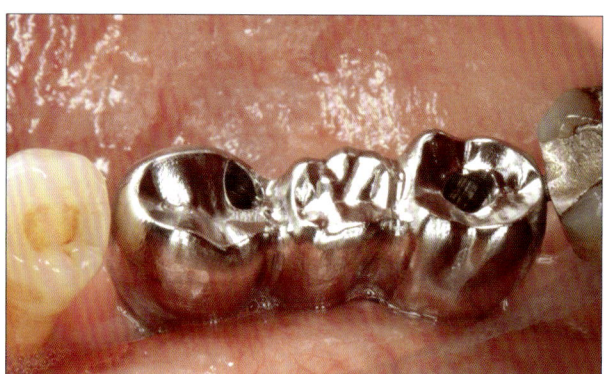

Fig 28   *Non-precious framework verified for clinical fit.*

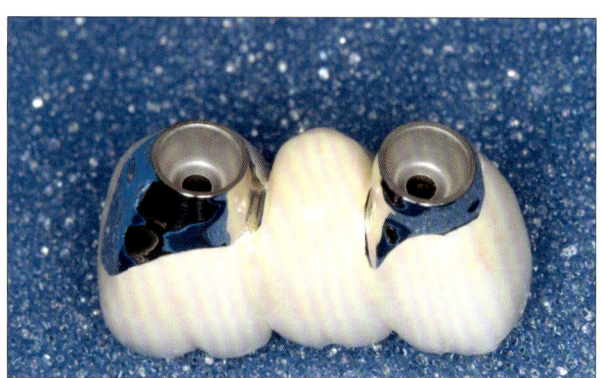

Fig 29   *Definitive ceramic veneering of the non-precious framework.*

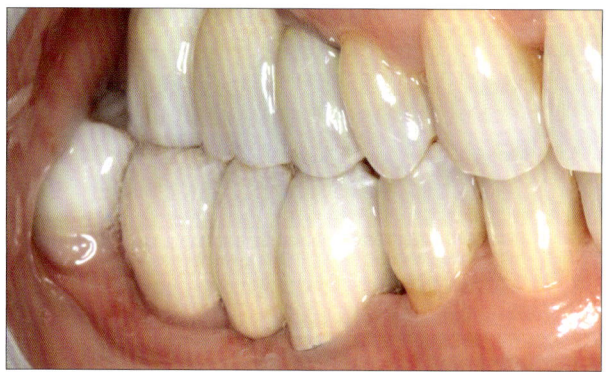

Fig 30   *Delivery of the definitive metal-ceramic restoration.*

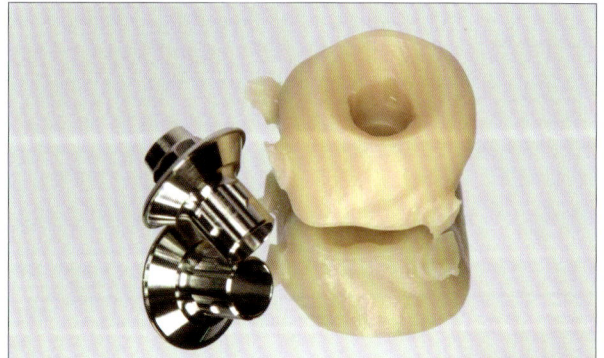

Fig 31   *Milled wax model ready for casting using the conventional lost-wax technique.*

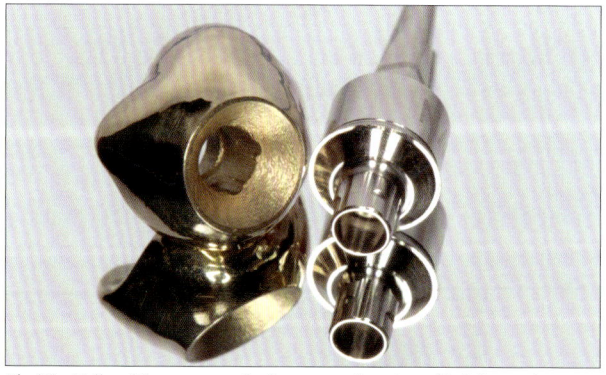

Fig 32   *Full gold crown ready for connection to a Variobase abutment (Institut Straumann AG, Basel, Switzerland).*

10.3 Zirconia

Zirconia is a polymorphic material that can have four different crystalline structures with properties that some authors consider optimal for dental use: superior toughness, strength, and fatigue resistance, low thermal conductivity, low corrosion potential, excellent wear properties, and biocompatibility (Della Bona and coworkers 2015; Nakamura and coworkers 2010; Guess and coworkers 2012).

Zirconia can be used for implant abutments, for frameworks for extended edentulous restorations, as copings for veneering restorations, or as a monolithic restoration. Early favorable clinical outcomes with zirconia-based implant-supported restorations and the increasing demand for esthetic restorations have driven the continued development and expanded use of zirconia as a restorative material (Zembic and coworkers 2012; Kapos and Evans 2014; Abdulmajeed and coworkers 2016; Shi and coworkers 2016).

At room temperature, zirconia remains in a monoclinic phase. On heating, the monoclinic phase is transformed into a tetragonal phase; however, the addition of stabilizing oxides such as ceria (CeO_2), yttria (Y_2O_3), alumina (Al_2O_3), or magnesia (MgO), alone or in combination, prevents the zirconia from returning to the monoclinic phase on cooling. It thus forms a multiphasic meta-stabilized structure, displaying stress-induced transformation-toughening attributes. If the material is subjected to mechanical stress, it undergoes a phase transformation to resist crack propagation. This transformation toughening involves a volume change, which closes the tip of the initial crack and produces compressive stresses within the material around the crack itself. The material can therefore effectively prevent fractures from opening within the zirconia material (Silva and coworkers 2010; Della Bona and coworkers 2015; Nakamura and coworkers 2010).

Dental zirconia objects can be milled from two different kinds of blocks:

- **Presintered blocks.** Presintering, or "soft-milling," of cold-pressed (CP) zirconia is less taxing on the milling tools, with the material reaching its final physical properties after sintering. Presintered milling produces an oversized structure that undergoes approximately 20% volumetric shrinkage during sintering. Careful control of the technique is therefore required to ensure that the accuracy of fit is maintained. Structural flaws arising from the milling process can be revised during the sintering process.
- **Fully sintered blocks.** The milling of post-sintered (hot isostatically pressed, HIP) blocks or zirconia requires "hard-milling" tools capable of grinding the material. There will be no shrinkage, as the material does not require further sintering after milling. A high degree of accuracy can be attained; however, residual "tooling" flaws may remain within the final material structure, which could present mechanical weaknesses and increase vulnerability to fractures.

A unique feature of zirconia is its susceptibility to a phenomenon called low-temperature degradation (LTD), where the material undergoes a spontaneous change from the tetragonal or toughened phase to the weaker monoclinic phase, predisposing the material to fracture (Guess and coworkers 2012; Ferrari and coworkers 2015). LTD is a potential concern with monolithic zirconia restorations, which could benefit from a thin layer of glass ceramics to coat all surfaces exposed to the oral cavity.

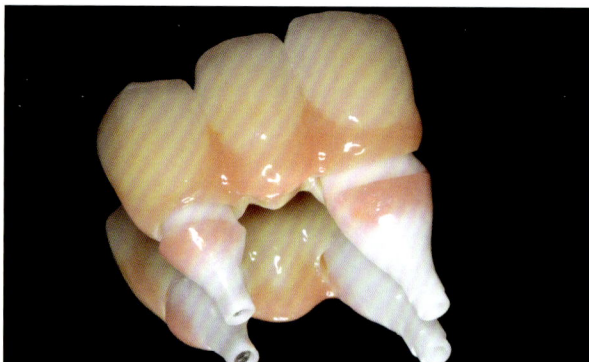

Fig 33a   Zirconia abutments designed to support a cemented implant-supported fixed dental prosthesis.

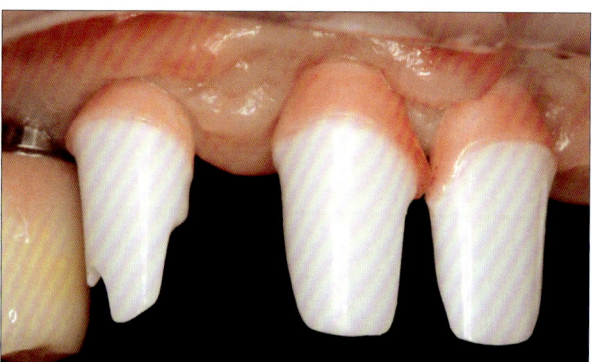

Fig 33b   The zirconia abutments are carefully inserted to avoid damage to the abutments themselves; pink ceramic has been fired onto the abutment surface to mask the pre-existing tissue loss in a patient who had been wearing a complete maxillary denture for 20 years.

10.3.1 Material Selection at the Abutment Level

The tissue response to zirconia appears to be similar to that seen with titanium. Early research found zirconia to be apparently superior to titanium in animal studies with regard to plaque accumulation; however, no clinical advantages were reported (Nakamura and coworkers 2010). More recently, several systematic reviews (Linkevicius and Vaitelis 2015; Sanz-Sánchez and coworkers 2018) have reported that zirconia abutments exhibit reduced bleeding on probing compared to titanium abutments and allow for a more natural soft-tissue color, which could be advantageous in the esthetic zone. If the peri-implant tissue is thinner than 2 mm, discoloration of the tissue due to the underlying titanium can be expected (Leticia and coworkers 2016; Lops and coworkers 2016). Zirconia may be used to eliminate this risk and ensure that, should peri-implant soft-tissue recessions occur after restoration, the appearance of visible metal will be avoided. Zirconia can be selected so as to match the value, hue, and chroma of the adjacent teeth, so the margins of cement-retained restorations can be placed supramucosally to prevent cement from contaminating the peri-implant soft-tissue collar.

All-zirconia abutments are milled from HIP zirconia and are not sintered after fabrication (Figs 33a-c). Special care must be taken at the technical stages to ensure the zirconia interface is not damaged and that no ceramic powder is inadvertently baked into the screw access hole. Tissue modeling using customized provisional restorations is advised prior to insertion of the prosthesis to avoid pressure from the tissue displacing the zirconia prosthesis laterally as the abutment is screwed into the implant.

Butt-joint screw interfaces are usually employed with zirconia abutments rather than tapered screw heads, to avoid lateral pressure on the abutment walls.

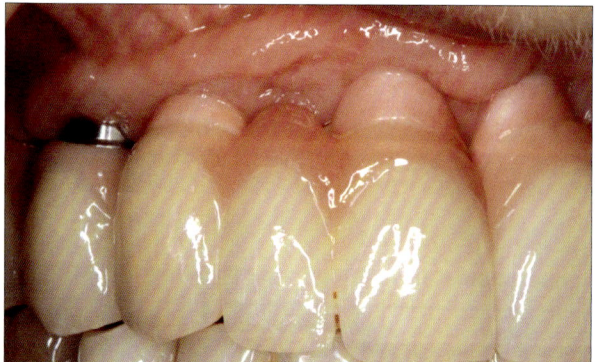

Fig 33c   Definitive cemented prosthesis with supragingival margins.

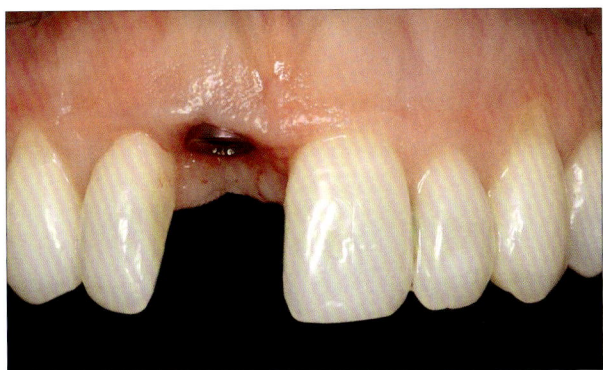

Fig 34a Implant ready for restoration following a staged treatment involving soft- and hard-tissue augmentation for a patient with a high smile line and thin tissue phenotype.

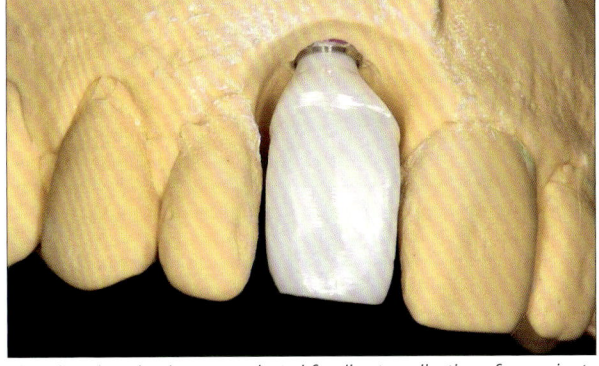

Fig 34b Zirconia abutment selected for direct application of ceramics to avoid tissue discoloration in the esthetic zone.

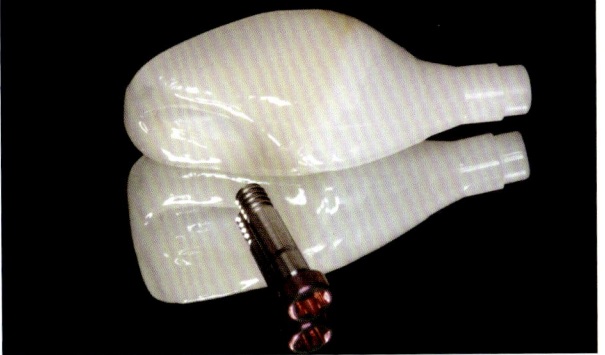

Fig 34c Completed screw-retained prosthesis, ready for insertion.

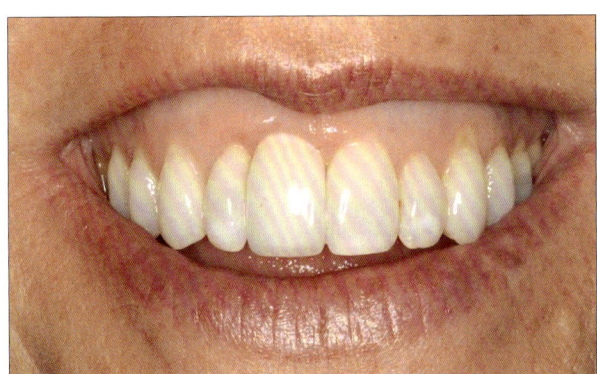

Fig 34d Twelve months after the insertion of the screw-retained zirconia crown 11.

Zirconia abutments engaging the dental implant directly have recently been shown to deposit titanium on the zirconia surface as a result of micromovement, which induces wear at the internal implant/abutment interface. This could potentially damage the implant interface and result in abutment misfit. Titanium has also been detected in the surrounding peri-implant tissue, which may also be explained by this micromovement. The rate of wear appears to be self-limiting, dropping off after some time, but the exact clinical implications, such as metallic deposits in the soft tissue or implant damage, are currently unknown (Klotz and coworkers 2011; Karl and Taylor 2016). If zirconia is considered for use in direct connection to the dental implant, genuine components that replicate the exact internal geometry of the implant/abutment connection have been shown to produce the most secure and reliable connection (Joda and Brägger 2015c; Truninger and coworkers 2012) (Figs 34a-d).

Concerns about possible damage to the implant caused by zirconia abutments can be addressed by using bonded titanium bases. Here, the zirconia abutment is bonded to a pre-machined titanium component that represents the implant/abutment connection. The design parameters of the abutment interface are loaded into the CAD file of the design software. Following the fabrication of the zirconia superstructure, the components are adhesively bonded to provide the definitive abutment or restoration. The zirconia is adhesively bonded after sandblasting using an adhesive containing 10-methacryloyloxydecyl dihydrogen phosphate (MDP) and resin cement. This technique can be used for single-tooth and multi-unit restorations. These composite structures can withstand loads within the anticipated clinical range (Joda and coworkers 2015) (Figs 35a-e).

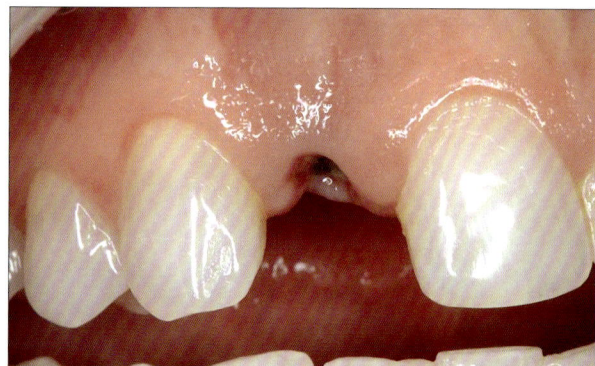

Fig 35a   Bone-level implant after integration showing partial tissue coverage of the healing abutment.

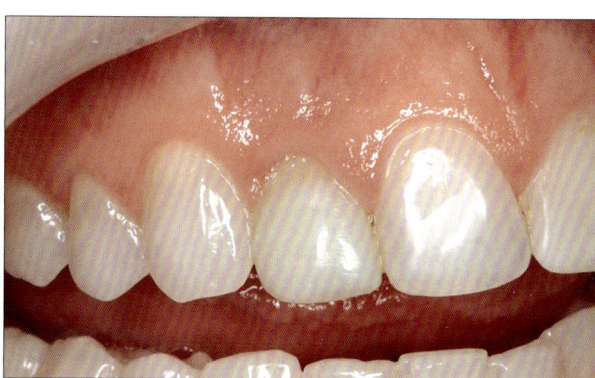

Fig 35b   The provisional restoration has sculpted the peri-implant mucosa.

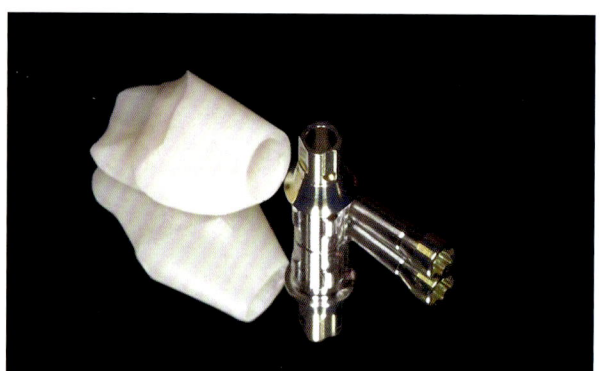

Fig 35c   Zirconia coping and Variobase abutment, avoiding the use of zirconia in directly contact within the implant. A zirconia shade can be selected to match the natural tooth shade.

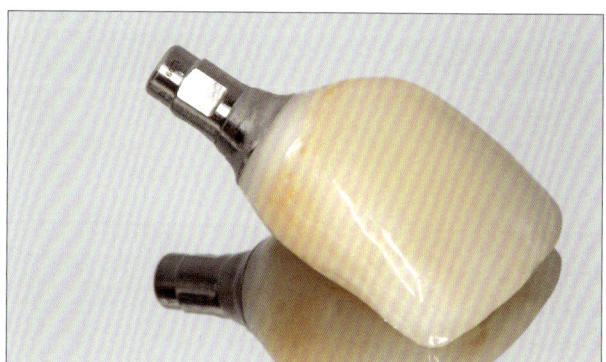

Fig 35d   After veneering the zirconia coping, it is adhesively bonded to the Variobase abutment extraorally using resin cement.

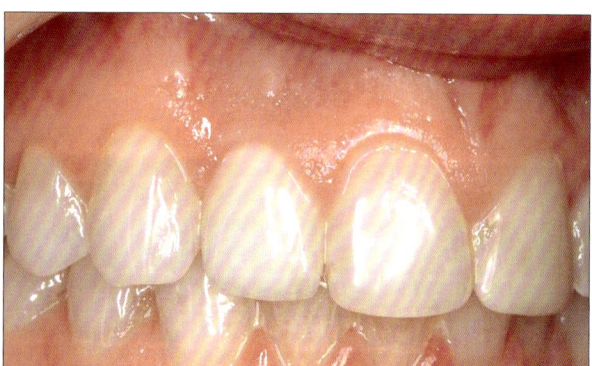

Fig 35e   Definitive result 12 months after delivery.

10.3.2 Material Selection at the Framework Level

Zirconia can be used in monolithic implant-supported restorations or as a framework for ceramic veneering (Figs 36a-b). If zirconia is to be used as a framework, care must be taken to reduce the incidence of ceramic chipping by:

- Ensuring uniform support of the veneering ceramic in the design process
- Carefully selecting the veneering ceramic to reduce any mismatch in the coefficients of thermal expansion
- Ensuring a slow cooling rate after firing or glazing the definitive veneer, allowing the framework to cool adequately
- Making careful occlusal adjustments with fine diamonds, followed by polishing (Guess and coworkers 2012)

To manage esthetic requirements, zirconia of increased translucency and a wide range of colors is commercially available, and color-graded blocks have recently been introduced.

Presintered ("soft-milled") monolithic frameworks can be stained prior to sintering, reducing the need to rely on traditional build-up techniques to produce esthetic restorations. Early clinical outcomes with such restorations have been favorable (Carames and coworkers 2015; Venezia and coworkers 2015). After finalizing these monolithic-style restorations, the zirconia must be bonded to a titanium base to provide the preferred metal-to-metal connection inside the dental implant. For external-connection implants, a zirconia-based restoration is available for direct single crowns; however, due to the need to provide a high precision of fit to the implant, a post-sintering milling process is required before the ceramic is built up on the framework (Figs 37a-g).

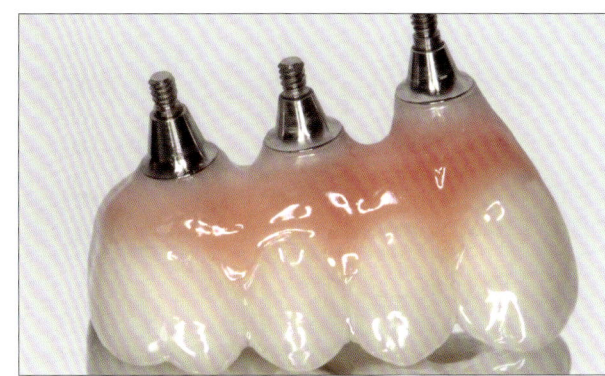

Fig 36a   Presintered zirconia framework stained prior to sintering to allow a mostly monolithic framework to receive a thin final glazing layer.

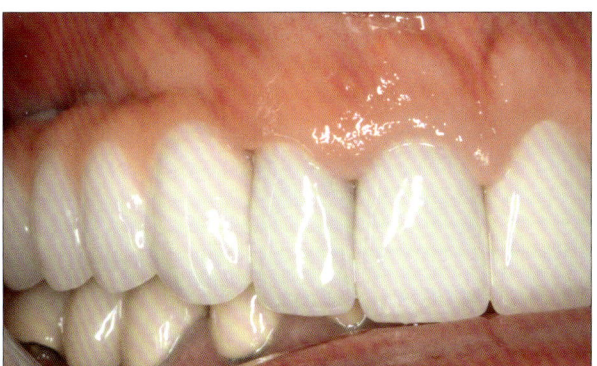

Fig 36b   The restoration in situ.

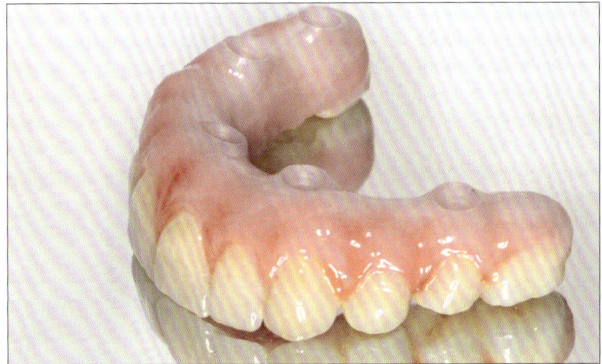

Fig 37a   Monolithic full-arch zirconia reconstruction milled in the presintered state and infiltrated with stains. A final glaze was applied to the surface.

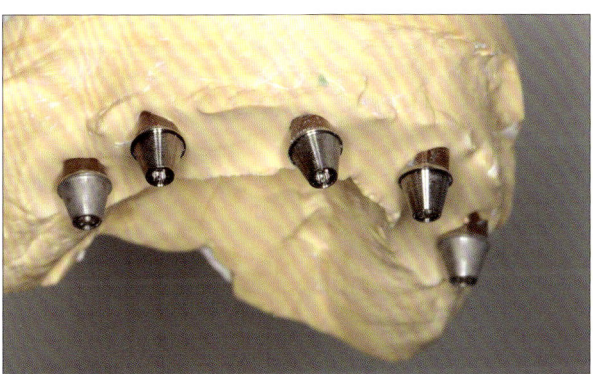

Fig 37b   Titanium bonding elements on the working cast.

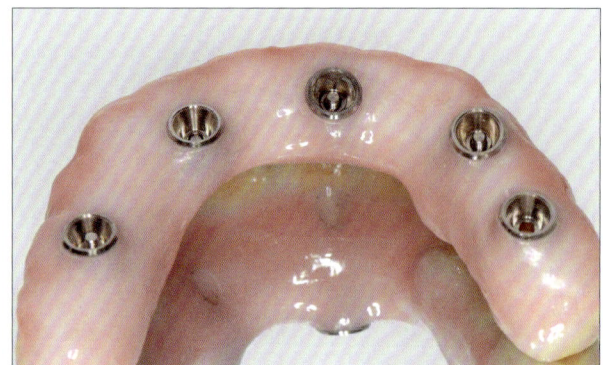

Fig 37c   Bonding of the titanium bases to the monolithic zirconia framework.

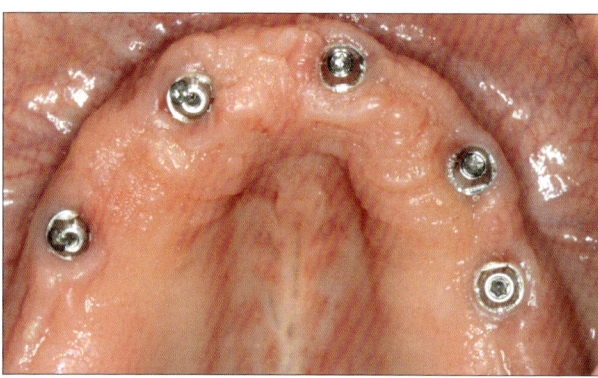

Fig 37d   Abutments in situ to support the prosthesis.

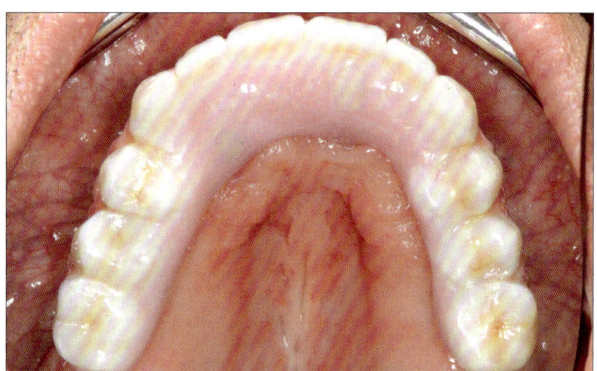

Fig 37e   Definitive prosthesis in situ (occlusal view).

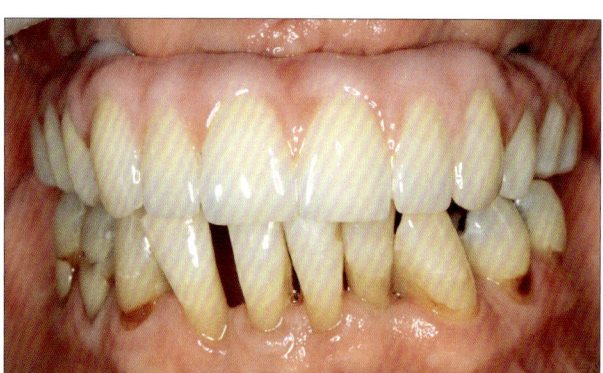

Fig 37f   Definitive prosthesis in situ (frontal view).

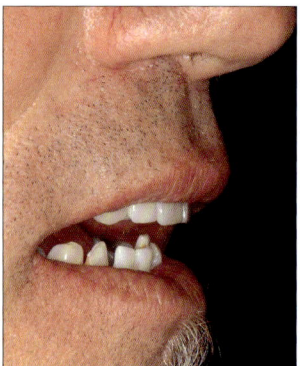

Fig 37g   Definitive prosthesis with patient smiling.

10.4 Lithium Disilicate

Lithium disilicate-based materials are best suited for single crowns. They are sold as precrystallized blocks that are blue-purple in color and can be prepared with diamond burs. A proprietary material designed for this use is IPS e.max CAD (Ivoclar Vivadent, Schaan, Liechtenstein). The material comes in small blocks fused to a holding pin that supports the material during grinding. A wide range of colors and translucencies are available.

IPS e.max is known for providing excellent esthetic results in a material of moderate strength. This material can be used as a monolithic material that receives a surface stain and glaze for finalization, or as a core to be veneered. It is possible to use IPS e.max CAD for crowns on a zirconia abutment or as a monolithic material on a titanium bonding base. Lithium disilicate infiltrated with zirconia is also available as a millable block (Figs 38a-h).

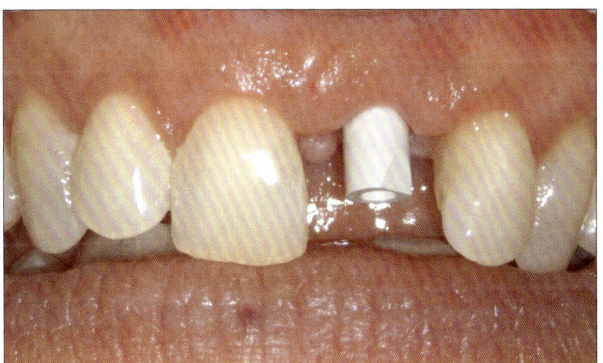

Fig 38a   Scanbody in situ for intraoral scanning of the implant position.

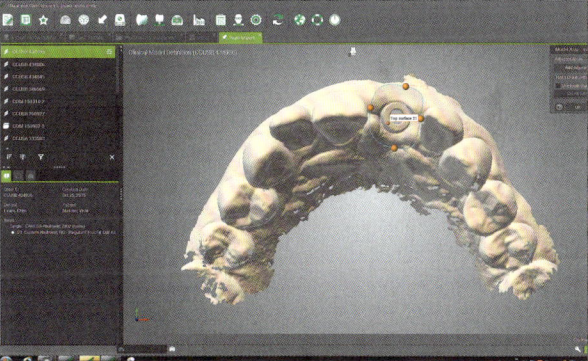

Fig 38b   Implant position from intraoral scan in the CAD software.

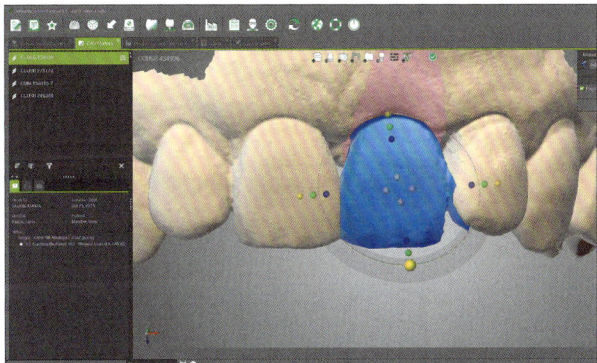

Fig 38c   Final position wax-up used to generate the abutment and restoration contours.

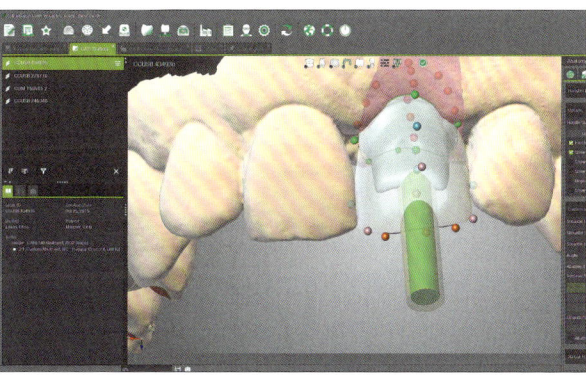

Fig 38d   CAD design of the zirconia abutment.

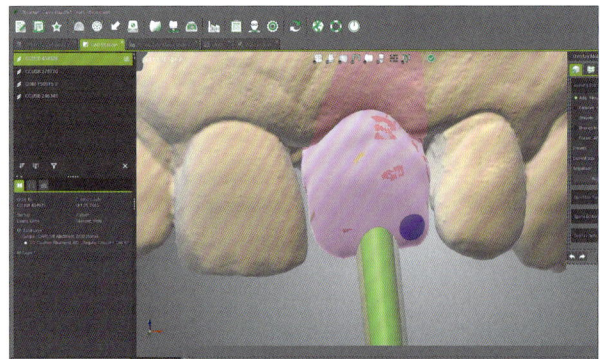

Fig 38e   Coping design for e.max CAD.

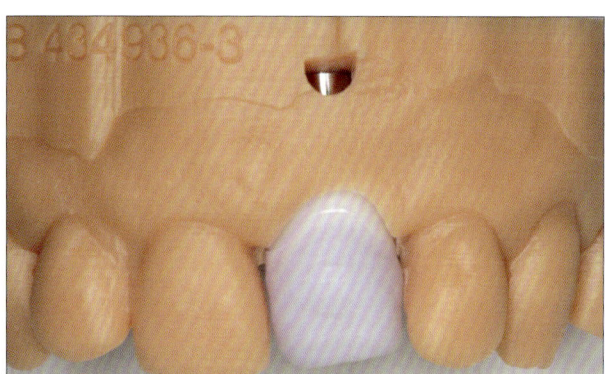

Fig 38f   Zirconia abutment on the 3D-printed model.

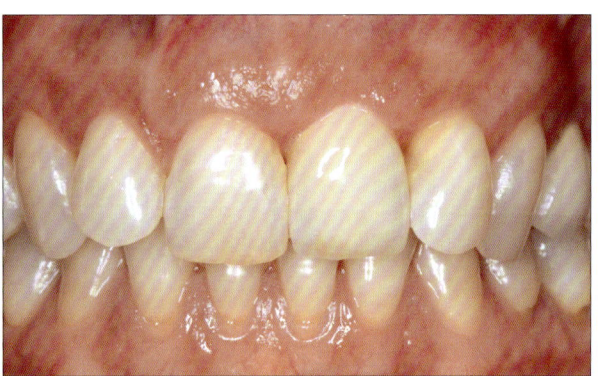

Fig 38g   Definitive restoration in situ.

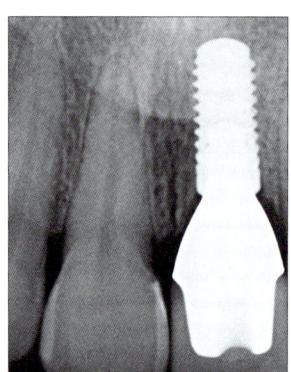

Fig 38h   Post-treatment radiograph showing stable crestal bone levels.

11 Complications and Technical Challenges

C. Evans

Technicians and clinicians who are used to working with physical models must firstly become accustomed to working with digital images and files. This may present a challenge to operators accustomed to handling conventional physical models.

Furthermore, the rapidly changing nature of digital workflows and associated software solutions potentially increases the risk of compatibility errors and complications during these processes. Digital workflows inevitably imply a need for ongoing re-education in terms of new workflows, new implant components, and new materials, as well as the training required to operate upgraded software packages.

A number of complications can occur in the different stages of the digital workflow. Table 1 presents a workflow checklist, outlining the individual process components

required for the clinician to commence working on a case with a complete digital workflow. If there is incompatibility between any of these stages, a fully digital treatment workflow may not be possible to complete.

Manufacturers increasingly offer open software systems that allow operators to move digital files between different software and design systems more readily. However, to realize a complete digital workflow, the clinician and technician sometimes need to overcome complications that may prevent the treatment being completed within a digital process.

In general, complications can be classified as either:

- Scanning-related complications
- Software integration complications
- Milling complications

Table 1   Checklist that the treatment team must consider for digital workflows.

Process components for the digital workflow	
CBCT	Available with a suitable software package
Surface scan technology	Available with a compatible file format
Scanbody	Recognizable design within the digital software library
Laboratory analog	Available and compatible with model-builder software
Digital implant library	Available with latest updates for the full range of implants in use
Digital prosthetic library	Genuine components compatible with the chosen implant
Implant components provided by manufacturers	Available for the selected digital prosthetic design and implant choice

11.1 Scanning-Related Complications

Digital scanbodies enables software to accurately record the actual implant position. They must have a unique shape that the software can recognize and accurately position a virtual implant replica within the digital surface scan. Surface scans rely on optical technology to capture the morphology of the scanbody. If the scanner is unable to visualize the full shape and contours of the scanbody, a complete digital image cannot be captured.

Intraoral scanning may be impeded by the size of the scanner tip itself, which may limit correct positioning of the scanner tip to enable full capture of the scanbody. Proximity of the scanbody to adjacent teeth may also prevent the scanner tip from registering the complete shape of the scanbody. Additionally, deeply placed implants may not expose the scanbody sufficiently for correct reproduction within the digital software (Fig 1).

Poorly placed implants that are too close to a neighboring tooth or to another implant may prevent the use of a scanbody and surface scanning as a whole. The scanbody must not be altered, adjusted, or changed in contour the way that a conventional impression coping may be modified; for the software to recognize the position accurately, the scanbody must remain unmodified. Misaligned implants may present situations where a digital workflow is impossible, and a conventional impression and analog workflow will then be necessary (Figs 2 to 4).

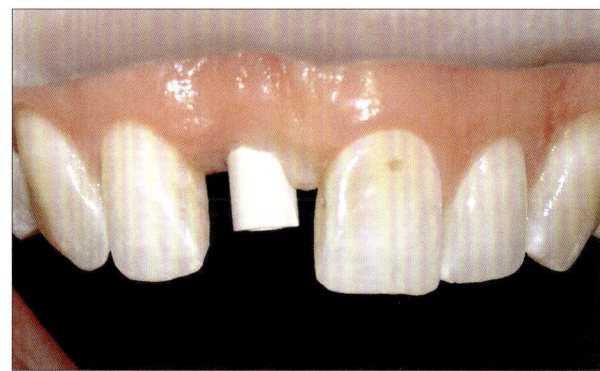

Fig 1   Insufficient scanbody exposure due to deep (apicocoronal) implant positioning.

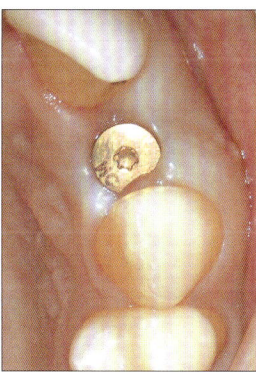

Fig 2   Implant malpositioning (mesiodistal dimension).

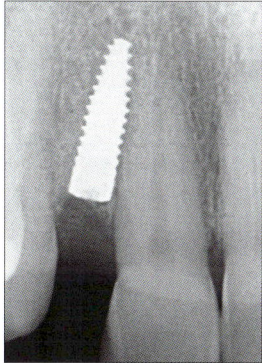

Fig 3   Radiograph showing the resulting angulation.

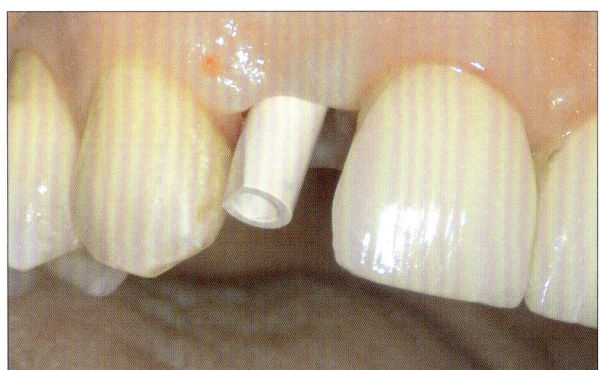

Fig 4   The scanbody cannot be seated because of the implant angle, resulting in contact with the adjacent tooth.

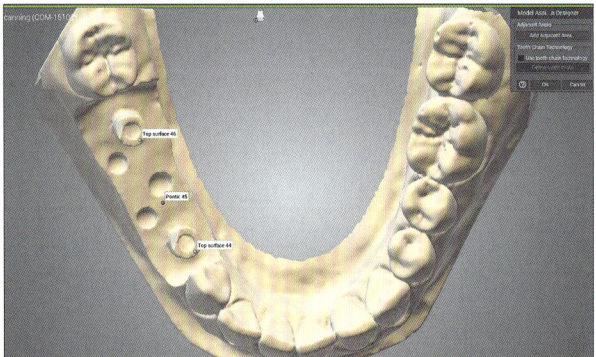

Fig 5   Scan of a model with tissue removed.

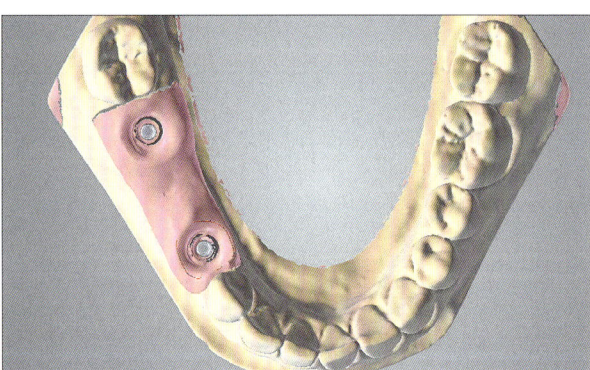

Fig 6   Final scan with gingival layer repositioned.

When scanning models with removable soft-tissue material, it is necessary to follow the correct scanning sequence to avoid layers being incorrectly placed in the virtual model.

Careful repositioning of the casts within the desktop scanner is necessary to avoid errors in recording the tissue height around implants, which can lead to metal or marginal interface exposure (Figs 5 and 6).

11.2 Software-Integration Complications

Integration complications occur when one software package cannot merge datasets obtained from other software packages.

Merging complications can occur:

- If there are not enough scanned reference points on either a scanbody or dental arch form to allow matched-point identification.
- In the event of changes in the surfaces being merged, such as new restorations or the presence of moveable tissue.
- If the scanbody selected by the clinician or technician is not supported by the software.

The alignment within the software begins with the scanbody being identified on the scan. The software then places a virtual implant by removing an area of the scan similar to a "punch hole," a data void, and inserting the virtual implant replica into this void.

If the implant has been placed in a narrow ridge or is angled, or insufficient gingival or mucosal data were captured during the intraoral scan, the "punch hole" void may overlap adjacent structures, such as the tooth or ridge outline (Figs 7 to 9).

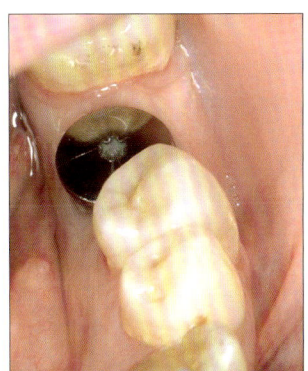

Fig 7   Clinical view of an implant 36 placed too far lingually.

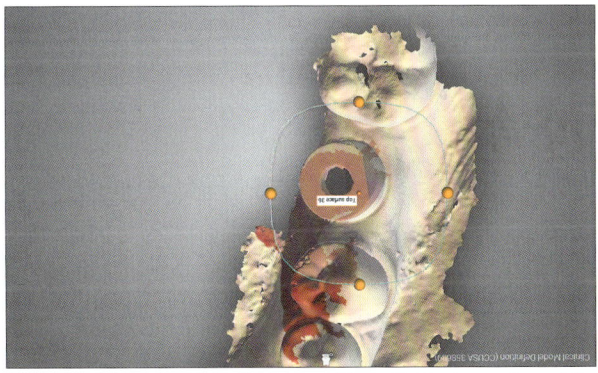

Fig 8   Intraoral scan of the implant position with the top surface of the implant located within the CAD software for virtual implant positioning.

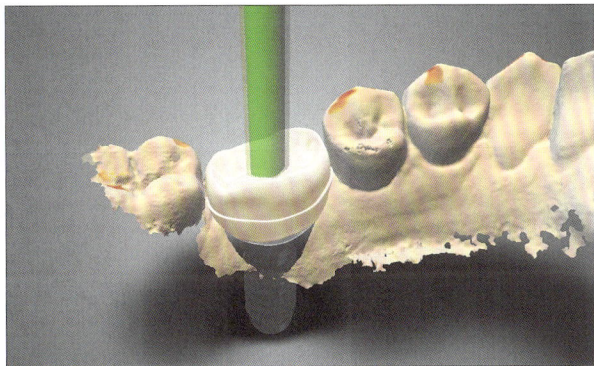

Fig 9   The virtual implant position has resulted in a lingual void in the dataset.

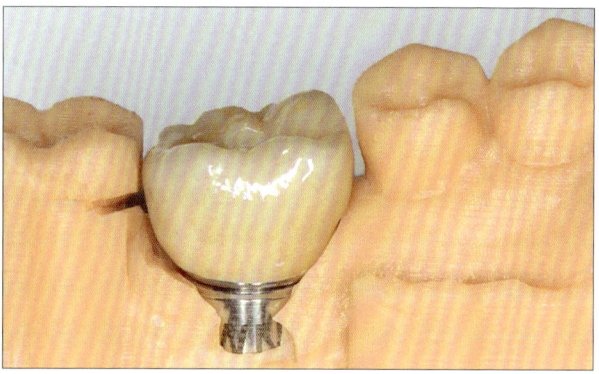

Fig 10   The 3D-printed model exhibits the same lingual void as the dataset, except that in this case it occurred in the molar area. This model was manually modified with acrylic resin to enable an analog to be placed at the site. The final restoration was adjusted for contact points and reseated on the model; however, the void had resulted in errors.

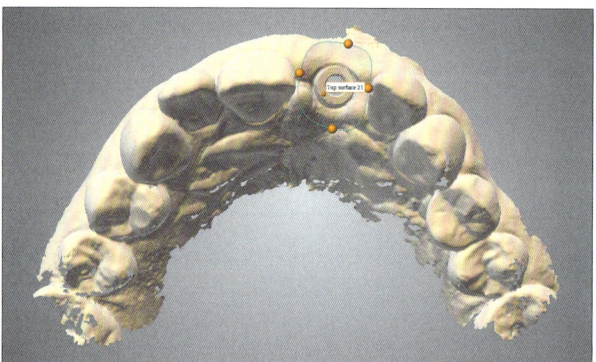

Fig 11   Imported scan with correct identification of the scanbody.

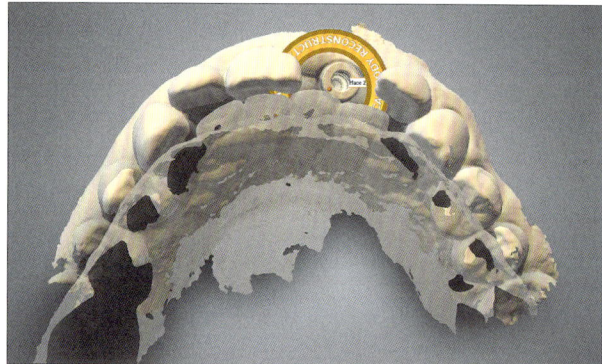

Fig 12   Following scanbody identification, the calculations create a "punch hole" in the scan.

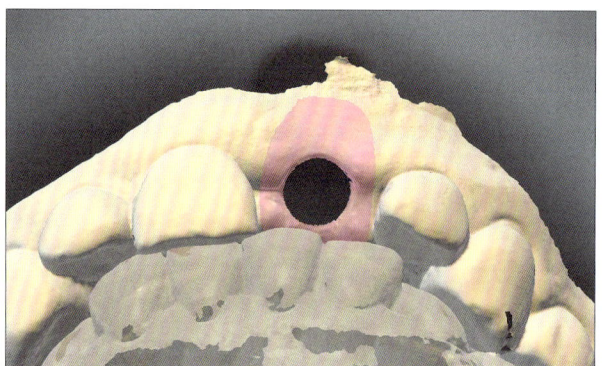

Fig 13   Correct punch hole within the scan.

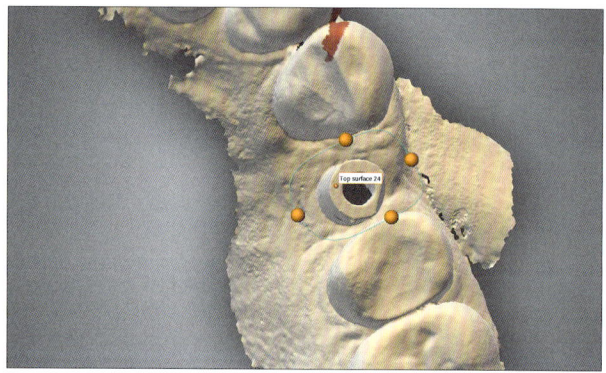

Fig 14   The aligned implant approximates the distally adjacent tooth.

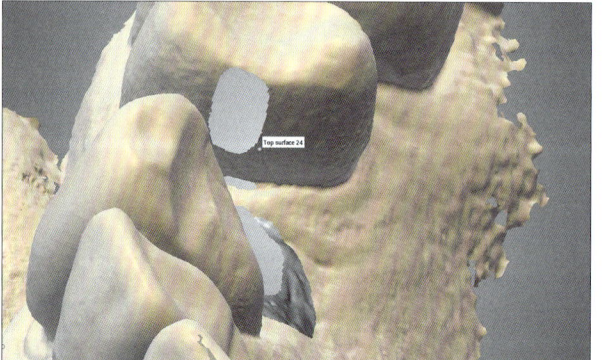

Fig 15   "Punch hole" deletes the contact point for the adjacent tooth.

For example, poorly aligned implants near the adjacent teeth may result in contact point detail being lost from the dataset. This can result in CAD errors, where the design software can generate odd shapes as the integrity of the data set is lost. Accurate production of 3D-printed models may prove difficult, as the material holding repositionable implant analogs will be compromised (Figs 10 to 15).

Aligning the occlusal scan with the arch scans within the software can be problematic if there are insufficient recognizable points between the antagonist arch and working model for correct merging. This can easily happen if only partial occlusion scans are made (Fig 16). Similarly, the use of only a unilateral occlusion scan when repositioning against a full arch scan is prone to rotational errors, which can result in poor occlusal alignment and errors in the prosthesis.

The scan must be "cleaned" of any aberrant scanning surfaces before processing the final design. Errant scanbody data points, or stray captures of movable mucosa or soft-tissue surfaces remaining after the "punch holes" are positioned can interfere with the CAD design (Figs 17 to 19). Recalculation of the restoration design will result in defects on the implant surface if the artifacts are left in place.

The presence of imaging artifacts or metallic scatter in a CBCT dataset may prevent the user from aligning the surface scan to the CBCT images. A CBCT of the area of interest with a limited field of view may also prevent the accurately merger of the surface scan with the CBCT due to a lack of common points of recognition. Even if the scan is free of scatter, the lack of suitable reference points around the arch may introduce an alignment error; this can result in implant malpositioning when using guided surgery for implant placement.

Users of this technology should be able to recognize limitations in the techniques that may create errors in implant positions, which could lead to esthetic complications or the risk of damage to adjacent anatomical structures (Figs 20 to 26).

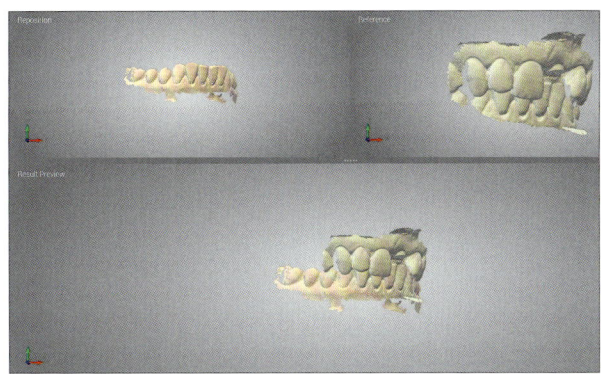

Fig 16   Partial-bite alignment of the arch without a full-bite scan can result in incorrect positioning of the arches.

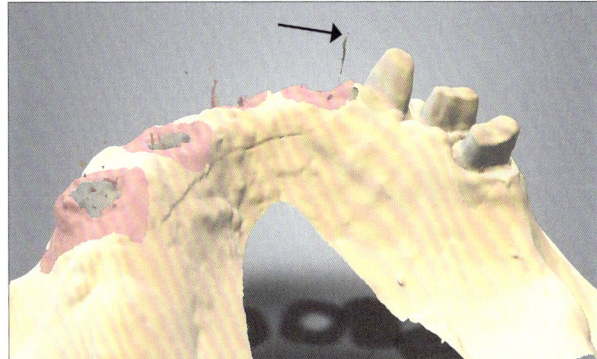

Fig 17   Residual scanbody surfaces after "punch hole" placement indicate alignment issues and can interfere with the design process.

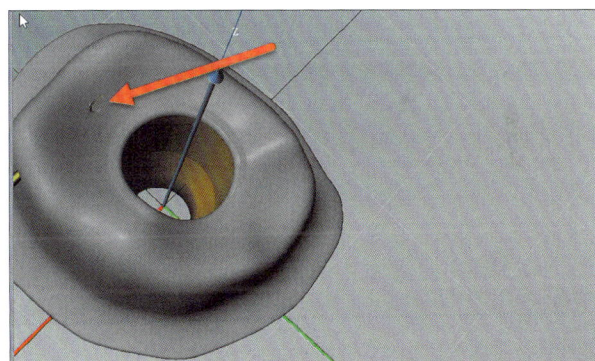

Fig 18   A defect in the abutment design identified by the red arrow due to a scanbody artefact left after "punching," preventing accurate abutment milling.

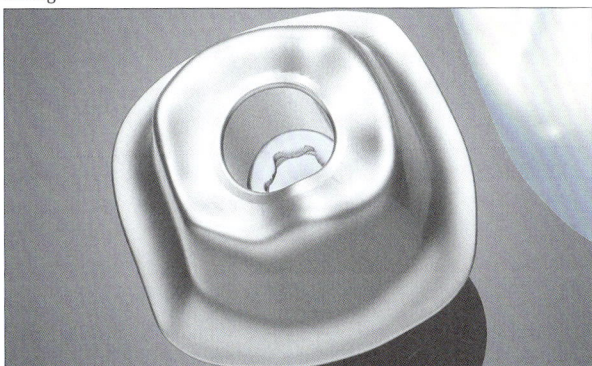

Fig 19   A correction of the scan helps create an abutment that is both correct and complete.

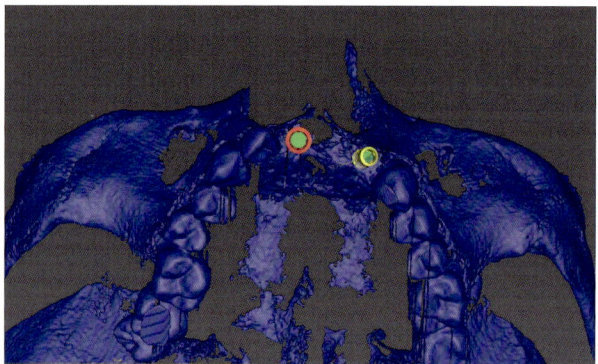

Fig 20 Correctly segmented CBCT with minimal metal artifacts, made with the teeth apart.

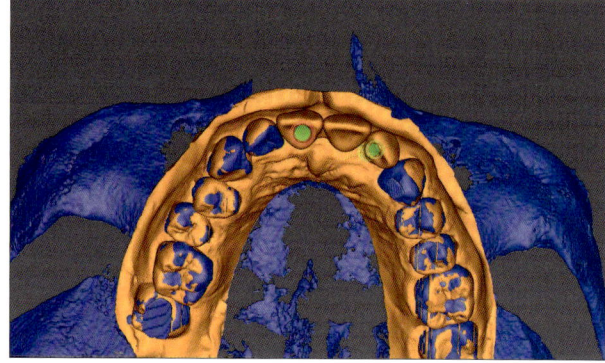

Fig 21 Correct and accurate alignment of the CBCT and surface scan due to the minimal scatter and correct segmentation.

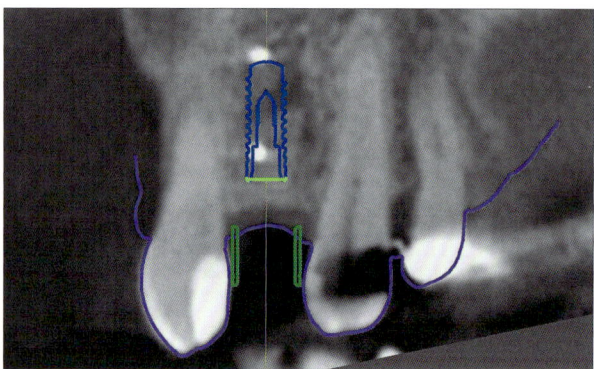

Fig 22 Correct alignment of the design proposal and implant position.

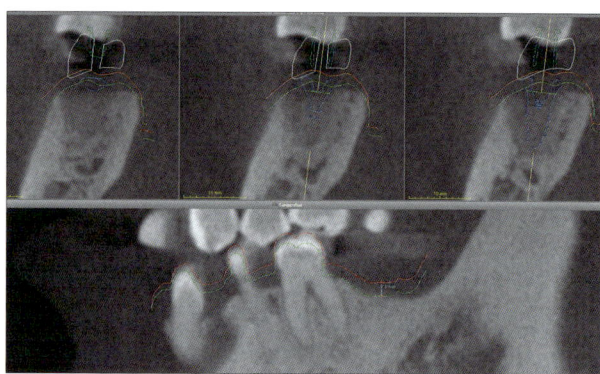

Fig 23 The patient moved during CBCT acquisition, resulting in an image artefact and a potential positional error because the surface scan cannot be accurately related to the CBCT.

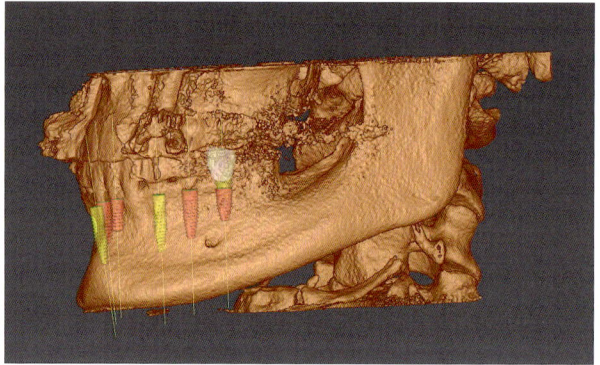

Fig 24 Poorly made CBCT with teeth occluding; artifacts from opposing metallic restorations make data segmentation difficult.

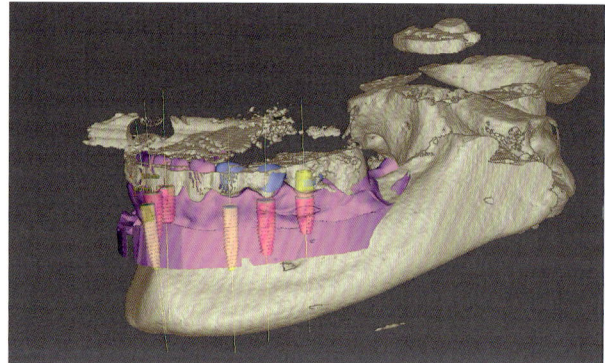

Fig 25 Alignment of the surface scan with the segmented CBCT dataset requires multiple manual manipulations.

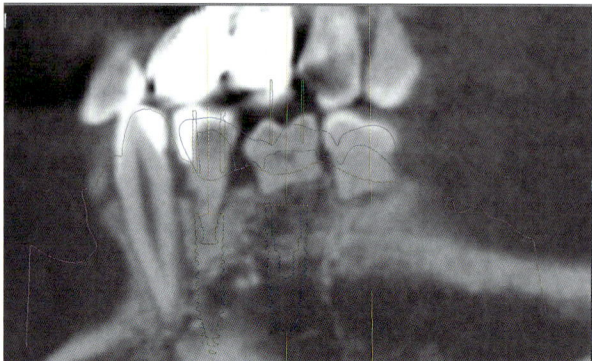

Fig 26 Unsuccessful alignment of the surface scan with the CBCT dataset.

11.3   Milling Complications

Before milling the restoration, the design must be nested within the material block to ensure that the block size will adequately contain the designed restoration. Block sizes vary according to the material selected. Figure 27 shows a restoration fitting well within the contours of the block.

For restorations where there is excessive restoration height, as a result of loss of the soft and hard dental tissues, the block size may be inadequate for the production of the proposed structure. Figures 28 and 29 demonstrate a case where the incisal edges of the restoration could not be incorporated into the milling block even into a block 25 mm in height. As a result, the restoration needed to be redesigned to allow for more layering ceramics, increasing the risk of a mechanical complications over time such as ceramic fracture. Alternatively, the restoration may have to be manufactured using a conventional lost-wax metal-ceramic technique.

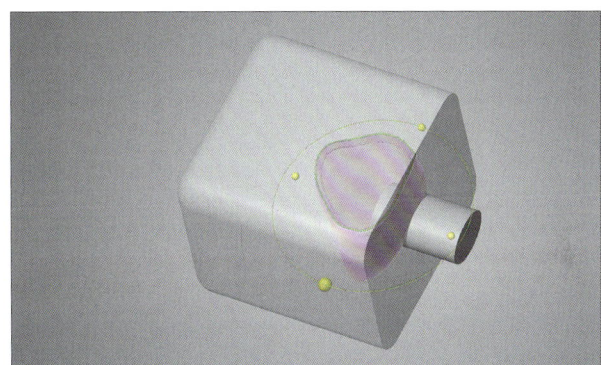

Fig 27   The restoration fits into the milling block.

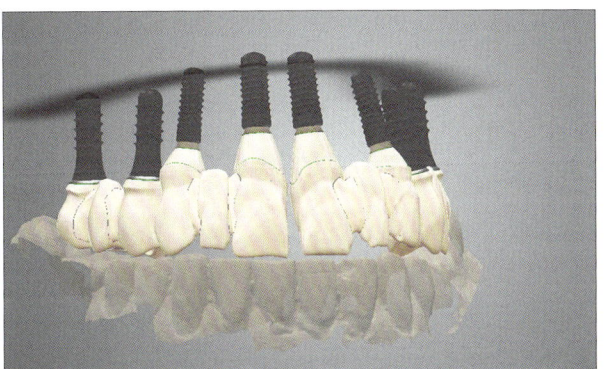 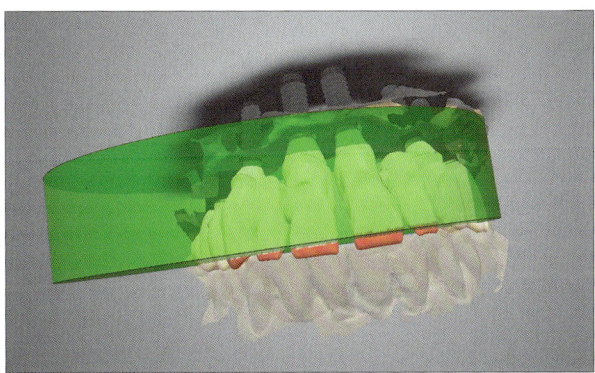

Figs 28 and 29   A full-arch restoration designed for ceramic veneering to be supported within the occlusal scheme—but the 25-mm milling disc is too thin for milling the entire restoration.

12 <u>Future Developments and Challenges</u>

A. Tahmaseb, D. Wismeijer

As digital technologies are rapidly embraced by the dental profession and are becoming part of the dental workflow, there are some factors that should be taken into consideration when thinking about future developments in digital implantology.

Digitization in dentistry can be seen as a disruptive innovation. Bower and Christensen (1995) defined a disruptive innovation as one that creates a new market and a new value network that eventually disrupts an existing market and value network, displacing established market leaders and alliances. This results in the industry players trying to position themselves such that they can harness new technologies and maintain their market share. It becomes difficult for large companies to create alliances with competitors in order to implement digital technologies in a standardized way. We see many implant manufacturers and implant-related companies developing their own digital technologies or creating alliances with non-competitor companies to help them integrate these technologies into their product offerings. We also see small companies creating specific digital tools that can only be used in one of the steps of the digital workflow.

Consequently, many digital devices available today must be considered standalone products, making communication with other devices in the digital workflow difficult, if not impossible. As most of the companies involved in developing the digital workflow create their products in their own system-specific or "closed-source" fashion, communication with devices and systems produced by other companies becomes a difficult undertaking.

Then there is the continuum of innovation, where every company marketing a digital device is already developing the next device or changing and upgrading the software used in the digital chain.

It is obvious that an open system, based on a universal format, could be beneficial for both developers and users (and especially perhaps for researchers). But is that in the interest of the industry?

There are of course unified software standards. DICOM (Digital Imaging and Communication in Medicine) can be considered a universal standard in digital radiography, the standard used for the transmission of radiographic images and other medical information between computers and various devices that acquire images, and also between devices and software systems produced by different manufacturers.

The American Dental Association joined the DICOM Committee in 1996, and dentistry has been actively participating in the development of DICOM standards. A DICOM image file contains an x-ray image or series of images (such as a multiple-slice CBCT imaging study) and other patient related information selected from a "library" of pre-selected standardized terms (patient name, identification number, and acquisition mode, to name but a few). Imaging devices in general and dental CBCT devices in particular produce so-called "raw data." These raw data contain the X, Y, and Z spatial coordinates of each voxel and its grayscale value, which is then reconstructed by the software of the CBCT device to create a DICOM file. Therefore, DICOM data from one device can be different from DICOM data from another device, but the actual file format is the same and can be universally read by software.

Moreover, the DICOM library is extensive and continually updated to reflect changing identification standards. But these continuous updates are not applied within every device. There are thus different "dialects" of the DICOM "language," which can lead to misconceptions when DICOM is used to export image data from one machine to another.

Other 3D devices in the digital workflow, such as intraoral or facial scanners, export their data as STL (Surface Tessellation Language) files. However, STL files usually have a system-specific extension that may not be compatible with software from a different developer; the STL file generated by a certain machine may only be recognized by other "accepted machines," reducing the number of machines, or brands of machines, that can be employed in a specific workflow.

In addition, CBCT images (DICOM) need to be converted to STL format in order to be merged with other 3D data. If you want to merge CBCT data (bone) with a scan of the teeth, this will have to happen in STL format; at present this is still a very time-consuming process. However, with self-learning computer systems, this process might be performed much faster in the future.

Today, most dental imaging companies that sell commercial software packages for storing, viewing, or retrieving digital images offer products based on DICOM standards. However, numerous improvements are needed before dentistry will be fully integrated into the DICOM world. For example, guidelines for the standardization of digital photography are sorely needed for its full integration into the dental workflow. Moreover, the integration of both intraoral and extraoral projections, the creation of templates for secure reports, and surgical workflow issues within DICOM in oral implantology needed to be addressed.

Farman (2005) stated that image format and attribute interoperability should give comfort to the users of digital diagnostic equipment and to their patients, meaning that images acquired on equipment purchased today should still be viewable into the future. Upgrades to newer equipment must not automatically mean a loss of important diagnostic information. Furthermore, diagnostic images should be portable and readable by professionals who may use digital imaging equipment from a different vendor. Also, DICOM images need to be integrated with the many dental record software products currently available. Dental imaging equipment working according to the DICOM standard, such as CBCT units, should be automatically updated whenever DICOM standards are upgraded.

PACS (Picture Archiving and Communication System) is a medical imaging technology that provides economical storage and convenient access to images from multiple source-machine types using different imaging modalities. This system offers the option of combining all patient information, including 3D data, in one universal file. This would mean that the files have to be transformed to DICOM or that the system must be transformed to accept more than just DICOM files. This could at least homogenize the process of image reconstruction within different systems. It also opens up ways to export data to third parties such as dental laboratories, medical specialists, or referring practitioners, within the limits of to data protection laws. A problem with cloud-based PACS is the risk of data leaks. As information is exchanged, it must be clear what part of the data is being transmitted and that the patient agrees to the sharing of those data; it must also be clear who has permission to use which part of the data and how the data is protected from misuse.

A further difficulty that prevents dental professionals from fully embracing these novel technologies is the everlasting issue of upgrades and improvements. A device that uses today's most advanced technology will be old news tomorrow. Technology is developing so rapidly that it is extremely challenging for the clinician to pick the right moment to "go digital." These developments have a direct impact on the precision and accuracy of the devices, their usability, and the treatments they can be used for. Producers of digital devices should recognize these facts and facilitate the necessary upgrades where these are beneficial for patient safety or for the quality of treatment outcomes, at reasonable cost.

From a technical point of view, intraoral scanners appear to offer promising accuracy in both partially and fully edentulous situations, at least according to measurements carried out in a model study (Papaspyridakos and coworkers 2016; Amin and coworkers 2017). However, in clinical situations, the interference of soft tissue such as the cheek or tongue can make intraoral scanning more difficult and reduce accuracy.

A rather old technology, photogrammetry, appears to be attracting new interest in the field of oral implantology. Photogrammetry is the science of making measurements based on photographs, especially for the purpose of recovering the exact positions of surface points. Photogrammetry is as old as modern photography, dating from the mid-19th century; in the simplest application example, the true distance between two points on a plane parallel to the photographic image plane can be determined by measuring their distance on the image, provided the scale of the image is known. This technology has been widely used in the automotive industry to calculate or simulate impact damage during a crash test.

In the dental field, scanbodies with numerous dots as targets are screwed into implants. The camera captures scanbodies on multiple implants. Special software calculates average angles and distances between the implants from these photographs, obtaining the accurate relative position of each implant in vector format. These data contain all the information on implant positions, geometries, connections, etc., later required by CAD/CAM software (Peñarrocha-Oltra and coworkers 2014). This promising technology might solve the issues surrounding digital "impression-taking" where multiple implants are involved.

We believe that the use of digital technology should be integrated into the undergraduate dental curriculum, but of course this means that the mindset of educators needs to be adjusted in that direction. Understanding the technology, its benefits and shortcomings, and gaining experience in its use and limitations, should be part of modern dental education. Zitzmann and coworkers (2017) conducted a randomized controlled trial where inexperienced dental students' perceptions of the difficulty and applicability of digital and conventional implant impressions as well as the students' preferences and performance were analyzed. They concluded that dental students with no clinical experience were very capable of using digital tools, indicating that digital impression techniques can be introduced early in the dental curriculum to help students keep abreast of ongoing developments in computer-assisted technologies used in oral rehabilitation.

In another study that evaluated students' and clinicians' perception of digital and conventional implant impressions, Lee and coworkers (2013) concluded that conventional impressions were more difficult to take for the student group than the clinician group; however, the difficulty level for taking digital "impressions" was the same in both groups. The study also found that the student group preferred the digital technique as the most efficient, while the clinician group was evenly split on preferences and on the efficiency of impression techniques.

However, a later study by Wismeijer and coworkers (2014) showed that for experienced treatment providers, the time involved in taking full-arch impressions of dental implants and the opposing arch and perform bite registration, was the same, regardless of whether they used an intraoral scanner or analog procedures. This may be one of the reasons why the digitization of implant-prosthetic treatment has not found greater favor with established restorative dentists.

DICOM has standardized the exchange of medical information and facilitated the cost-effective interconnection of different medical systems. This has made the DICOM standard superior to other standards developed by manufacturers of medical equipment and has also helped avoid problems when patient moves from one clinic to another. The fact that all medical specialties support DICOM makes it comprehensive, transparent, and easy to use. DICOM takes up less space for digital storage and digital data and is easy to transmit over great distances.

Analog data can suffer from degradation caused by the limited durability of the recording media—something that is not the case with digital data. DICOM allows a conversion of analog data to the digital DICOM format, providing data fields (required or optional) to provide all necessary patient information. A disadvantage of the DICOM standard is actually that there may be too many optional fields available. This disadvantage manifests itself in the form of inconsistencies when attempts are made to complete all data fields. Some images turn out to be incomplete because some fields are left blank and others contain incorrect data.

At this time, the digital workflow contains several imaging devices such as CBCT and intraoral scanners, software packages used to analyze the acquired data and to design a treatment, and 3D printers or milling units for additive or subtractive manufacturing. Various software packages use different approaches and incorporate different tools to make a system usable. In the future, we may expect software packages to become increasingly user-friendly, recognizing structures more easily and performing the necessary merging of data in a more autonomous fashion. The time spent on importing data,

cleaning up files, or merging different files to analyze the digital "structure" of the patient could be reduced, perhaps with the incorporation of image-recognition software.

Navigation packages used in performing implant surgery are a step toward "robotizing" the surgical aspect of the digital workflow. A camera tracks the patient's movement, and a robot arm drills the osteotomy guided by the planning software using the STL and DICOM information that has been generated from the patient. The role of the implant dentist may then be reduced to that of a technician doing the planning.

However, considerable challenges remain to be conquered. As we implement these digital technologies into the implant workflow, new questions and potential problems arise. One of the questions is: who owns the data? Is it the device manufacturer? If, for instance, an intraoral scan is taken of a patient, or even of an analog model of a patient, and this is transferred to the cloud, who will be responsible for that data, and who owns it? How long can the data be stored? What if the data is lost or corrupted, or even worse, is used by third parties, for instance in data-mining research? If the patient is the owner, then what tools does he or she have to protect the data?

What if the device is not as accurate as the manufacturer has promised? Or if it develops some flaws in function? If a drill guide or a prosthesis has been designed and produced based on corrupted information, who is responsible?

Then there is the software developer. Software is used to design and create surgical guides and temporary and definitive restorations. Who owns the designs? Who owns any design or adjustment to a design made either by the treatment provider or the dental technician, who has also played a role in the design process? Who is responsible for the final design? Has this person been trained according to standards that have been agreed on by some form of legal body?

Then we have the milling units and 3D printers in the workflow. Are they compatible with the software used? If the software gets updated, does this affect any stages of the workflow, and is the update then tested for all the units in the digital workflow? Who is responsible for the update, and will software developers that have their software incorporated into the units in the workflow have enough information to adjust their software in time for the coming update? Is it clear which materials can be used in the 3D printing process, and have all these materials been validated? Who is responsible for the quality of these materials, and how are these responsibilities laid down in the form of protocols to protect our patients?

Another development is the design and manufacture of custom implants. With the digital data acquired from the patient, an individual customized implant fitting the site-specific bone volume and anatomy could be designed and manufactured. The restoration will then be an integral part of this design and can be manufactured at the same time.

Barriers to such developments include cost and legislation. If implant dentists have to become implant manufacturers, which is what (European) legislation says they are when they design and develop individual implants, this process will only advance at a snail's pace.

The technology is developing rapidly, but its implementation in the dental field is being delayed. The most significant reason for this could be the many different platforms, which are developing in isolation and do not communicate. An open system design can contribute to homogenizing development and research, which in the end can benefit the industry, the clinicians, and—most importantly—our patients.

13 Clinical Case Presentations: Implant-Supported Restorations Using Guided Surgery and CAD/CAM in a Digital Workflow

13.1 Replacing a Mandibular Second Premolar with a Chairside-Fabricated Crown

T. Joda

A 32-year-old male patient was referred to our department for a single-tooth replacement with an implant-supported crown. The patient was diagnosed with tooth agenesis at site 45 after extraction of the retained deciduous tooth (85, primary second molar) by his general practitioner. At baseline, the full-mouth plaque score (PI) was 21%; probing pocket depths (PPD) ranged from 1 to 3 mm, and bleeding on probing (BoP) was 17%.

The implant treatment including all surgical and prosthodontic steps was planned and performed in a complete digital approach, using static computer-aided implant surgery (sCAIS; Fig 1):

1. Digital data acquisition
2. Virtual treatment planning
3. Guided implant placement surgery
4. Digital impression-taking (surface scanning)
5. Computer-aided design (CAD) of the implant crown
6. Computer-aided production (CAM) of the implant crown
7. Post-production crown processing
8. Delivery of the final restoration

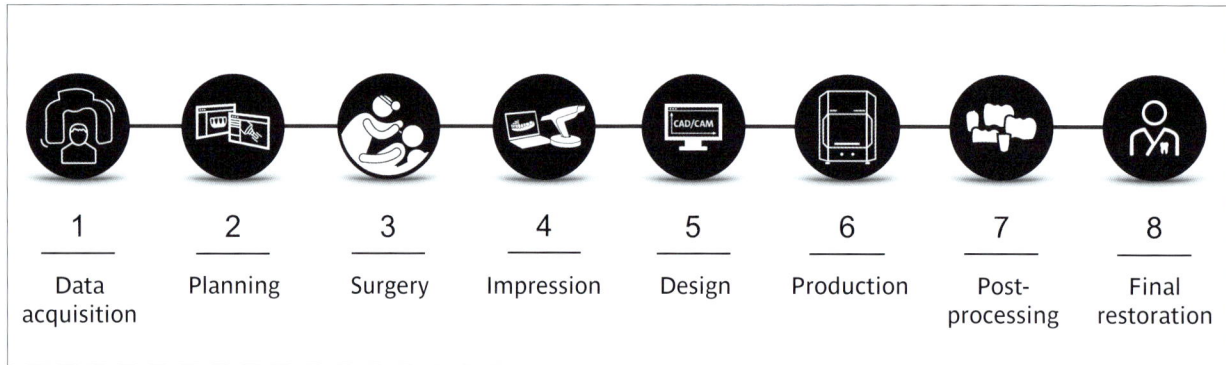

1	2	3	4	5	6	7	8
Data acquisition	Planning	Surgery	Impression	Design	Production	Post-processing	Final restoration

Fig 1   Iconized flow-chart showing the step-wise treatment protocol for posterior single-unit implant restorations in a complete digital workflow.

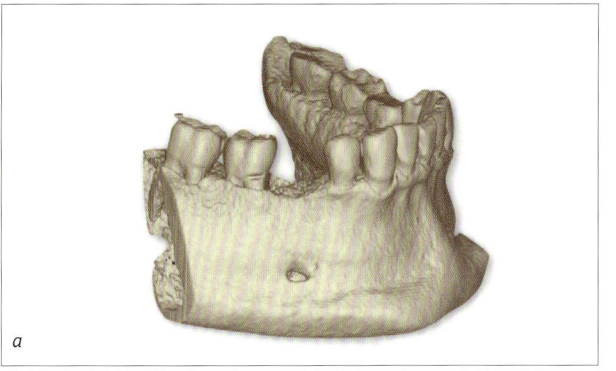
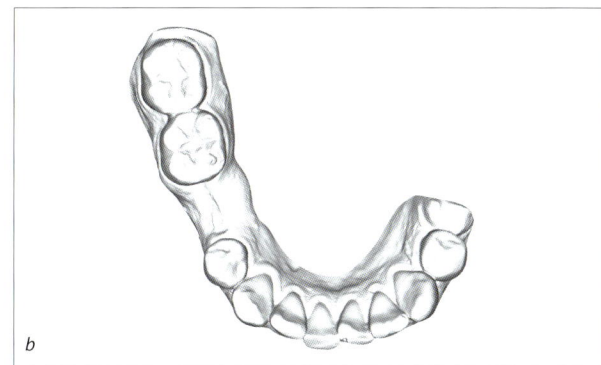

Figs 2a-b   DICOM file from the CBCT depicting a 3D rendering of the mandible with missing tooth in position FDI 45 (a) and interpolated mesh-structured surface of the STL file from the IOS (b).

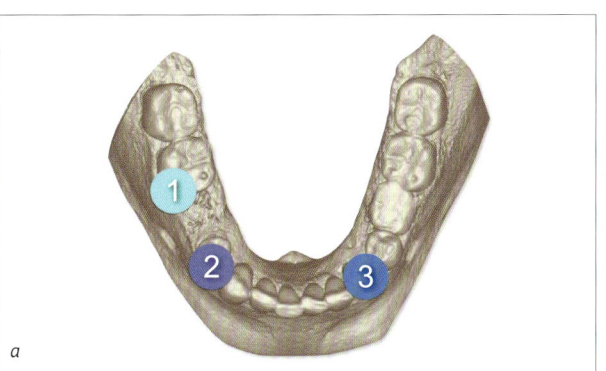
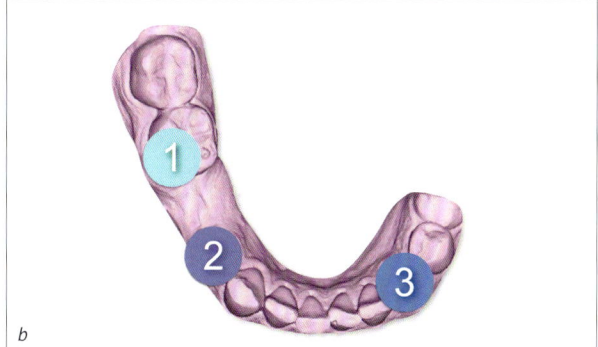

Figs 3a-b   Superimposition of DICOM and STL datasets using virtual implant-planning software.

Data acquisition

After clinical assessment, cone-beam computed tomography (CBCT) and intraoral optical scanning (IOS) were performed to digitize the clinical situation, and to generate the DICOM and STL files. Neither a physical model nor a radiographic template was necessary during the phase of digital data acquisition (Figs 2a-b).

Planning

The DICOM file was transferred to the virtual implant-planning software (coDiagnostiX; Dental Wings, Montreal, Quebec, Canada). The software settings were adjusted for the individual patient coordinates and the panoramic curve, and the 3D visualization of the inferior alveolar nerve was prepared.

Next, the STL file of the pre-operative intraoral situation was imported. Based on superimposition of suitable identifiable landmarks, the datasets were merged using the built-in software algorithm (Figs 3a-b).

A virtual set-up was then made of the prospective optimal 3D implant position, using the accepted prosthetically driven backward-planning concept and allowing for local anatomical considerations. From this, a surgical guide was designed in the software, also using the STL file from the IOS. On completion of these software steps, a 3D printer was used to produce a surgical guide using rapid-prototyping techniques, without the need for physical models. Finally, the implant-planning software delivered a case-specific drilling protocol with an appropriate instrument sequence for correct, safe and predictable 3D implant placement (Figs 4a-b).

Surgery

The surgical treatment protocol involved a fully guided approach for the drilling sequence and the placement of a tissue-level dental implant (TL RN 4.1 × 12 mm; Institut Straumann AG, Basel, Switzerland). The virtual planning facilitated a safe, predictable, and streamlined workflow using guided implant surgery. Prior to implant placement, the 3D printed surgical guide was checked intraorally for accuracy of fit. Buccal and lingual viewing windows were provided adjacent to the implant site for better clinical control.

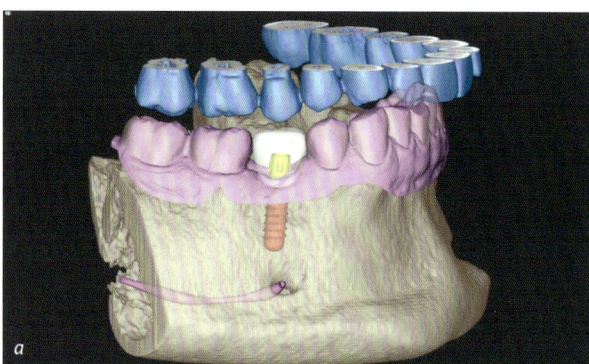 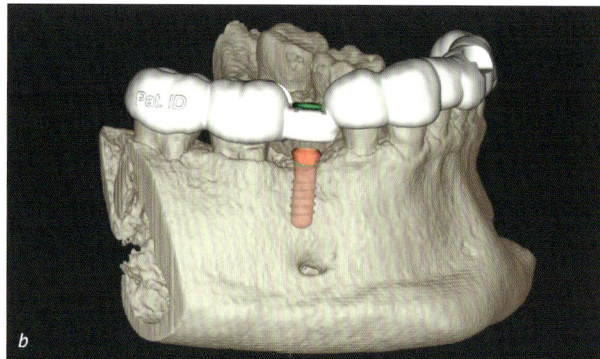

Figs 4a-b   Prosthetically driven backward planning with simulation of the crown using a tooth library provided by the implant-planning software, including visualization of the implant and abutment selection (a) and virtual design of a surgical drill guide for transfer of the 3D implant position (b). Proposed implant: TL RN 4.1 × 12 mm (Institut Straumann AG, Basel, Switzerland).

After anesthesia, the surgical guide was used for initial site marking through the mucosa, and a full-thickness mucoperiosteal flap was elevated (Figs 5a-d).

The implant bed was prepared using successive specialized guide sleeves and corresponding spiral drills (Figs 6a-d).

An implant depth gauge was placed to verify the position of the osteotomy. Any positional errors can be detected at this stage, permitting manual correction of the proposed implant position if necessary. The tissue-level implant was placed with full guidance via the integrated 5-mm drill sleeve (TL RN 4.1 × 12 mm; Institut Straumann AG) (Figs 7a-d).

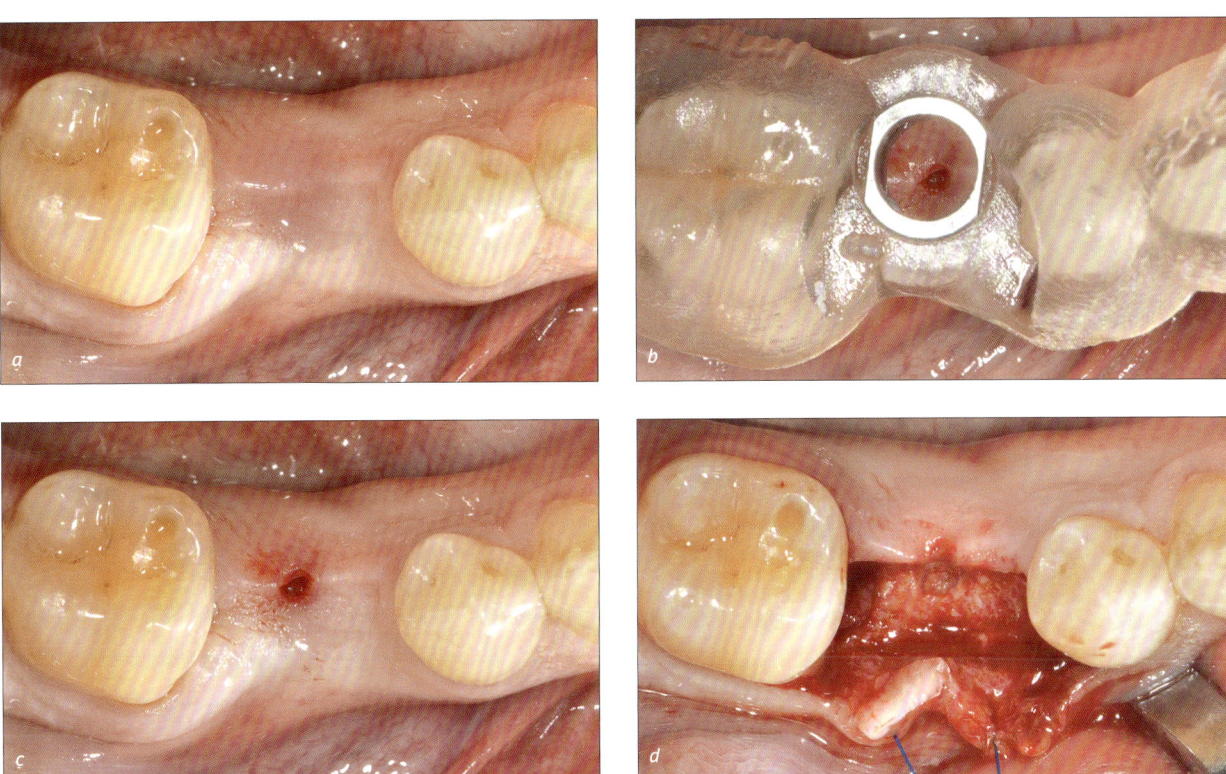

Figs 5a-d   Occlusal view of initial clinical situation showing the partially edentulous gap at site 45 (a). Try-in of the 3D plotted surgical guide with marking through the center of the sleeve (b). Visual blood spot indicating the prospective implant position (c). Full-thickness mucoperiosteal flap (d).

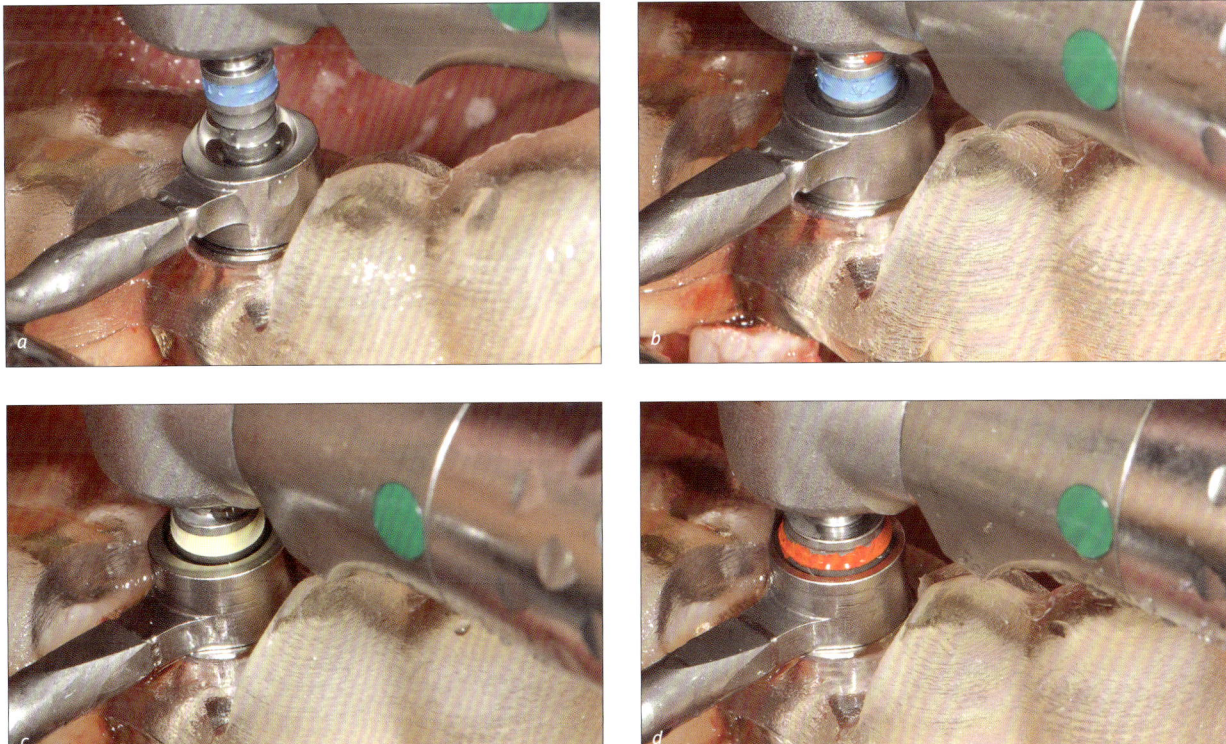

Figs 6a-d   Surgical sequence for fully guided implant bed preparation using a 3D printed guide with specific drills in a standardized protocol.

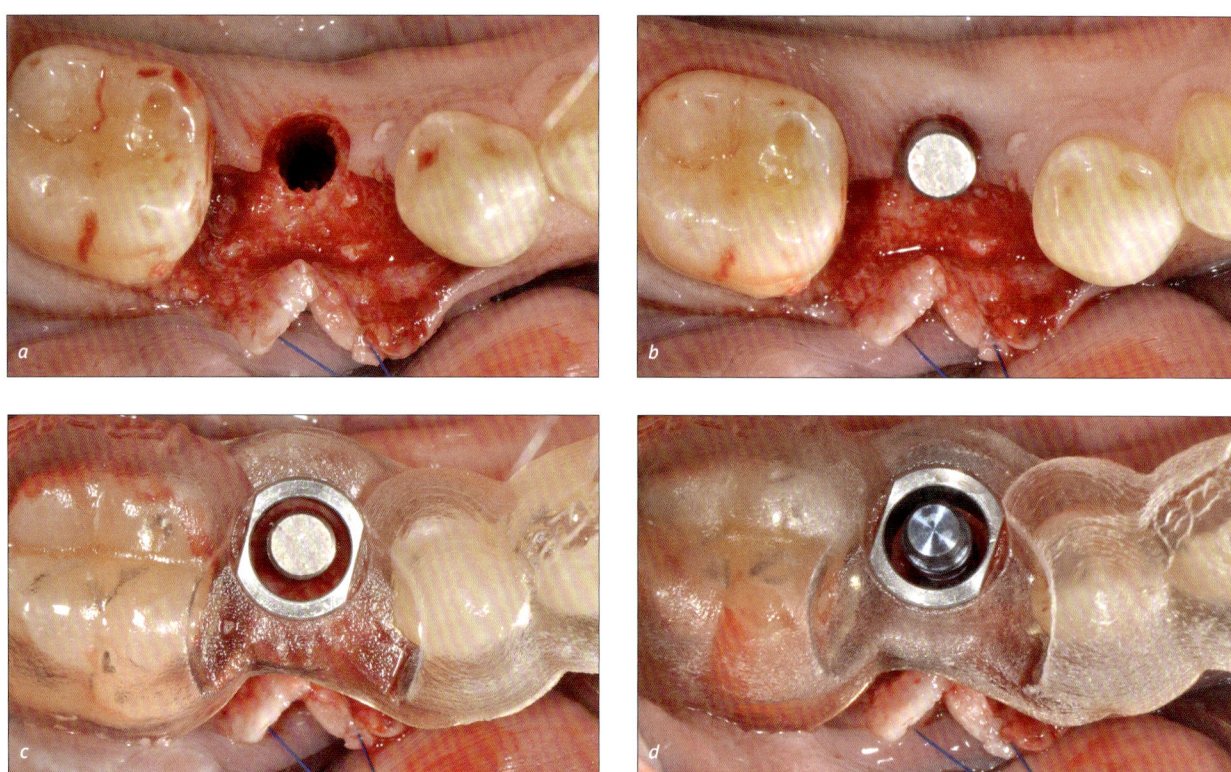

Figs 7a-d   Occlusal view of prepared implant bed (a). Depth gauge in situ without (b) and with (c) 3D printed guide. Fully guided implant placement through the surgical guide (d) – TL RN 4.1 × 12 mm (Institut Straumann AG).

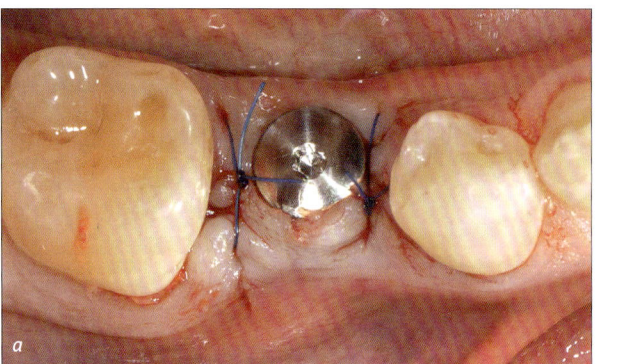
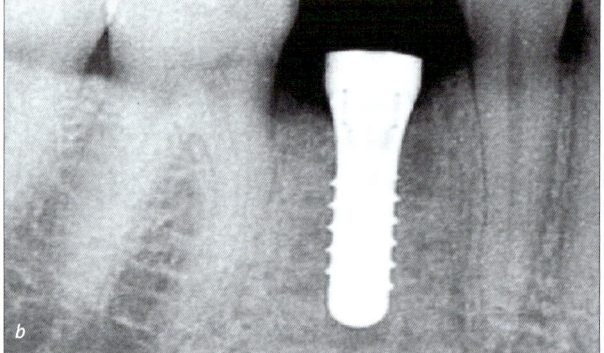

Figs 8a-b   Inserted healing cap and suturing for transmucosal healing (a). Control radiograph (b).

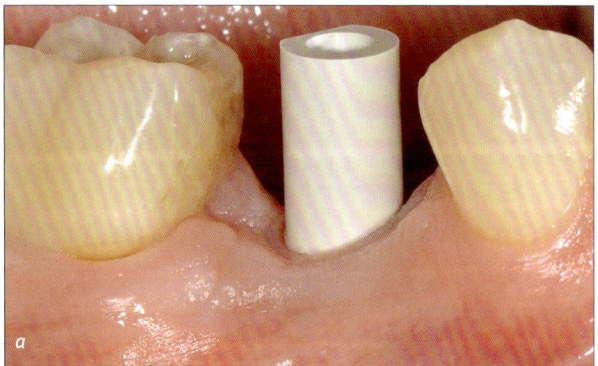
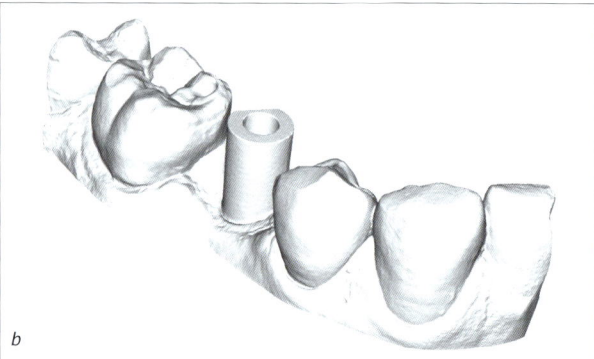

Figs 9a-b   Clinical situation with screwed-in monotype scanbody for digitization of the implant at site 45 using IOS (a). Screenshot of the interpolated mesh-structured surface produced from the IOS STL file, with soft-tissue emergence profile and adjacent dentition (b).

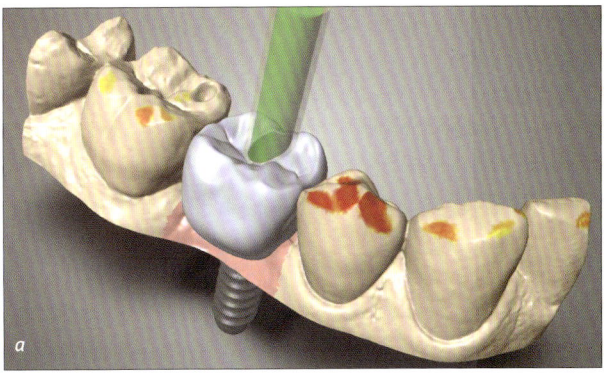
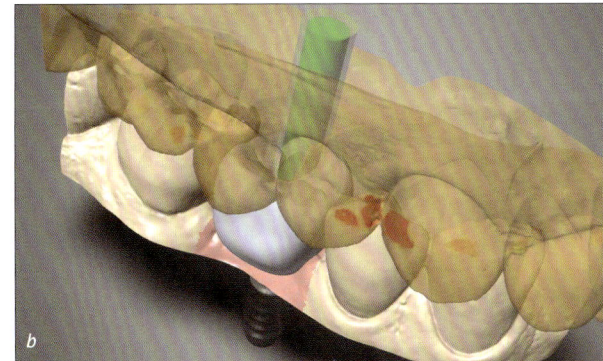
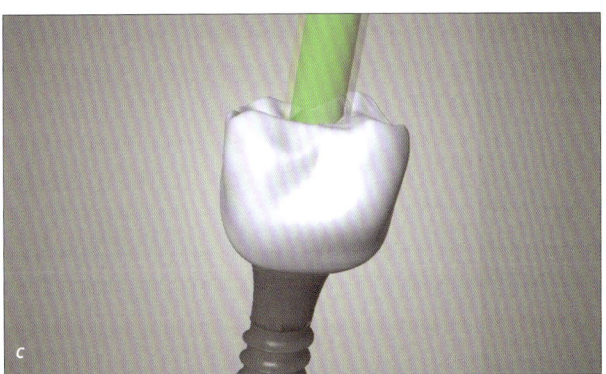
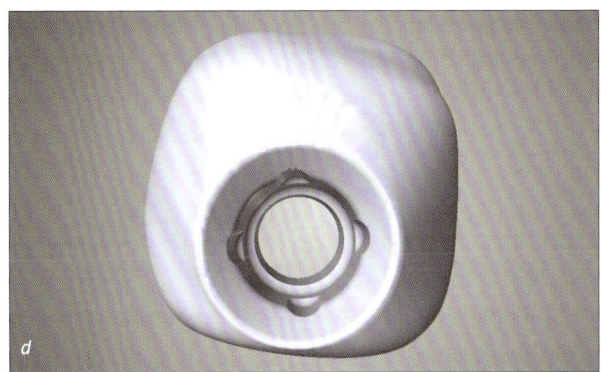

Figs 10a-d   Virtual design of a screw-retained fully contoured crown 45 accounting for the individual occlusal situation.

The postoperative clinical situation and related radiograph showed the prosthetically correct 3D position of the implant, keeping some safety distance from the inferior alveolar nerve and adjacent teeth (Figs 8a-b).

Digital impression

The prosthodontic and technical steps followed a digital approach including IOS (TRIOS Pod; 3Shape, Copenhagen, Denmark) and used CAD/CAM and a prefabricated titanium abutment (Variobase RN; Institut Straumann AG).

After guided implant placement, a second IOS captured the peri-implant mucosal architecture and neighboring teeth. A scanbody was inserted into the implant and the 3D implant position was scanned. The opposing arch was also scanned and the bite registration digitally transferred (Figs 9a-b).

Design

The final implant crown was planned as a screw-retained monolithic restoration made from a lithium disilicate (LS$_2$) CAD/CAM blank (Nice CAD; Institut Straumann AG) bonded to a prefabricated titanium abutment (Variobase RN; Institut Straumann AG).

Based on the IOS STL file, the anatomically correct contour of the crown was designed and produced using a completely digital process without physical casts. The interproximal and occlusal contacts were defined virtually using integrated software tools (CARES C-Series; Institut Straumann AG) (Figs 10a-d).

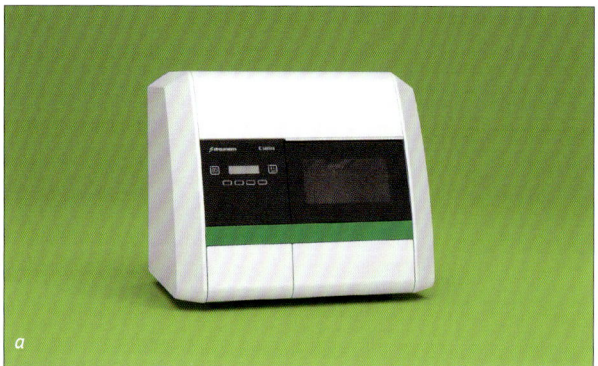
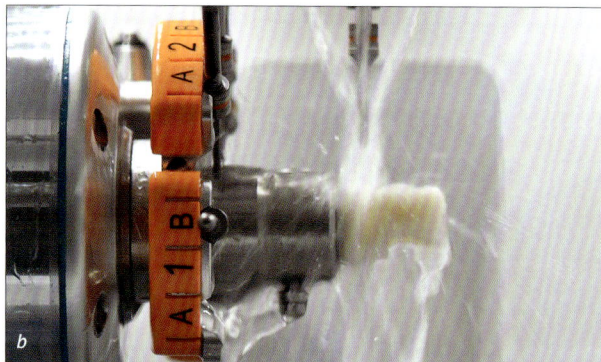

Figs 11a-b   Chairside milling of the implant crown.

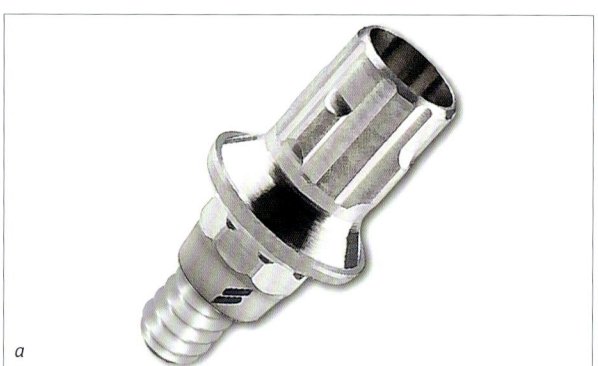
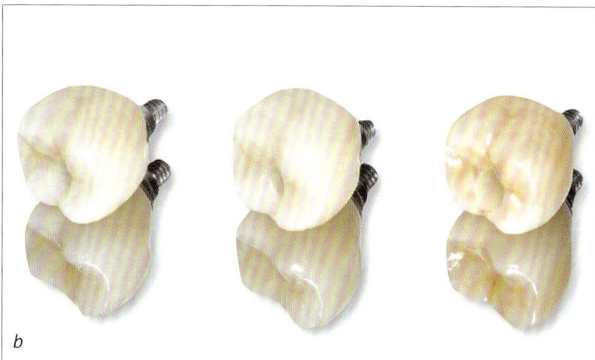

Figs 12a-b   Pre-fabricated titanium abutment (a). Post-processing sequence showing the different fabrication steps for finalization of the LS$_2$ crown—immediately after milling, after polishing, and after individual characterization (b).

Production

The virtual crown design was processed and the restoration produced in a 4-axis wet milling and grinding unit (CARES C-Series; Institut Straumann AG) for in-house manufacturing of the crown from a monolithic LS$_2$ CAD/CAM blank (Nice CAD; Institut Straumann AG) (Figs 11a-b).

Post-processing

Once the monolithic LS$_2$ crown had been milled, the restoration was cleaned with 95% ethanol, polished, and individually characterized. The prepared LS$_2$ crown was directly bonded (extraorally) to a prefabricated titanium abutment (Multilink Implant; Ivoclar Vivadent, Schaan, Liechtenstein; and Variobase RN; Institut Straumann AG) (Figs 12a-b).

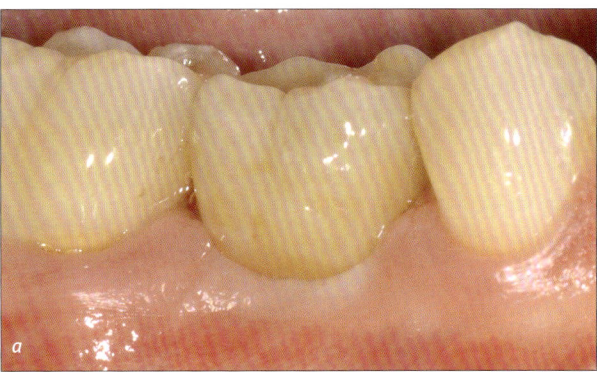 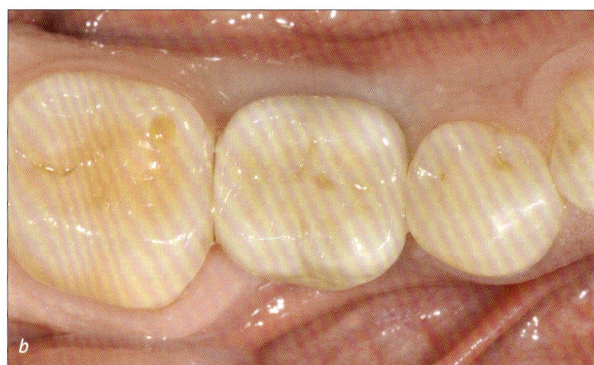

Figs 13a-b   Final implant-supported monolithic LS$_2$ crown 45, lateral (a) and occlusal (b) view. The screw access hole was closed with composite resin.

Final restoration

The crown was tried in to verify marginal and interproximal fit. The mesial and distal contact points were checked for equivalence using dental floss. The occlusal scheme was checked statically and dynamically to achieve light occlusal contacts in centric without excursive interferences. The monolithic restoration was screw-retained with a controlled torque of 35 Ncm, following to the implant manufacturer's recommendations. The screw access hole was sealed with PTFE tape and composite resin. The full-mouth score for PI was 19%, PPD was 1 to 3 mm, and BoP was 15% (Figs 13a-b and 14).

Discussion

Prosthetically driven implant placement is a key factor for successful implant therapy. In this context, sCAIS offers a powerful instrument for treatment planning, surgical implant placement, and prosthodontic rehabilitation in an interdisciplinary approach.

The present clinical case illustrates the chairside treatment sequence for a posterior single-unit implant-supported crown using a completely digital workflow. The surgical and prosthodontic treatment stages and the technical fabrication of the prosthesis are integrated seamlessly in a validated protocol using original implant components for in-house production of the restoration (Joda and coworkers 2017a).

A prerequisite for completely digital implant treatment is the use of monolithic CAD/CAM restorations combined with prefabricated abutments, based on prosthetically driven implant positions determined by 3D radiographic imaging and optical surface scanning to guarantee a predictable outcome. This simplified prosthodontic protocol avoids traditional laboratory steps and ensures streamlined production, with specific advantages arising from using materials of standardized quality (Joda and coworkers 2014).

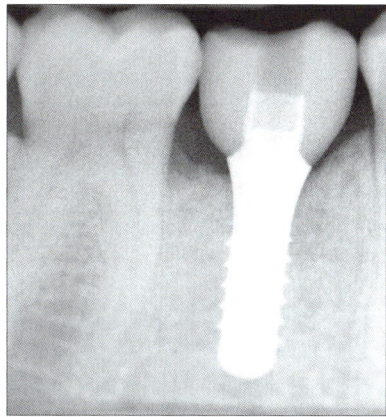

Fig 14   Intraoral 2D radiograph after delivery of the definitive implant-supported crown.

Initial randomized controlled clinical trials have indicated that a complete digital workflow is superior to conventional techniques in terms of cost efficiency, particularly given the reduction in overall production time (Joda and coworkers 2016). As for the cost to the patient, the economic analysis reveals reduced overall treatment costs for first-line therapy, including laboratory costs, for implant crowns produced using quadrant IOS with CAD/CAM technology (Joda and coworkers 2015a).

Furthermore, the need for chairside corrections such as secondary adjustments and polishing can be minimized, or even eliminated, using a fully digital protocol and monolithic restorations. This reduces working time but may also decrease the risk of cracks and chipping associated with veneered ceramic restorations (Joda and coworkers 2017b).

13.2 Replacing a Mandibular First Molar with a Crown Following Soft-Tissue Modeling

A. Kökat

A 35-year-old female patient was referred to the clinic for the prosthetic restoration of a tissue-level dental implant placed at the mandibular right first molar site (site 46).

The tooth had been extracted due to an untreatable carious lesion (Fig 1). Four months after the extraction, cone-beam computerized tomography (CBCT) scans of the edentulous site were obtained (Figs 2 and 3). The placement of a Straumann implant (Standard Plus RN, diameter 4.8 mm, length 12 mm; Institut Straumann AG, Basel, Switzerland) was planned. The implant was placed in a submerged approach, with primary closure due to the level of the crestal bone. The patient then relocated and was referred back to our clinic after the first surgical phase. The referring surgeon provided the preoperative periodontal indices for the two teeth 47 and 45 as 1.5 (Löe and Sillness 1963).

A SAC assessment of the case indicated a straightforward restorative phase (Table 1).

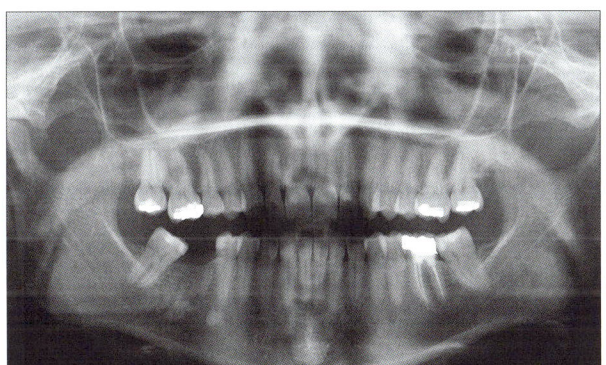

Fig 1   Preoperative panoramic view.

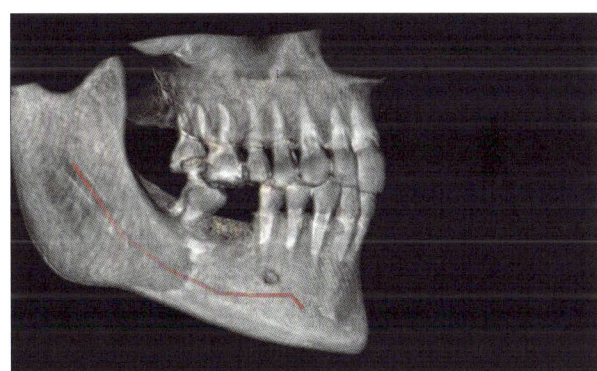

Fig 2   Preoperative CBCT scan of the area.

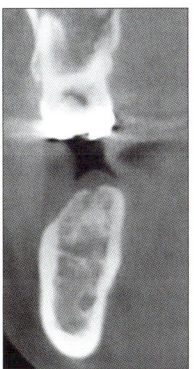

Fig 3a   CBCT scan adjacent to premolar area, sagittal view.

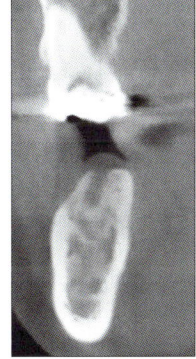

Fig 3b   CBCT scan adjacent to second-molar area, sagittal view.

Table 1   SAC assessment.

Patient Name:	N Yalcin	
Patient ID:	2014-10-AMKTL-212	
Date:	03.03.2018 07:43:21	**ITI** International Team for Implantology

Restorative Assessment: Single-Tooth Restoration in the Posterior Zone

Defining characteristics:	One missing tooth to be replaced by an implant-borne crown.
Tilted 47 requires papillar formation and soft tissue management around 46	

Basic Indication	Single-tooth gap
Zone Selection	Posterior
Tooth	Molar
Visibility of Treatment Area upon Smiling	No
Inter-Arch Distance	Ideal tooth height +/- 1 mm
Mesio-Distal Space (Molar)	Anatomic space corresponding to the missing tooth +/- 1 mm
Loading Protocol	Conventional or early
Bruxism	Absent
Provisional Implant-Supported Restoration	Restorative margin < 3 mm apical to mucosal margin
Interim Restoration during Healing	Fixed
Retention	Cemented, with restoration margin < 3mm submucosal

Normative SAC Classification	**Straightforward**

Additional Complexity/Risk based on Modifiers	Low	Medium	High

Restorative Assessment: Single-Tooth Restoration in the Posterior Zone

Defining characteristics:	One missing tooth to be replaced by an implant-borne crown.
Tilted 47 requires papillar formation and soft tissue management around 46	

Modifiers

Patient's Expectations	Craniofacial/Skeletal Growth
Low (Low)	Completed (Low)
Oral Hygiene and Compliance	Access
Good (Low)	Adequate (Low)

Additional Complexity/Risk based on Modifiers	Low	Medium	High

Four months after the implant placement, the implant was exposed and a 3-mm healing abutment was placed. At the time of reentry, there was minimal bleeding on probing for both adjacent teeth. The probing pocket depth of the neighboring teeth was 3 mm.

The emergence profile of dental implants is not only important in anterior sites for esthetic reasons, but it is also related to the maintenance of healthy peri-implant mucosal conditions. Tooth 47 was mesially tilted and a gap would have occurred after the restoration if the correct emergence profile of tooth 46 had not been not achieved. Achieving a natural anatomical form and emergence profile for the implant-supported crown was important to help the patient with effective interproximal plaque control. This is secondary to esthetic objectives, which are of less importance in the posterior zone. However, function follows form, and by recreating natural crown contours, we would be able to provide the optimal peri-implant soft-tissue contours for optimum oral hygiene and to prevent the creation of a stagnation area for plaque accumulation. The distally tilted second molar had the potential to result in an unfavorable contact point and an unnatural interdental gap, presenting a risk for future peri-implant disease.

Tarnow (2000) showed almost 100% successful papilla formation in cases where the distance between the alveolar crest and the contact point was less than 5 mm. With unnatural contours, it might be quite challenging for the patient to clean the area with interdental brushes or dental floss. Therefore, the decision was to create a molar with a predominantly natural shape to obtain proper embrasures and help the patient keep the peri-implant tissue as healthy as possible.

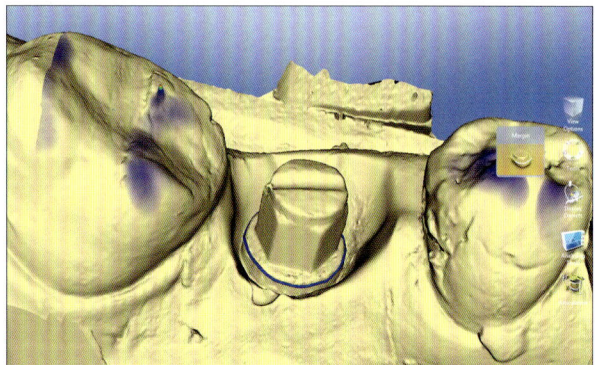
Fig 4   Digital model of the transfer mount used for provisionalization.

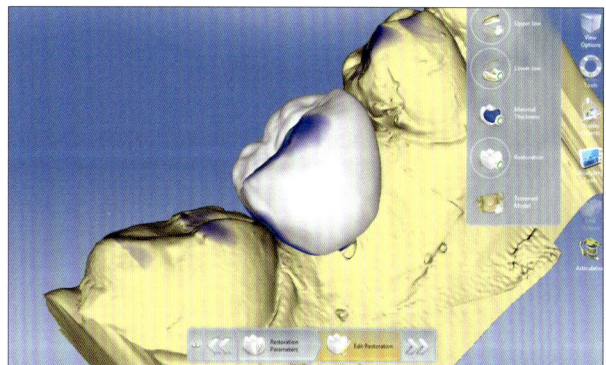
Fig 5   Provisional crown designed on Cerec software.

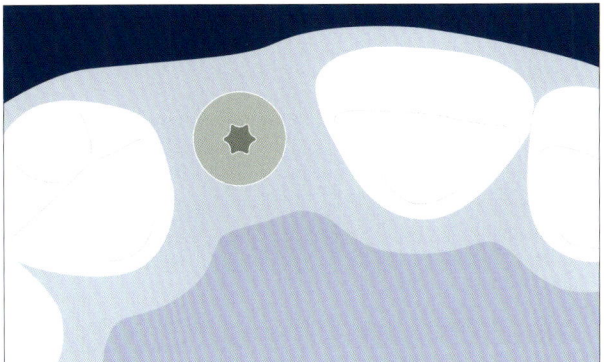

Fig 6   Diagrammatic representation of a typical situation with healing abutment in place.

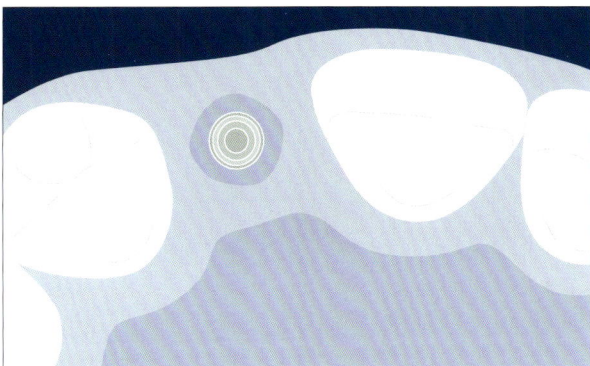

Fig 7   A typical gingival profile created by a healing abutment.

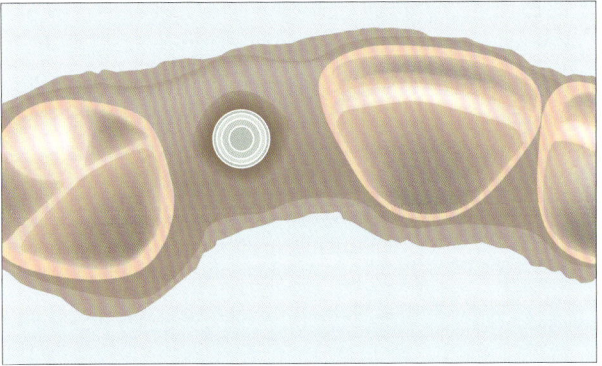

Fig 8   Scan data image without healing abutment.

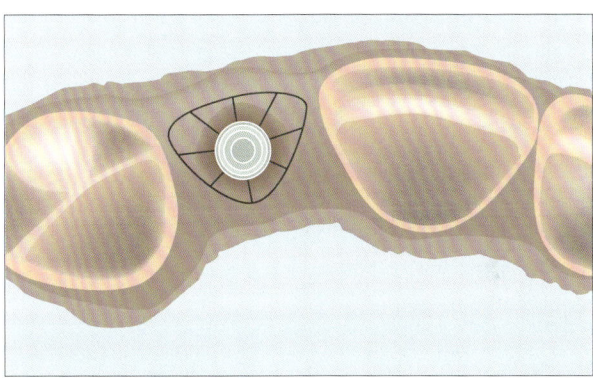

Fig 9   Desired emergence profile of the final restoration as drawn in the software.

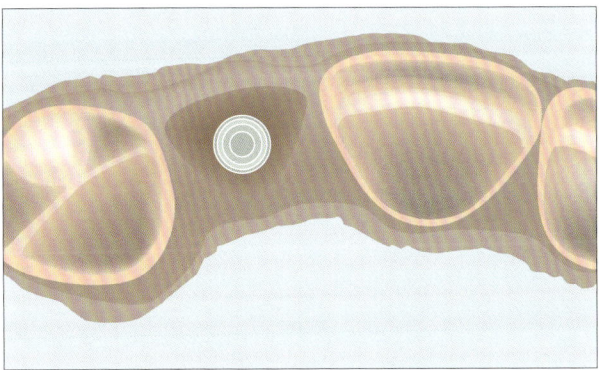

Fig 10   Virtual emergence profile created by editing scan data.

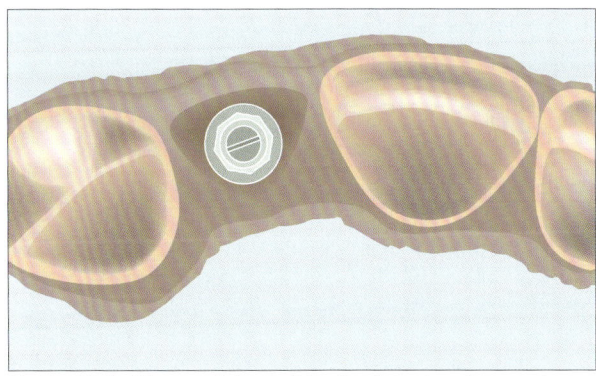

Fig 11   Meshed images of the provisional and the virtually created emergence profile.

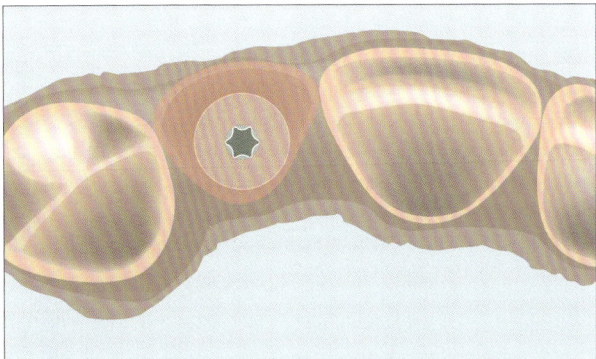

Fig 12   Provisional crown design to fit the new emergence profile.

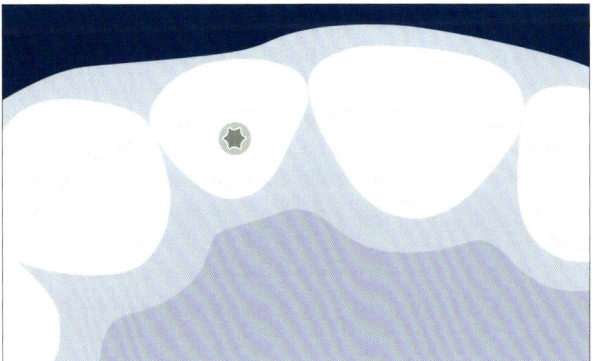

Fig 13   Provisional crown milled and placed on implant.

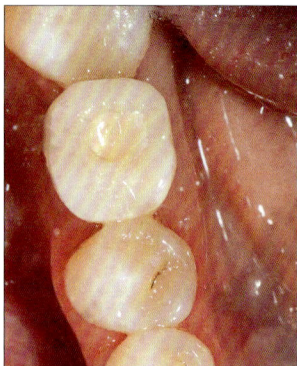

Fig 14   Screw-retained provisional crown, occlusal view.

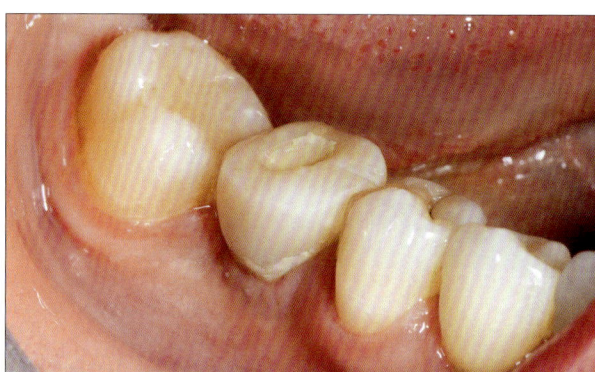

Fig 15   Screw-retained provisional crown, buccal view.

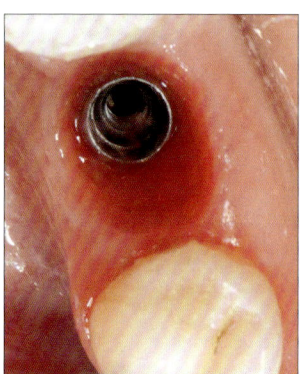

Fig 16   Peri-implant soft-tissue modeling, occlusal view.

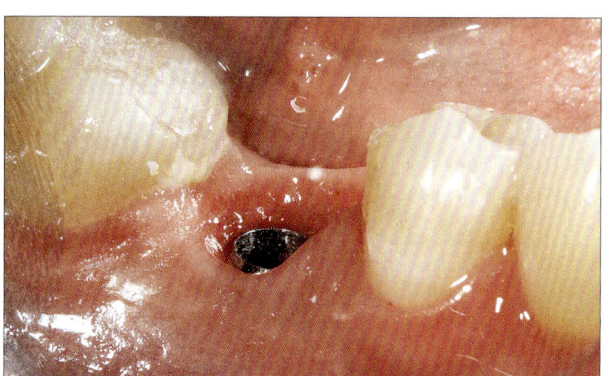

Fig 17   Peri-implant soft-tissue modeling, buccal view.

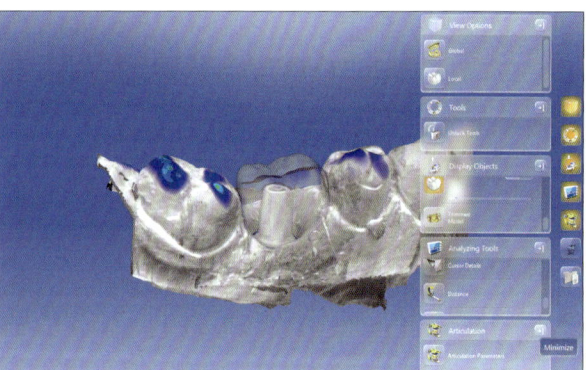

Fig 18   Digital design of the crown with a favorable emergence profile.

To achieve a good emergence profile, it was decided to make a provisional crown using the technique described by Kökat and Akça (2013). A progressive approach was chosen to shape the architecture of the mucosa around the molar to represent the cervical anatomy of the natural tooth. As a starting point, the implant transfer mount was adjusted. The screw of the transfer mount was customized with a separating disc. A slot was created in the custom screw and placed on the implant. Then an intraoral scan was made (Cerec BlueCam; Dentsply Sirona, York, PA, USA) (Figs 4 and 5).

The emergence profile was designed digitally on the virtual model and a provisional crown was produced (Telio CS C&B; Ivoclar Vivadent, Schaan, Liechtenstein) using the workflow illustrated (using the example of an incisor) in Figs 6 to 13. The provisional crown was created with an occlusal access hole to facilitate removal and replacement for further tissue contouring (Figs 14 and 15). For that purpose, the external contour of the crown in the horizontal plane was drawn on the 3D image in the software.

The gingival part between the external border and implant shoulder was removed and smoothed to shape the emergence profile on the virtual model using the editing tools of the software. The provisional crown was designed to fit the new gingival shape and produced on a milling machine. A screw access hole was provided on the occlusal surface of the provisional. The transfer mount of the implant was sandblasted to increase the retention of the luting resin and cemented to the provisional crown. The access hole in the provisional crown was cleared immediately and the assembly was tried in intraorally for proximal and occlusal adjustments.

The provisional crown was unscrewed, reshaped with flowable composite, polished, and refitted every 3 to 5 days. Once the final form of the desired emergence profile had been achieved (Figs 16 and 17), a SynOcta cemented abutment (Straumann) was placed and secured at 20 Ncm of torque, and another intraoral scan was taken. A lithium disilicate crown was designed and produced with Cerec software to support the created emergence profile (Fig 18). After sintering, polishing, and glazing, the lithium disilicate crown was cemented using a dual-cure resin cement (RelyX U200; 3M ESPE, St. Paul, MN, USA) after torqueing of the abutment to 35 Ncm.

The mucosa showed no signs of pressure and had formed a papilla between the natural teeth and the implant-supported crown (Figs 19 and 20). A control radiograph showed a good fit of the crown and favorable peri-implant bone levels (Fig 21).

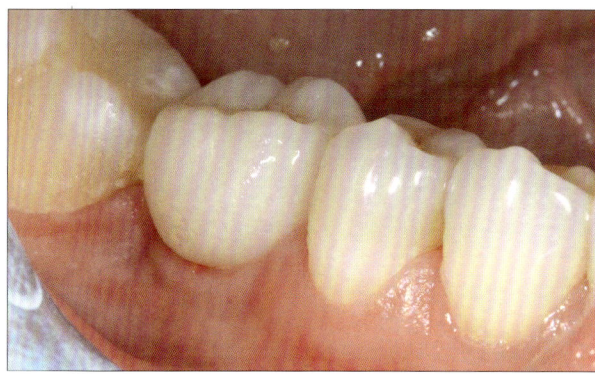

Fig 19   Definitive crown in situ.

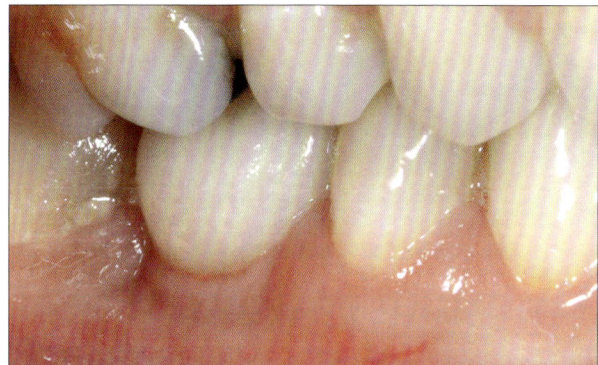

Fig 20   Definitive crown in situ. Good peri-implant tissue conditions and recreated papillae between the restoration and the adjacent teeth.

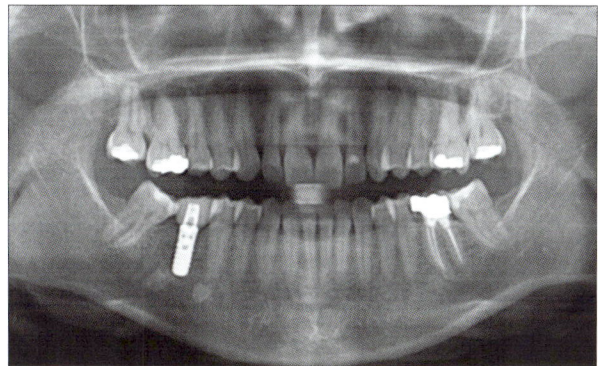

Fig 21   Panoramic radiograph at the time of crown delivery.

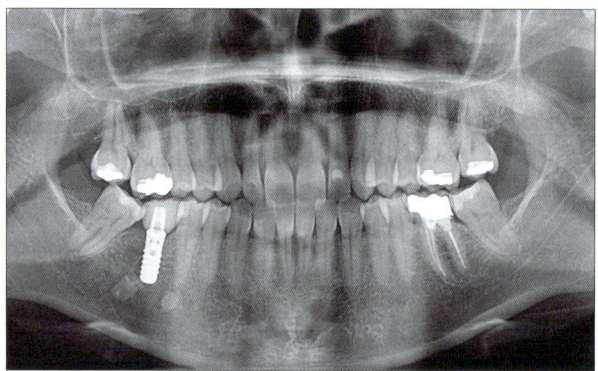

Fig 22   One-year panoramic radiograph.

At the one- and two-year follow-ups, it was found that the interdental papilla and stable mesial and distal bone levels had been maintained (Figs 22 to 26). The peri-implant plaque index for the first year was 1, and for the second year, 1.25. There was no bleeding on peri-implant probing at either follow-up. Peri-implant probing depths were a maximum of 3 mm on the proximal and 2 mm on the buccal and lingual aspects.

Acknowledgments

Surgical procedures
Prof. Erdem Kılıç – Istanbul, Turkey

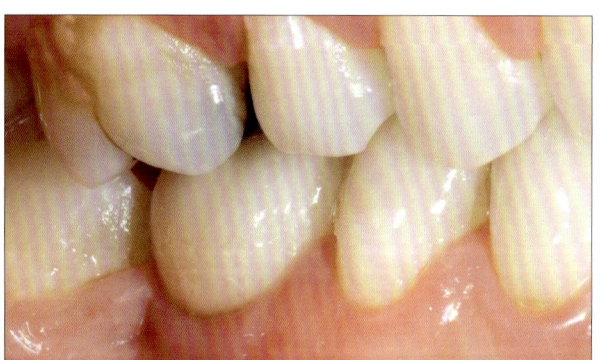

Fig 23   Two-year follow-up, buccal view.

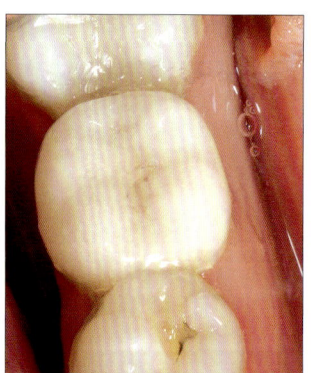

Fig 24   Two-year follow-up, occlusal view.

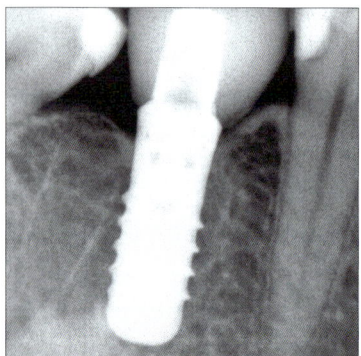

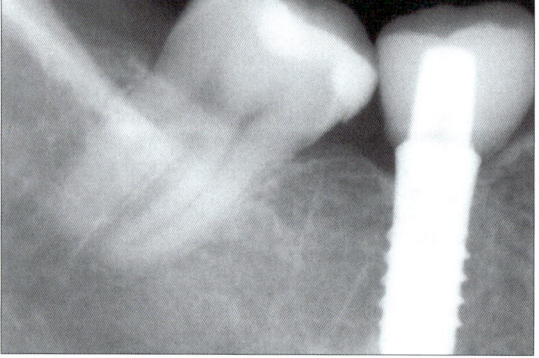

Figs 25 and 26   Two-year periapical radiograph showing a bone levels and an optimal fit of the crown.

13.3 Immediate Loading of a Premolar Implant with a Provisional Restoration

C. Fijnheer

Assessment of case complexity

A 47-year-old healthy female patient, a non-smoker, was referred to our department for implant therapy. All maxillary second premolars had been extracted as part of previous orthodontic treatment. A course of periodontal therapy had produced stable outcomes over seven years. Five years previously, tooth 14 had been removed because of an untreatable carious lesion (Fig 1).

The clinical examination revealed a single-tooth gap with limited crestal width due to the loss of the buccal cortical plate. Tooth 15 had been heavily restored with composite; tooth 13 had also been restored with composite on its distal aspect (Figs 2 to 8).

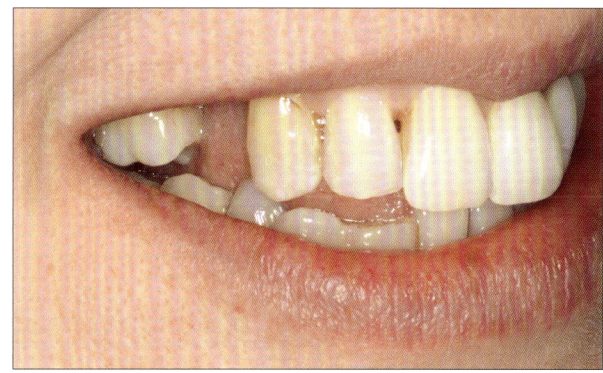
Fig 1   Lateral photograph with missing first premolar.

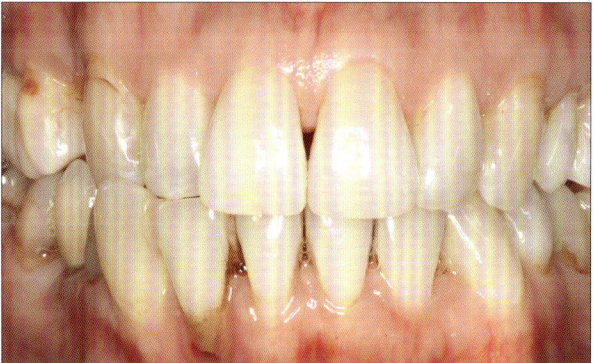
Fig 2   Frontal view in occlusion.

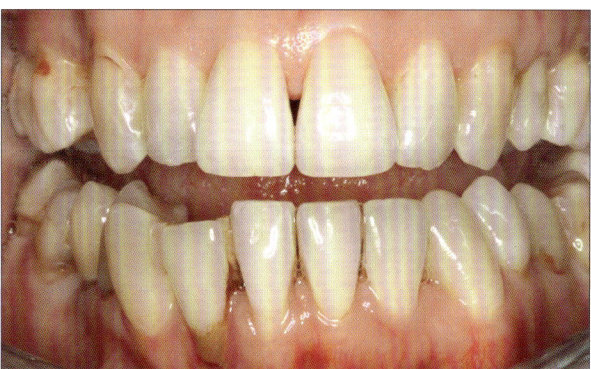
Fig 3   Frontal view in disclusion.

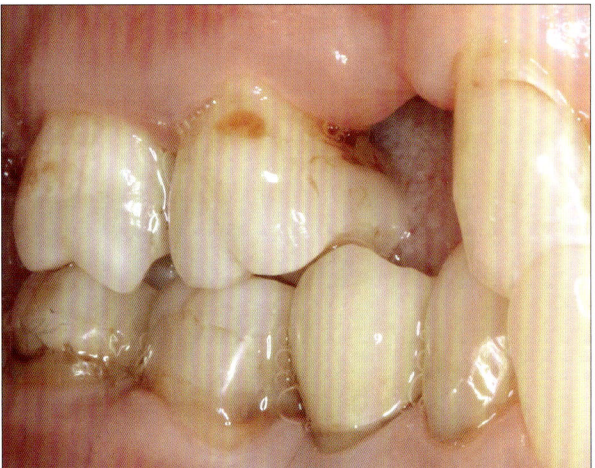

Fig 4   Right lateral view.

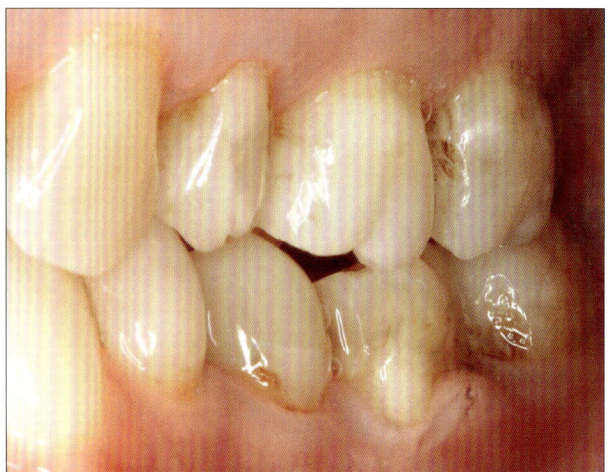

Fig 5   Left lateral view.

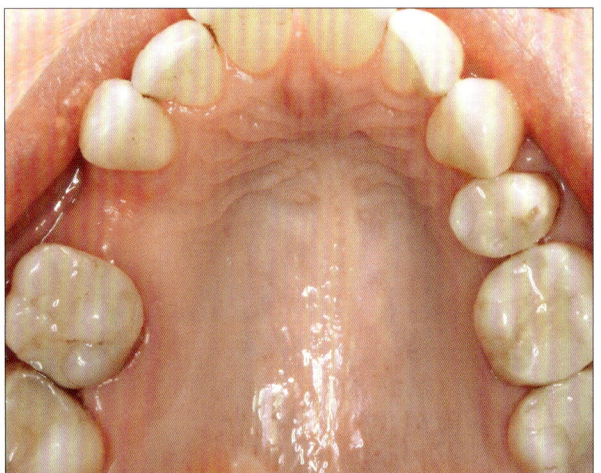

Fig 6   Maxillary occlusal view.

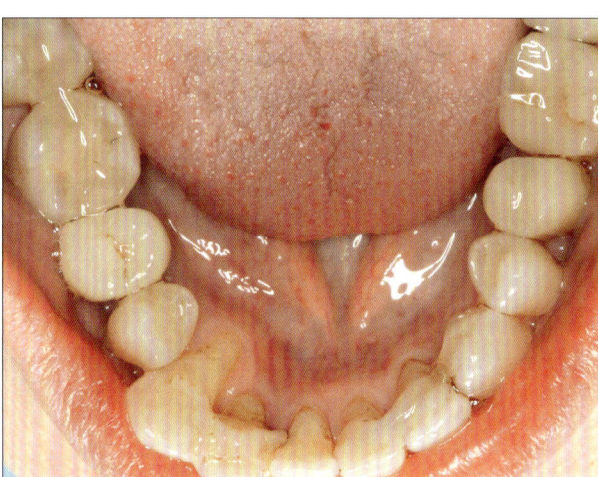

Fig 7   Mandibular occlusal view.

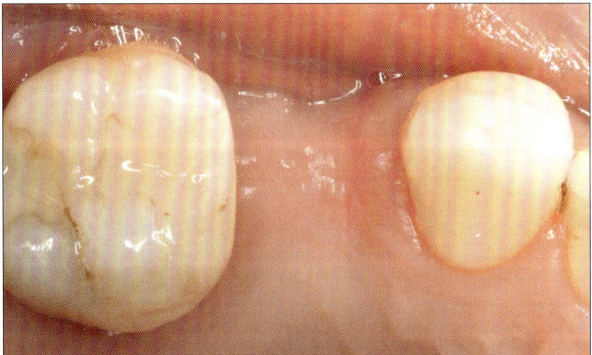

Fig 8   Single-tooth gap.

Case analysis, pre-operative planning, and implant selection

A CBCT scan revealed limited loss of the buccal cortex. The digital implant-planning software (coDiagnostiX; Dental Wings, Montreal, Quebec, Canada) found the bone supply to be adequate for correct prosthetically driven implant placement (Fig 12). After matching an intraoral scan with the CBCT scan, the hard- and soft-tissue data were combined for prosthetically driven implant planning (Figs 9 to 11).

A surgical drill guide was designed and milled in a chairside milling unit (DWX-4; Roland DGA, Irvine, CA, USA) (Figs 12 to 14). By adding a virtual scanbody, the planned implant position was transferred to the prosthetic design software (DWOS; Dental Wings) (Fig 15).

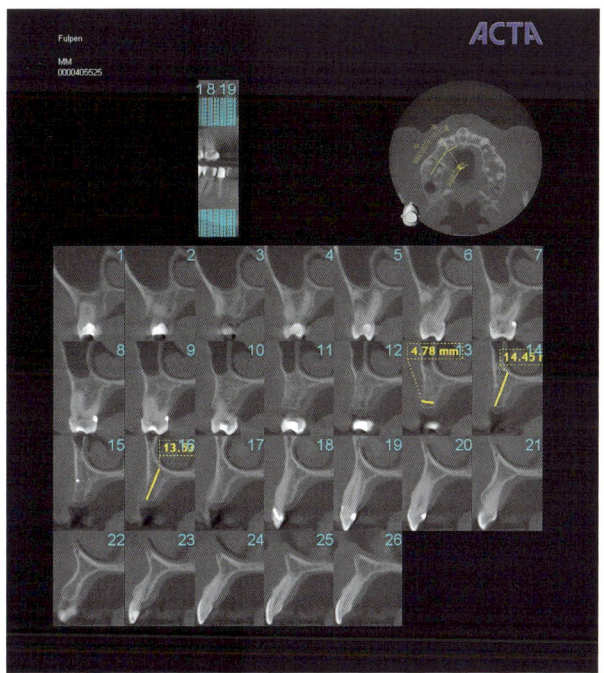

Fig 9   CBCT scan.

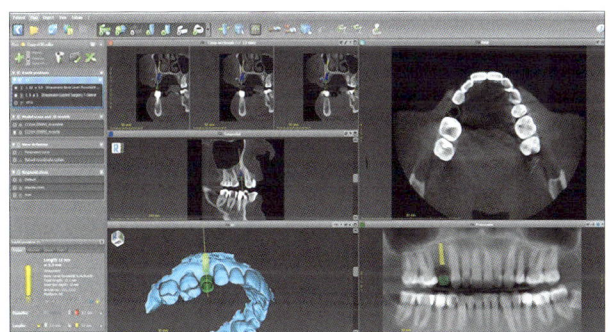

Fig 10   Implant and prosthetic planning in coDiagnostiX.

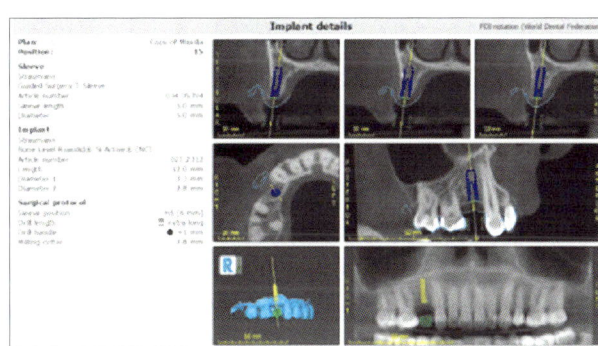

Fig 11   Guided-surgery protocol.

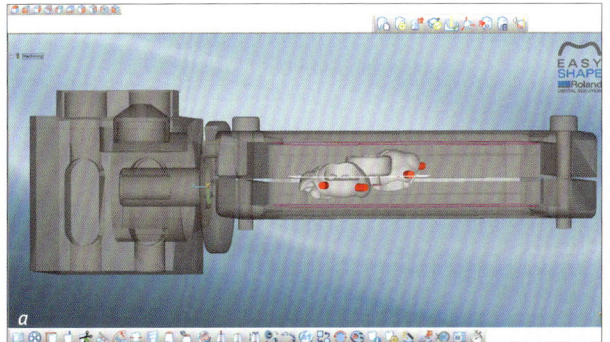

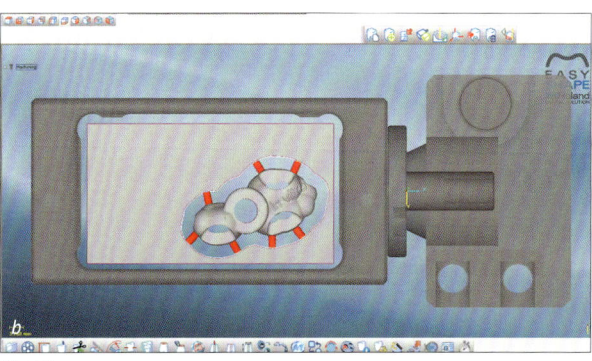

Figs 12a-b   Virtually developed surgical guide as implemented in the milling software.

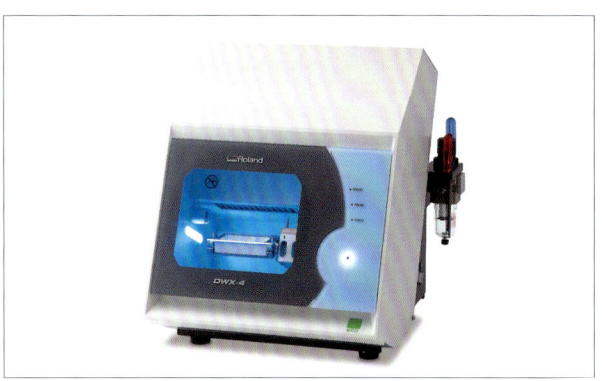

Fig 13   Chairside milling unit (DWX-4).

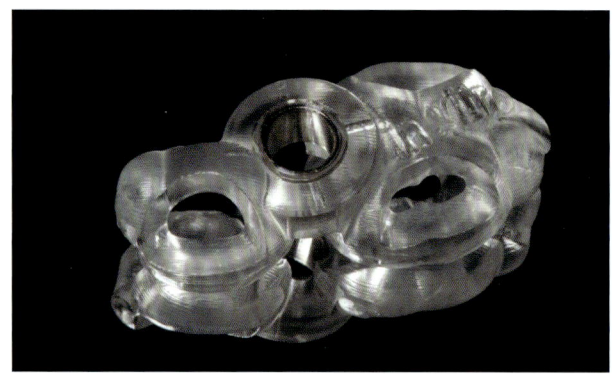

Fig 14   Milled surgical guide.

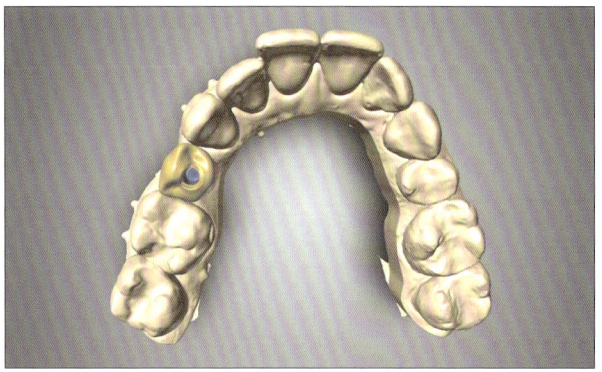

Fig 15   Prosthetic design based on the virtually planned implant.

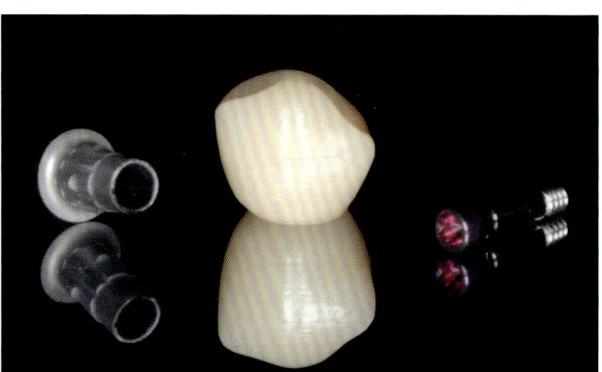

Fig 16   Variobase abutment with pre-designed milled crown.

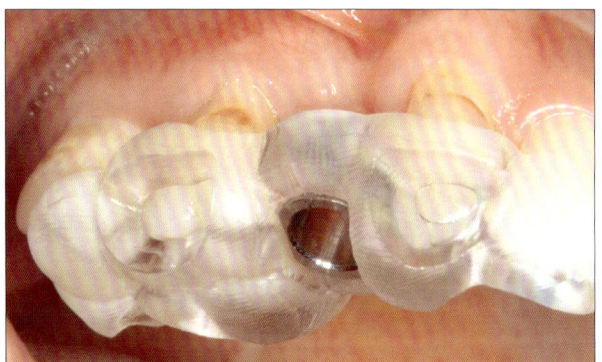

Fig 17   Fitting of the surgical guide.

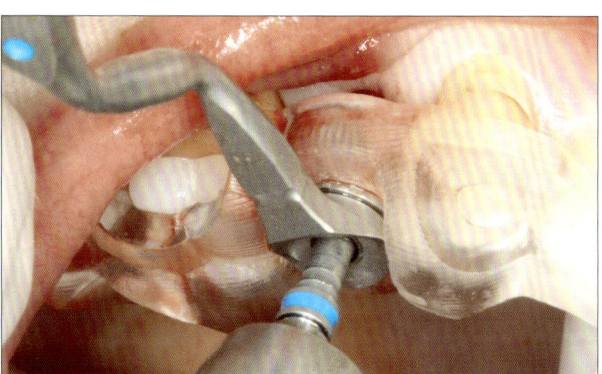

Fig 18   Drill handle and pilot drill, diameter 2.2 mm.

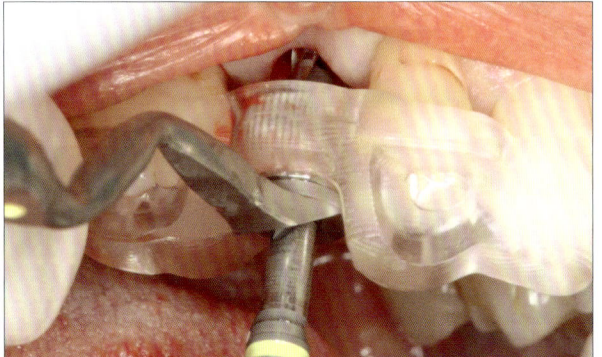

Fig 19   Drill handle and twist drill, diameter 2.8 mm.

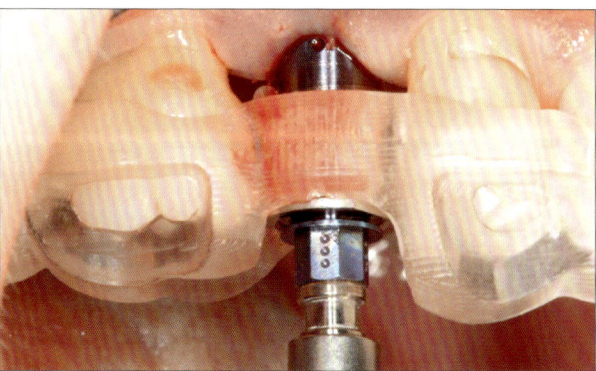

Fig 20   Guided implant insertion.

A crown was designed and milled based on the virtual implant position (Fig 16). A screw-retained Vita Enamic crown (Vita Zahnfabrik, Bad Säckingen, Germany) was milled using the DWX-4 and cemented with Multilink Automix (Ivoclar Vivadent, Schaan, Liechtenstein) on a standard Variobase abutment (Institut Straumann AG, Basel, Switzerland).

Guided surgery

Implant surgery was performed under local anesthesia and perioperative antibiotic prophylaxis (Amoxicillin 2 g p.o. one hour before surgery). Flapless surgery was performed and a bone-level implant (Bone Level BL NC, diameter 3.3 mm, length 12 mm; Institut Straumann AG) was successfully placed at site 14 following the guided-surgery protocol (Figs 17 to 21).

Immediate final restoration

Following implant placement, the pre-designed crown (Vita Enamic; Vita Zahnfabrik) was placed at a torque of 35 Ncm and the screw access hole was sealed with PTFE tape and a composite restoration (Filtek Supreme; 3M ESPE, St. Paul, MN, USA) (Figs 22 and 23). No adjustment of the contact points or the occlusion and articulation pattern was necessary. Six weeks later, baseline measurements (probing depth and bleeding on probing) were obtained at a clinical examination (Table 1).

Follow-up and maintenance

One year after implant insertion and immediate crown placement, a follow-up examination confirmed a stable peri-implant soft-tissue situation and stable crestal bone levels (Tables 1 and 2; Figs 24 to 26). Due to financial constraints, the provisional crown inserted immediately after implant placement will stay in situ for another year.

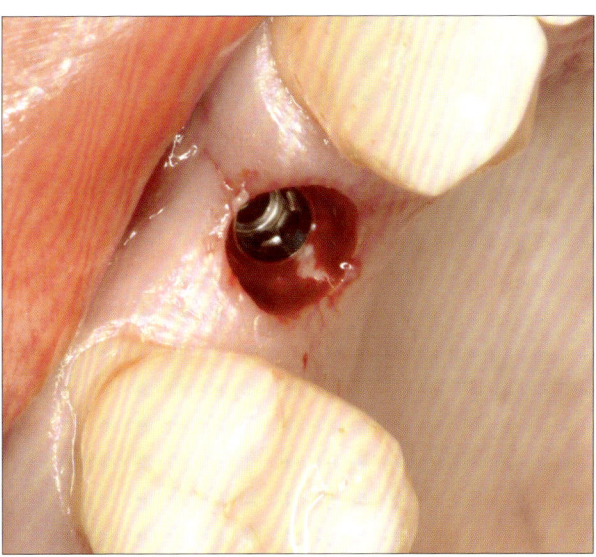

Fig 21   Flapless surgery.

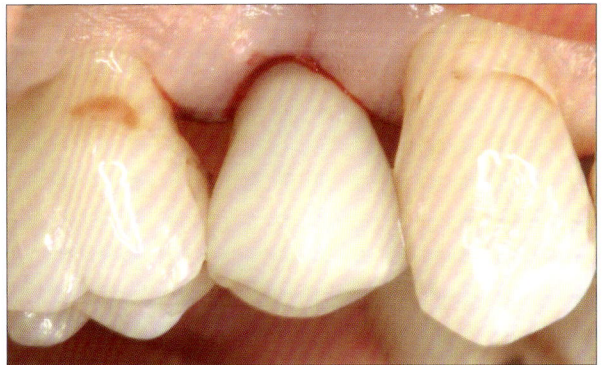

Fig 22   Immediate restoration with pre-designed crown.

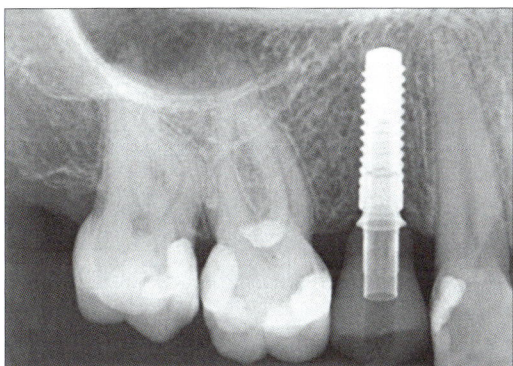

Fig 23   Periapical radiograph after insertion of the implant and crown.

Table 1   Probing depth (PD; in mm) and bleeding on probing (BoP; red) six weeks after implant insertion and placement of the immediate crown.

Distal	Buccal	Mesial
<u>**4**</u>	2	2
3	1	3
Distal	Palatal	Mesial

Table 2   Probing depths (PD; in mm) and bleeding on probing (BoP; red) one year after implant insertion and placement of the immediate crown.

Distal	Buccal	Mesial
4	2	3
<u>**4**</u>	2	3
Distal	Palatal	Mesial

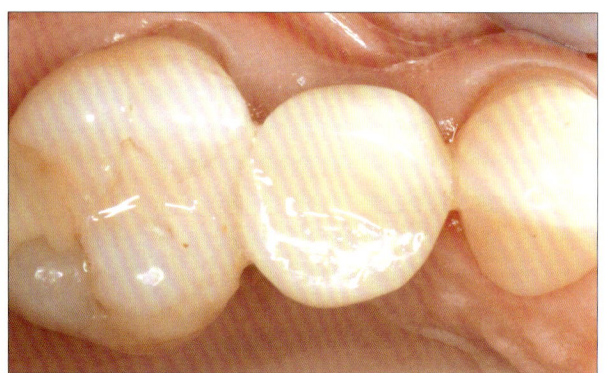

Fig 24   Intraoral situation after one year of function, occlusal view.

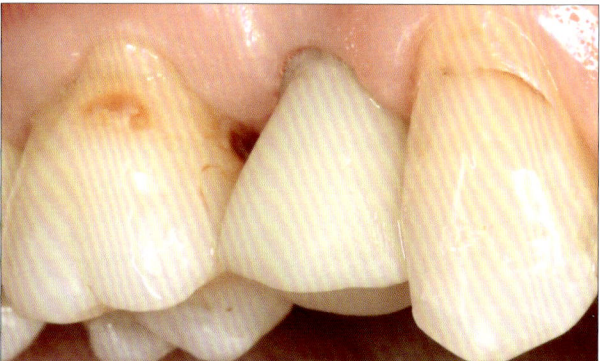

Fig 25   Intraoral situation after one year of function, lateral view.

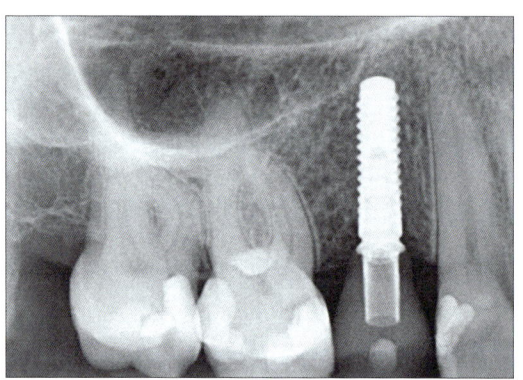

Fig 26   Periapical radiograph after one year of function.

Conclusion

The widespread availability of chairside equipment for computer-aided design and computer-aided manufacturing (CAD/CAM) have taken clinical practice into a new era. Immediate loading of a prefabricated CAD/CAM implant-supported crown is a novel concept, promising a reduction in the number of clinical steps required and total treatment time and potentially making treatment more efficient and acceptable for both patients and clinicians.

A complete digital workflow combining chairside scanning, fabrication of a surgical guide, and delivery of an immediate implant-supported crown by CAD/CAM can be successful. Based on this individual case, it appears that immediate loading of a virtually planned implant with a virtually planned restoration can be a one-stage procedure that need not require any additional interventions.

13.4 Replacing a Mandibular Second Premolar with a Chairside-Fabricated Crown

A. Hamilton, A. De Souza, S. Doliveux

A healthy 47-year-old male patient requested implant treatment for his missing maxillary left central incisor (tooth 21). The tooth had been avulsed due to trauma several years earlier. The patient had previously been provided with a removable partial denture but was unable to wear it due to restricted mobility of his upper limb, which made it difficult for him to insert or and remove the denture.

The patient had specific concerns regarding the esthetic outcome of implant treatment, including the appearance of the tooth and the peri-implant mucosa. He presented with a medium-high smile line and an edentulous space larger than the width of the contralateral central incisor; the patient agreed to accept a small midline diastema. The shape of the alveolar ridge appeared favorable, with only slight flattening of the labial contour (Figs 1a-d). An esthetic risk assessment (ERA) was completed during the examination and discussed with the patient as part of the consent process (Table 1).

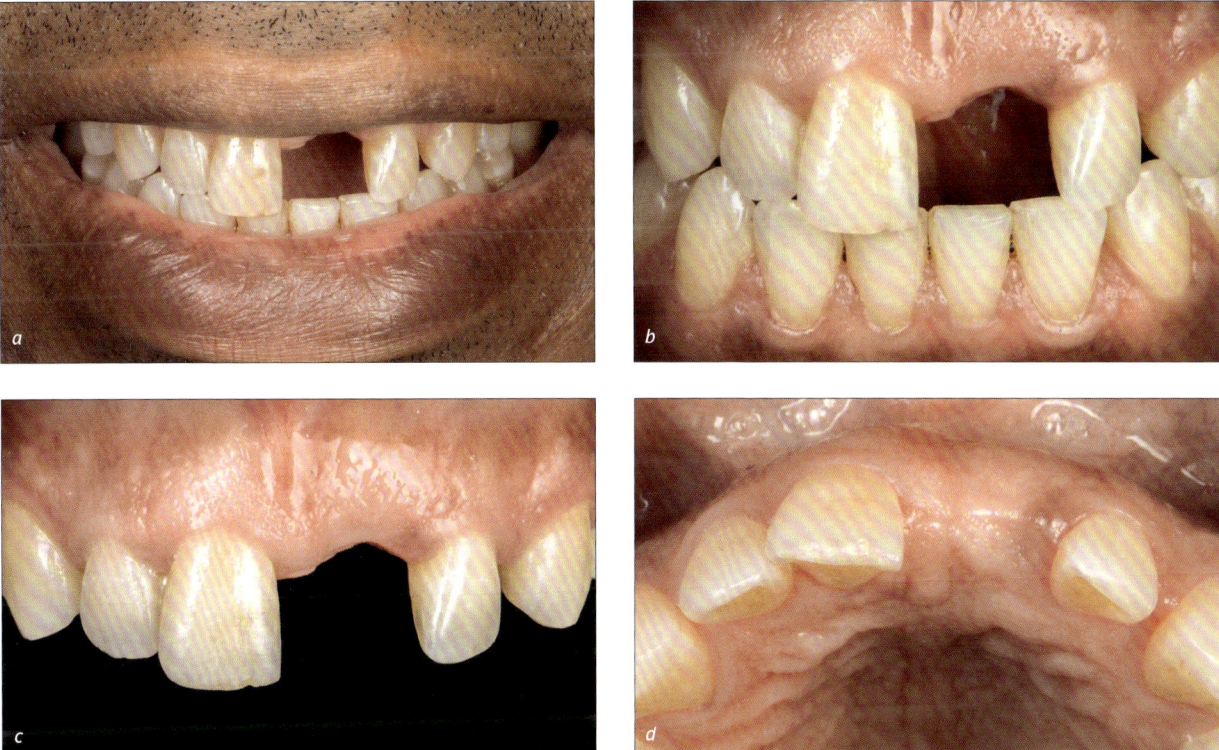

Figs 1a-d   Initial photographs showing the missing tooth 21 with favorable soft-tissue height and volume and a slight flattening of the alveolar ridge contour on the labial aspect.

Table 1   Esthetic Risk Assessment

Esthetic risk factors	Level of risk		
	Low	**Medium**	**High**
Medical status	Healthy, uneventful healing		Compromised healing
Smoking habit	Non-smoker	Light smoker (≤ 10 cigs/day)	Heavy smoker (> 10 cigs/day)
Gingival display at full smile	Low	Medium	High
Width of edentulous span	1 tooth (≥ 7 mm)[1] 1 tooth (≥ 6 mm)[2]	1 tooth (< 7 mm)[1] 1 tooth (< 6 mm)[2]	2 teeth or more
Shape of tooth crowns	Rectangular		Triangular
Restorative status of neighboring teeth	Virgin		Restored
Gingival phenotype	Low-scalloped, thick	Medium-scalloped, medium-thick	High-scalloped, thin
Infection at implant site	None	Chronic	Acute
Soft-tissue anatomy	Soft tissue intact		Soft-tissue defects
Bone level at adjacent teeth	≤ 5 mm to contact point	5.5 to 6.5 mm to contact point	≥ 7 mm to contact point
Facial bone-wall phenotype*	Thick-wall phenotype ≥ 1 mm thickness		Thin-wall phenotype < 1 mm thickness
Bone anatomy of alveolar crest	No bone deficiency	Horizontal bone deficiency	Vertical bone deficiency
Patient's esthetic expectations	Realistic expectations		Unrealistic expectations

* If three-dimensional imaging is available with the tooth in place
[1] Standard-diameter implant, regular connection
[2] Narrow-diameter implant, narrow connection

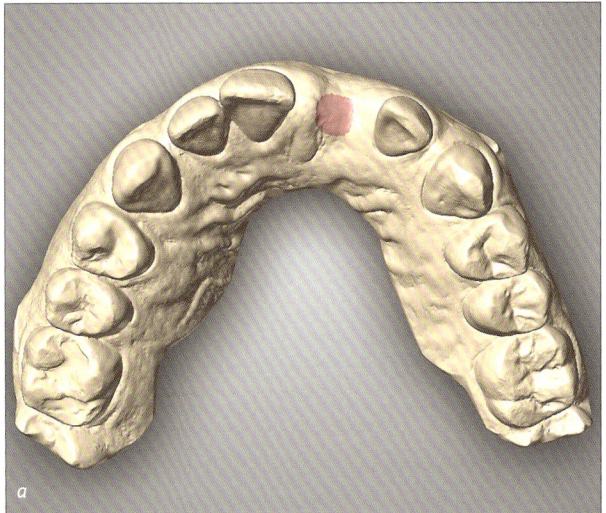
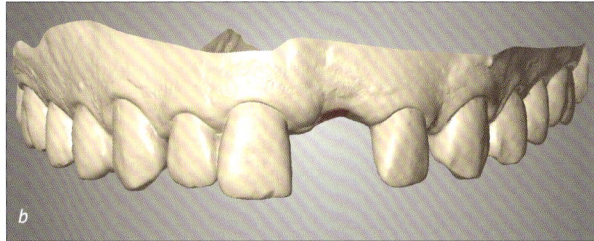
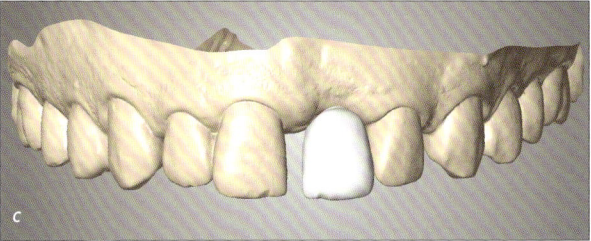

Figs 2a-c   Digital diagnostic casts imported into CAD/CAM software (a-b). Detailed digital diagnostic wax-up (c).

Digital diagnostic impressions were taken of the patient with an intraoral scanner (iTero; Align Technology, San Jose, CA, USA) (Figs 2a-b). The STL file was imported into computer-aided design (CAD) software (CARES Visual 9.0; Straumann, Andover, MA, USA) and a digital diagnostic wax-up was created that followed the tooth dimensions (width, length, thickness) and contours obtained from the adjacent contralateral tooth using a mirroring feature. This digital wax-up (Fig 2c) formed the basis of our implant-prosthodontic planning, an integral part of virtual treatment planning.

A cone-beam computed tomography (CBCT) image was acquired (i-CAT; Imaging Sciences, Hatfield, PA, USA) and imported into virtual implant planning software (co-DiagnostiX; Dental Wings, Montreal, Canada) as a DICOM file. Three-dimensional rendering and segmentation of the maxillary bone and tooth anatomy was carefully executed to isolate the areas of interest (Fig 3a). Threshold values must be appropriately selected and any scattering cleaned up to produce a segmentation that will allow accurate superimposition of the digital diagnostic casts (STL files) (Flügge and coworkers, 2017) (Figs 3b-c). This critical step significantly affects the accuracy of guided implant surgery.

The digital diagnostic casts and the digital wax-up were transferred between the CAD software and the planning software with a synchronization tool (Synergy; Dental Wings, Montreal, Canada). This tool registers datasets and transfers information such as the digital wax-up, abutment design, and implant position between the two

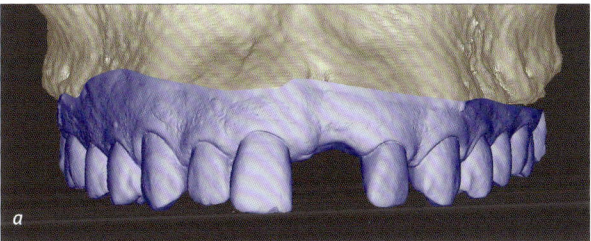
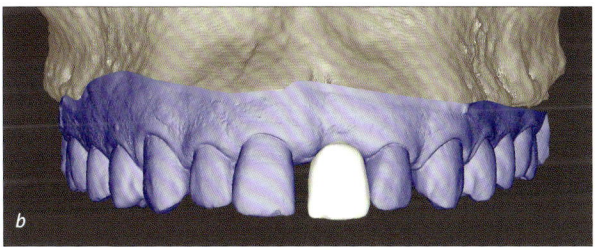
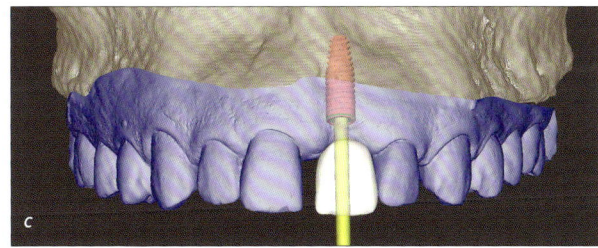

Figs 3a-c   Creation of a virtual patient by combining the data from the CAD/CAM wax-up and diagnostic casts with the CBCT dataset.

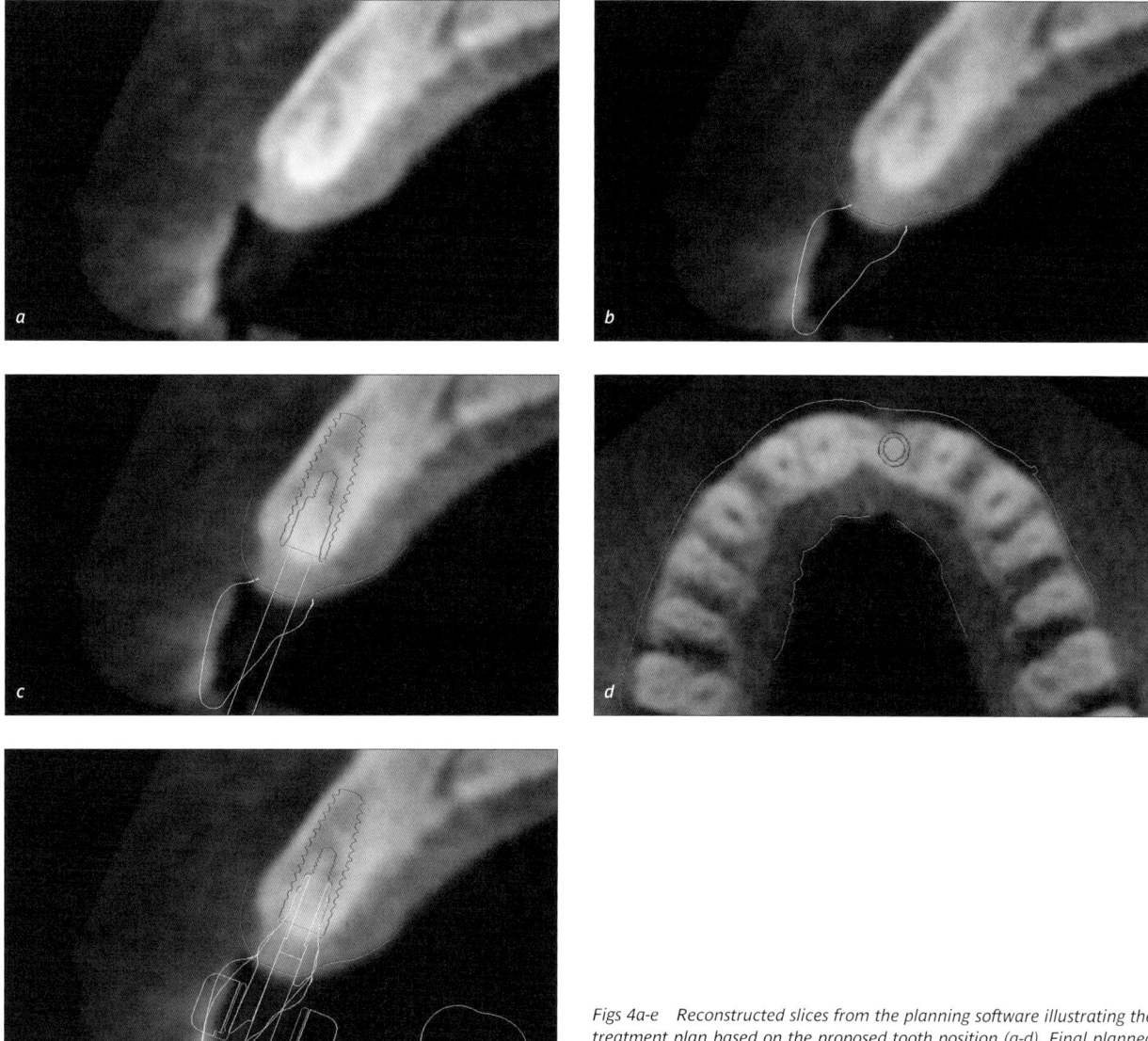

Figs 4a-e   Reconstructed slices from the planning software illustrating the treatment plan based on the proposed tooth position (a-d). Final planned implant position and visualization of the CAD/CAM abutment contours in the planning software (e).

software programs. Once the datasets were registered in the planning software, the ideal three-dimensional implant position for a screw-retained restoration was planned based on the digital wax-up and radiographic anatomical features. An implant (Bone Level Tapered, diameter 4.1 mm, length 10 mm; Institute Straumann AG, Basel, Switzerland) was planned, avoiding the need for bone grafting (Figs 4a-d).

The implant position was transferred from the planning software to the CAD software in real time so the dental technician could simultaneously assess and provide input on the planned implant position based on restorative

parameters. Once the planned implant position was finalized, a CAD/CAM custom zirconia abutment and PMMA provisional crown were designed in the CAD software based on the proposed implant position and sent to a centralized production center for manufacturing (Figs 5a-g). The synchronization feature also transmits the design of the abutment to the planning software, so that the abutment contours can be assessed according to anatomical and biological parameters (Fig 4e). The abutment and provisional crown were slightly undercontoured at the mucosal margin to minimize pressure on a subepithelial soft-tissue graft planned to be performed at the time of implant placement.

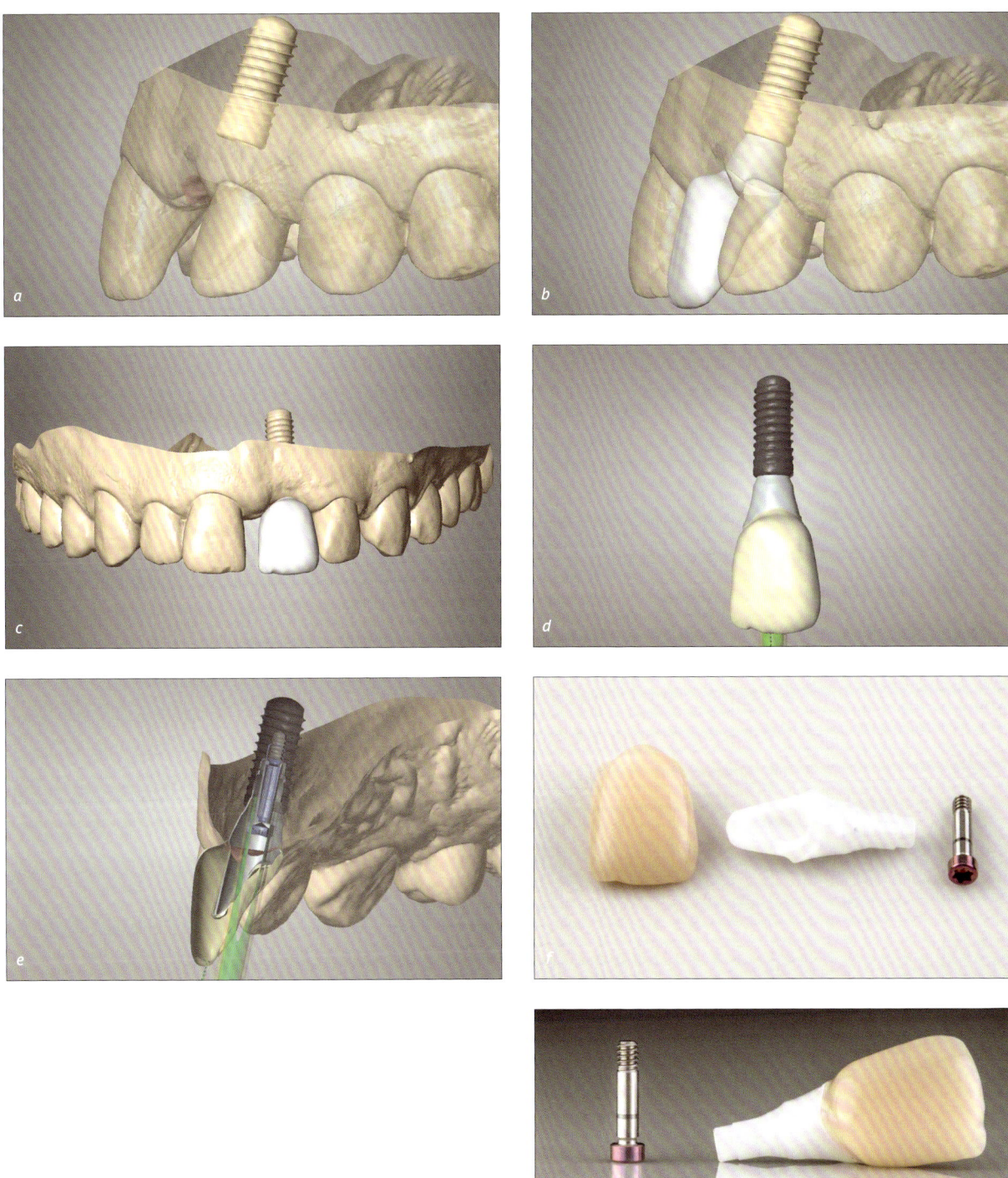

Figs 5a-g Transfer of the proposed implant position to the CAD/CAM software for the design and fabrication of a custom zirconia abutment (a-e) and an acrylic provisional crown (f-g).

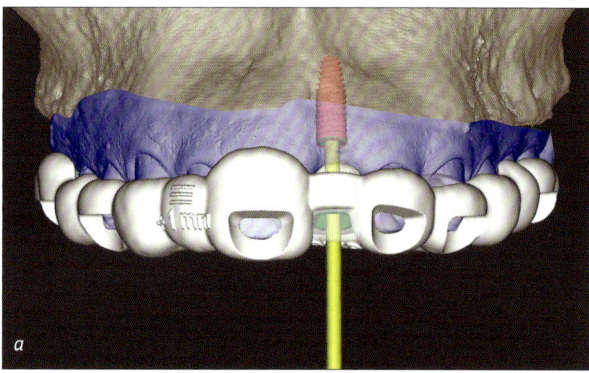

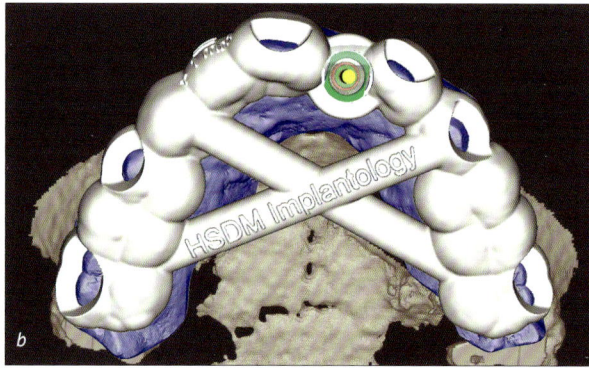

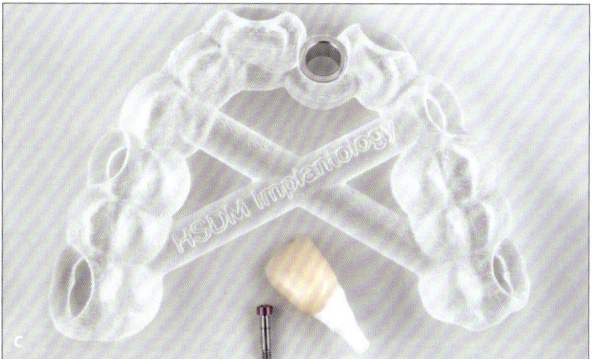

Figs 6a-c Surgical guide designed in the planning software (a-b). Surgical guide and prefabricated crown ready for the surgical appointment (c).

The surgical guide was designed in the planning software (Figs 6a-b). The occlusal support extended from tooth 16 to tooth 26. Six inspection windows were placed. A 3.5-mm wall thickness with a 0.15-mm offset between the surgical guide and the contact surface were established. The surgical guide design was exported as a STL file and printed on a PolyJet 3D Printer (Objet Eden260VS; Stratasys) (Fig 6c). The use of implant rotation markers is recommended to control the rotational position of the implant, as this permits accurate reproduction of the internal abutment-connection index; however, they were not used for this patient.

Based on the CBCT and the amount of keratinized tissue available, the patient was a good candidate for flapless implant placement (Figs 7a-f). Several research groups have demonstrated the predictability of flapless guided surgery using a tooth-supported surgical guide (Raico Gallardo and coworkers 2017; D'haese and coworkers 2017). To compensate for a facial soft-tissue deficiency, a subepithelial connective-tissue graft was performed at the time of implant placement (Figs 8a-e).

The surgical guide was placed and its seating verified visually through the inspection windows. The patient was anesthetized with facial and palatal local infiltration of xylocaine 2% with 1 : 100,000 epinephrine. A soft-tissue punch was used first, followed by a combination of surgical drills and handles according to the prescription provided by the planning software. The implant was placed with an insertion torque above 35 Ncm.

A conservative split-thickness flap was elevated on the facial aspect of the implant site and extended beyond the mucogingival junction using a micro scalpel blade (Fig 8a). A periosteal microsurgery instrument ensured that the dimensions of the site were adequate to receive the soft-tissue donor graft. A subepithelial connective-tissue graft was harvested from the palate using the technique described by Lorenzana and Allen (2000). A single horizontal incision extending from the distal of the canine to the mesial of the first molar was created approximately 3 mm from the gingival margin. A split incision was then made within the first incision, and a periosteal elevator was used to release the tissue graft from the bone. The connective-tissue graft was prepared and immediately placed at the implant site. Two interrupted sutures stabilized the soft-tissue graft. The immediate provisional crown had been designed to develop the soft-tissue contours (Figs 9a-b).

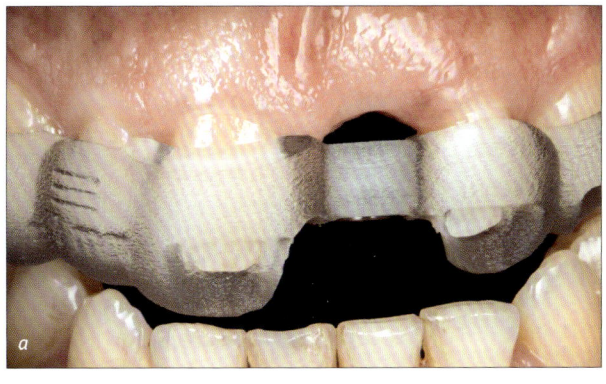 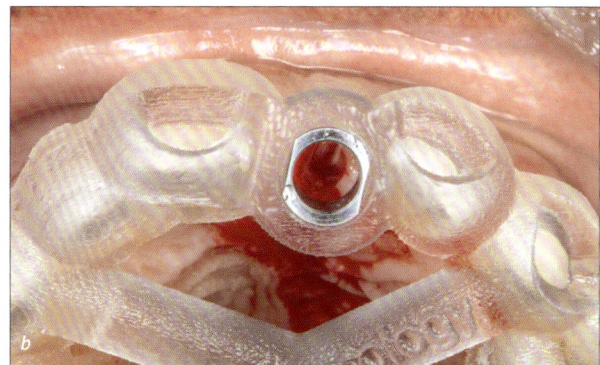

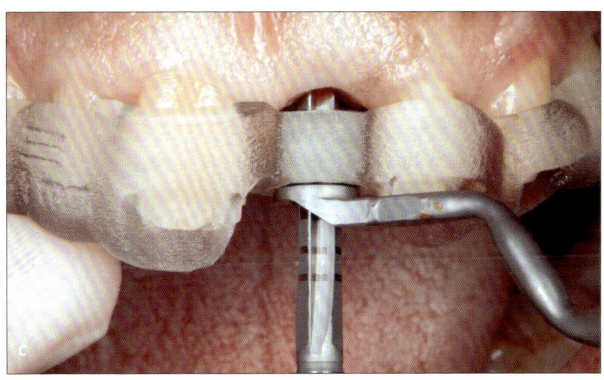 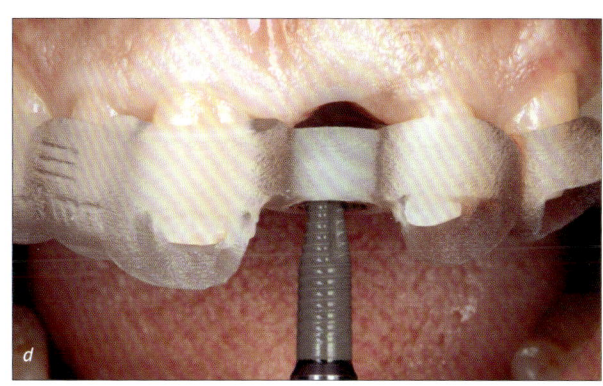

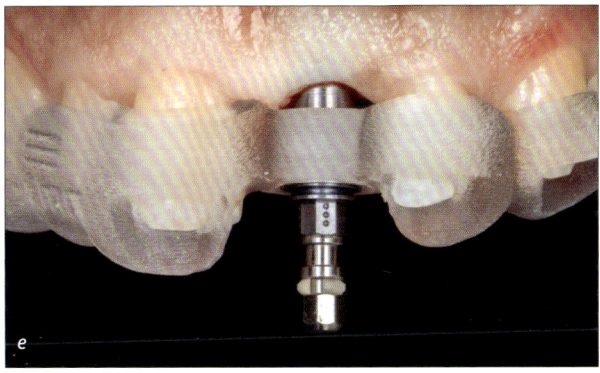 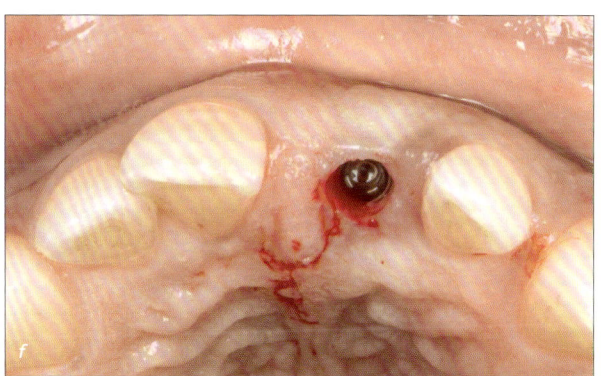

Figs 7a-f Flapless guided implant surgery with guided implant placement. Clinical assessment of the fit of the template through the inspection windows (a-b). Guided osteotomy preparation (c). Guided implant placement (d-e). Soft-tissue contours immediately after implant placement and prior to soft-tissue augmentation and contouring with the provisional restoration (f).

After eight weeks of healing, the provisional crown was removed. The osseointegration of the implant was tested at 35 Ncm; the peri-implant soft tissue was found to be perfectly healthy. The provisional crown was modified to shape the emergence profile and change the position of the labial mucosal margin to better match the marginal tissue level of the contralateral tooth.

After twelve weeks of functional loading, the peri-implant soft tissue appeared esthetic and healthy (Figs 10a-b). A digital impression abutment (Mono scanbody; Institut Straumann AG) was inserted (Figs 10c-d) and a final digital impression taken with the intraoral scanner (iTero) (Figs 11a-b).

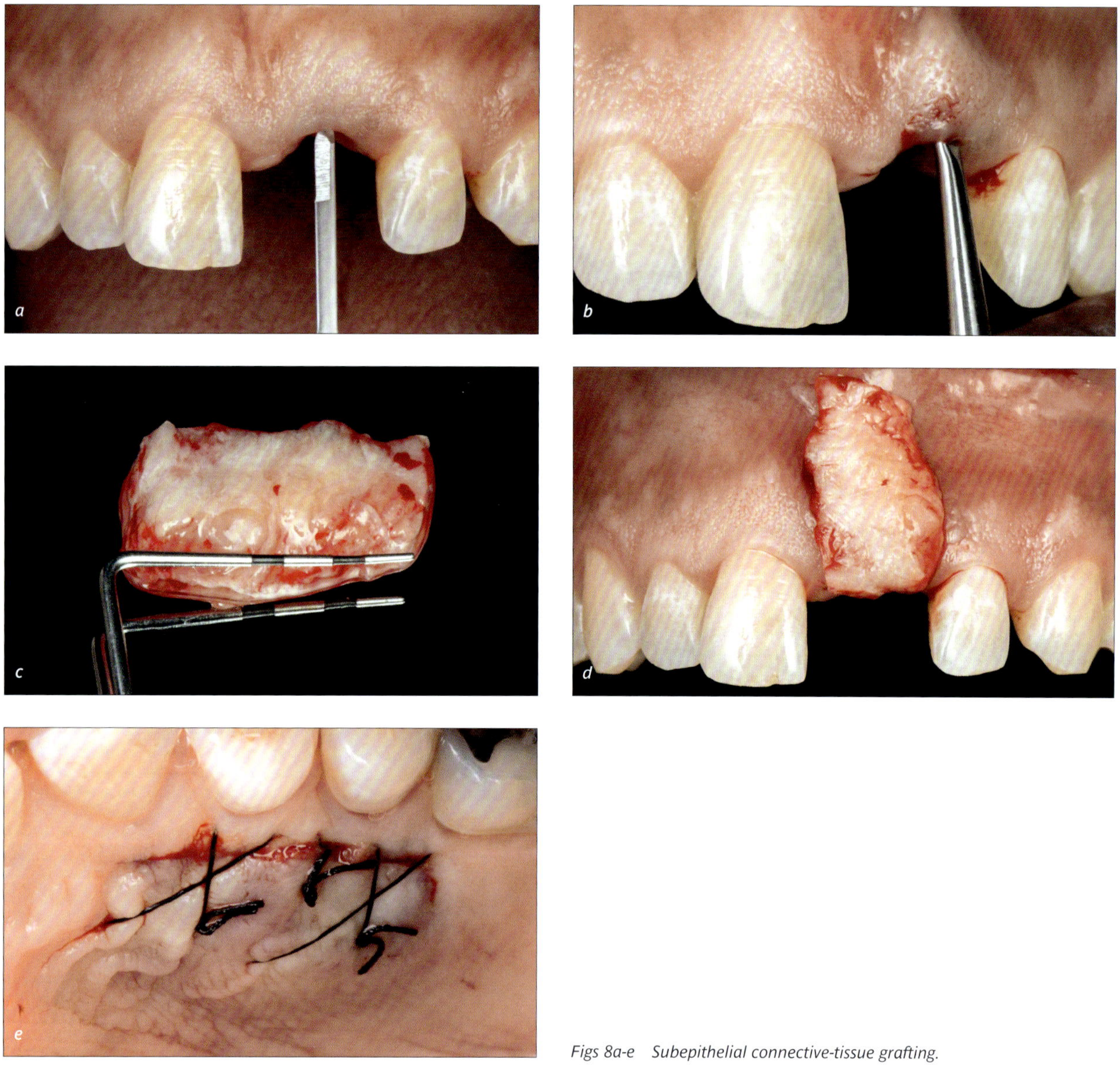

Figs 8a-e   Subepithelial connective-tissue grafting.

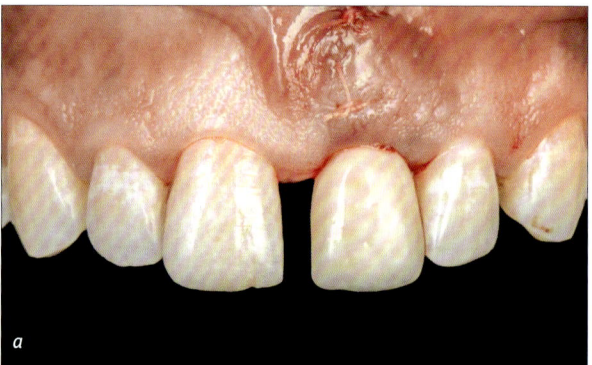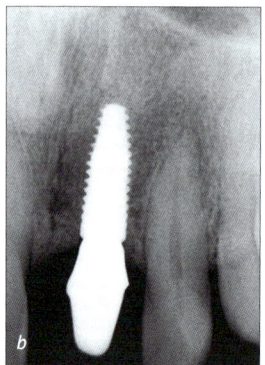

Figs 9a-b   Provisional restoration immediately after insertion on the day of implant placement (a). Postoperative radiograph (b).

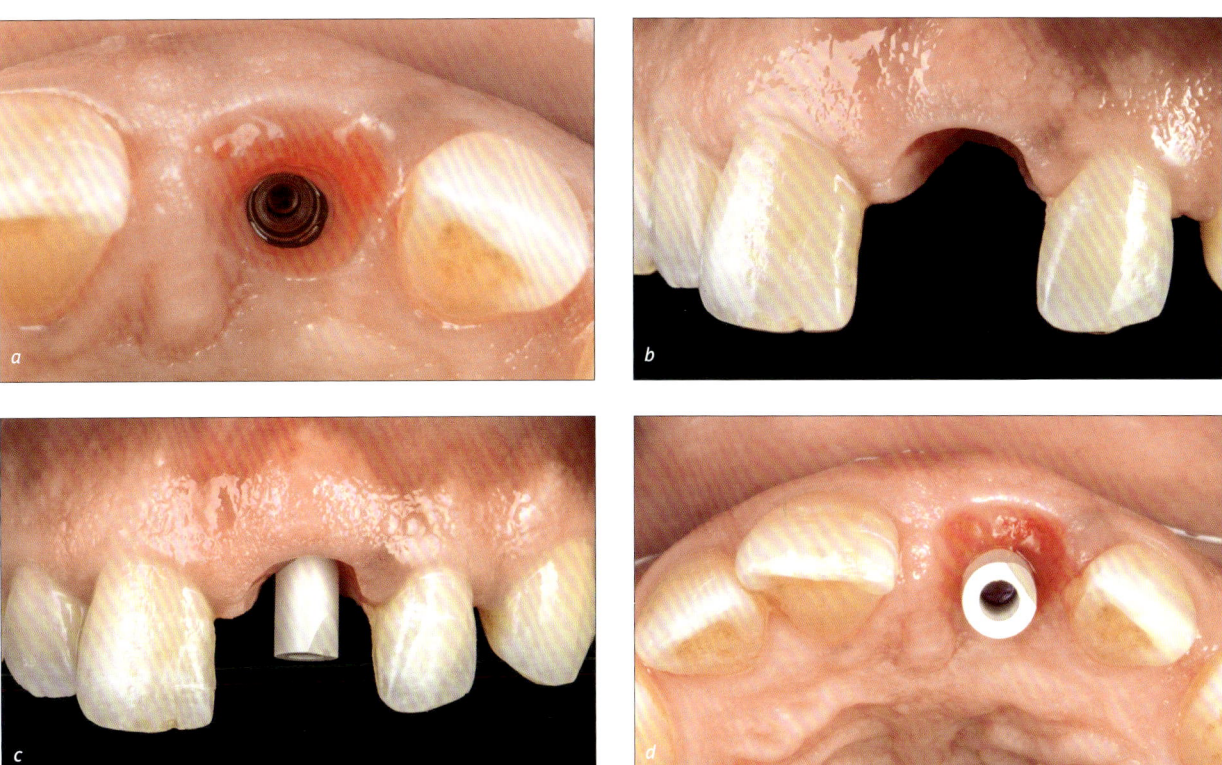

Figs 10a-d   Soft-tissue profile after healing (a-b). Surface scan with digital scan coping (c-d).

The maxillary and mandibular models were milled from the surface-scan STL files with a receptacle for a repositionable implant analog to replicate the implant position. The models were used for the wax-up, ceramic build-up, and finishing of the restoration. Following the preference of the master dental technician, the abutment was custom-waxed onto the milled model (Figs 12a-b), placed in an abutment scan holder (Fig 12c), and scanned with a laboratory scanner (3Series; Dental Wings). The design was verified in the CAD software (Figs 12d-e) and digitally sent to a centralized milling center for fabrication of the zirconia abutment (Straumann Manufacturing; Arlington, VA, USA) (Figs 13a-c).

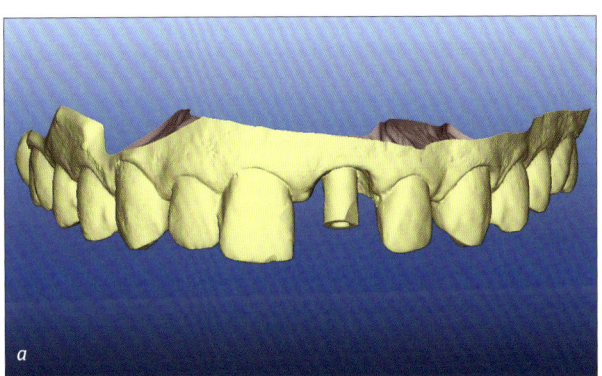
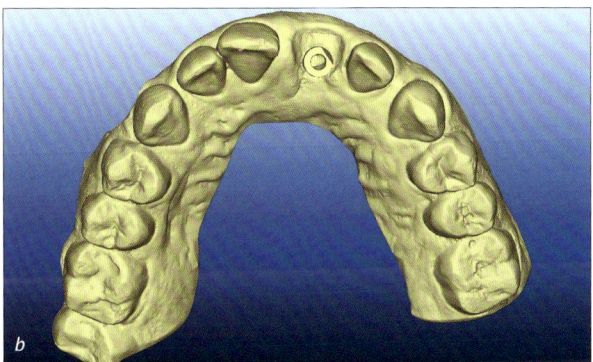

Figs 11a-b   STL file representation from surface scan used for digital model fabrication.

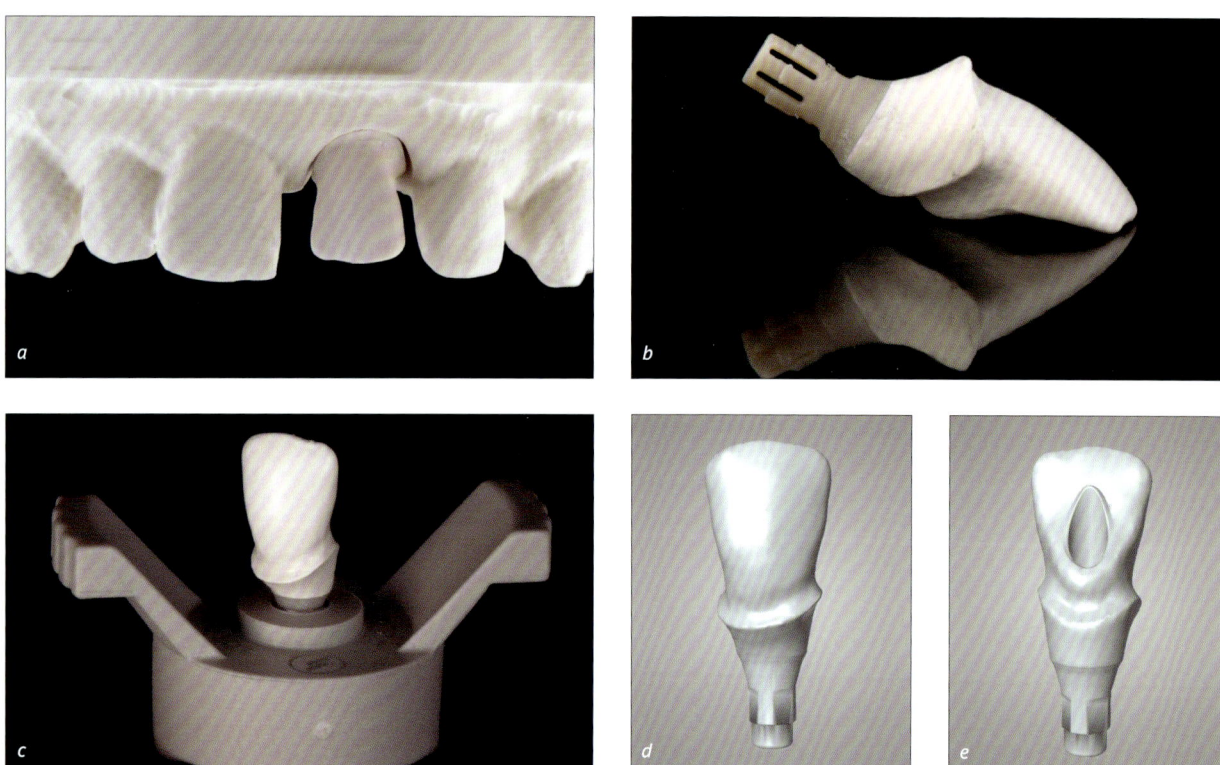

Figs 12a-e   Conventional wax-up of a custom abutment (a-b), scanned (c) to provide a digital abutment design for CAD/CAM manufacturing (d-e).

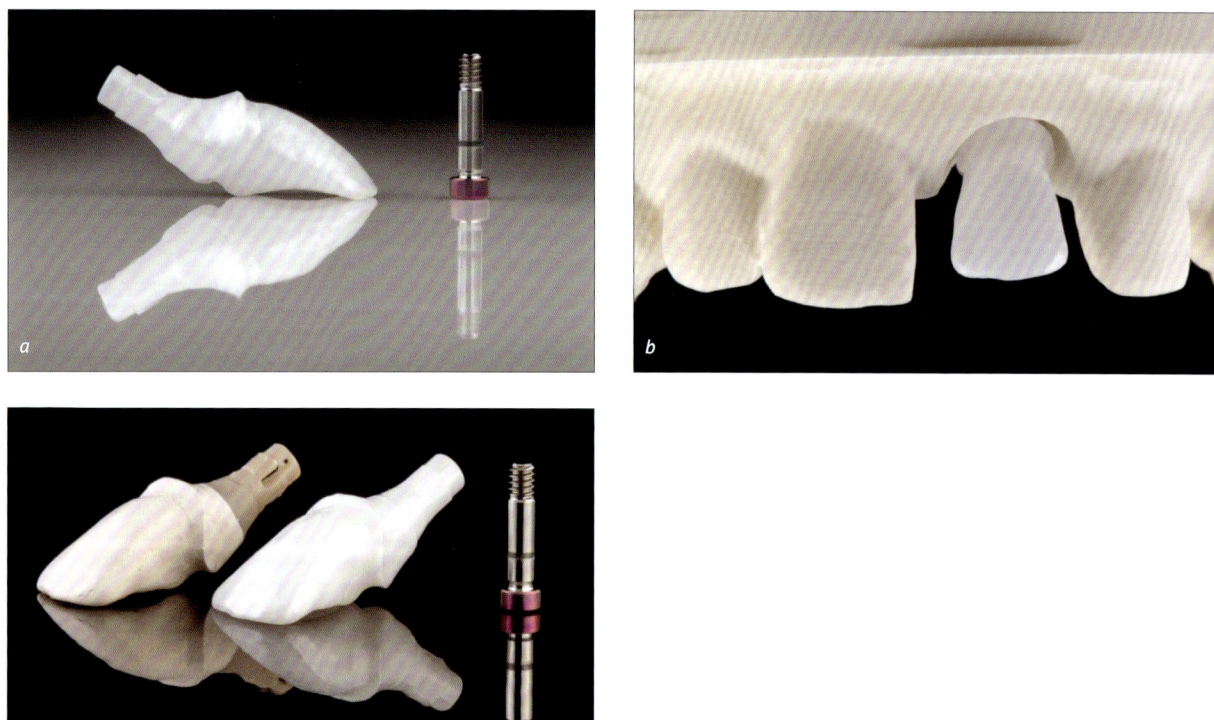

Figs 13a-c   CAD/CAM custom zirconia abutment (a-b), which exactly copied the conventional wax-up (c).

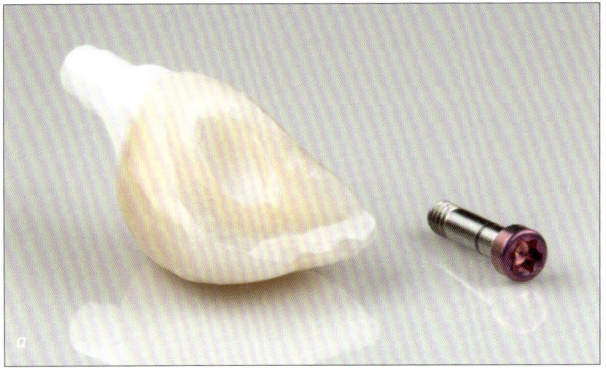
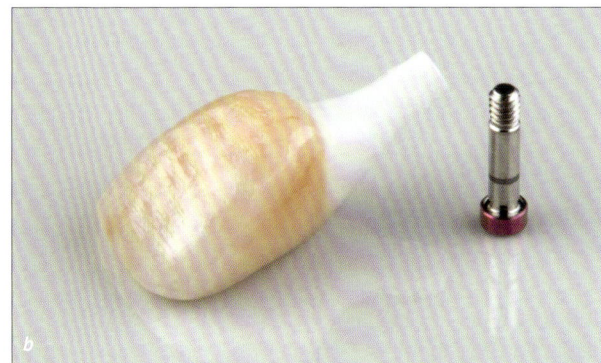
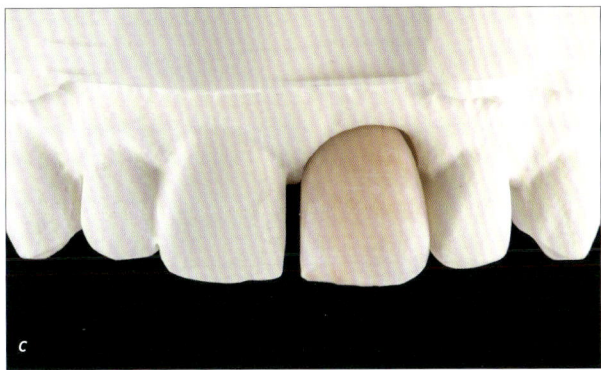
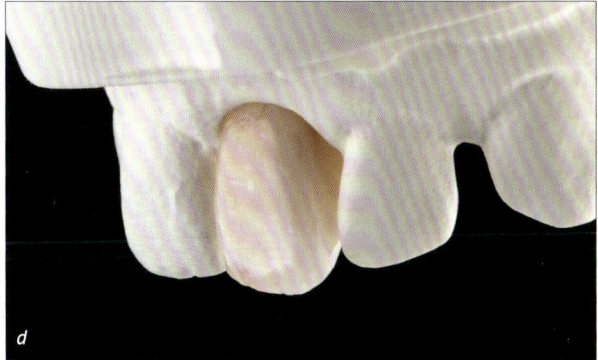
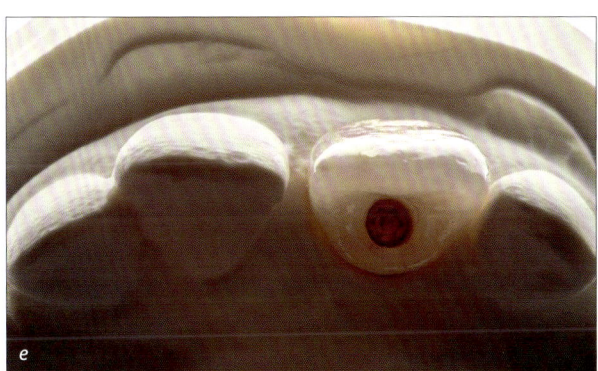

Figs 14a-e   Screw-retained final restoration with feldspathic ceramics built up on the CAD/CAM zirconia abutment by a master dental technician.

The wax-up step may be substituted with a full digital workflow using CAD software to digitally design the abutment. The technician preferred a conventional abutment wax-up to be copy-milled, as he perceived this to be faster and felt he had more control over the abutment shape in providing ideal support for the feldspathic ceramic material. A full zirconia abutment was chosen for its excellent biological soft-tissue response and to maximize the potential of the pink and white esthetics (Linkevicius and Vaitelis 2015).

The presence of a favorable occlusion helped ensure a low risk of mechanical/technical complications with all of the material choices available. A zirconia abutment cemented onto a prefabricated titanium base could have been chosen as an alternative to avoid having zirconia within the implant-abutment connection. Feldspathic ceramic material was applied to the abutment to produce a one-piece screw-retained implant-supported restoration (Figs 14a-e).

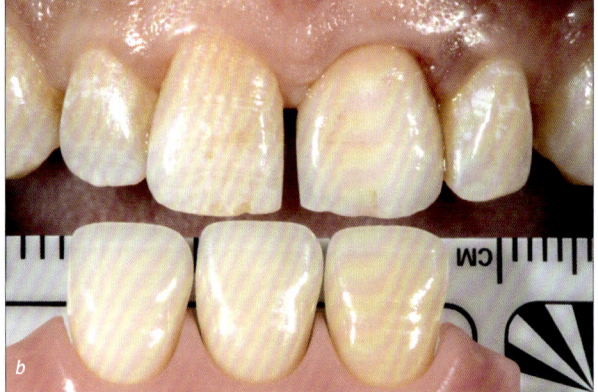

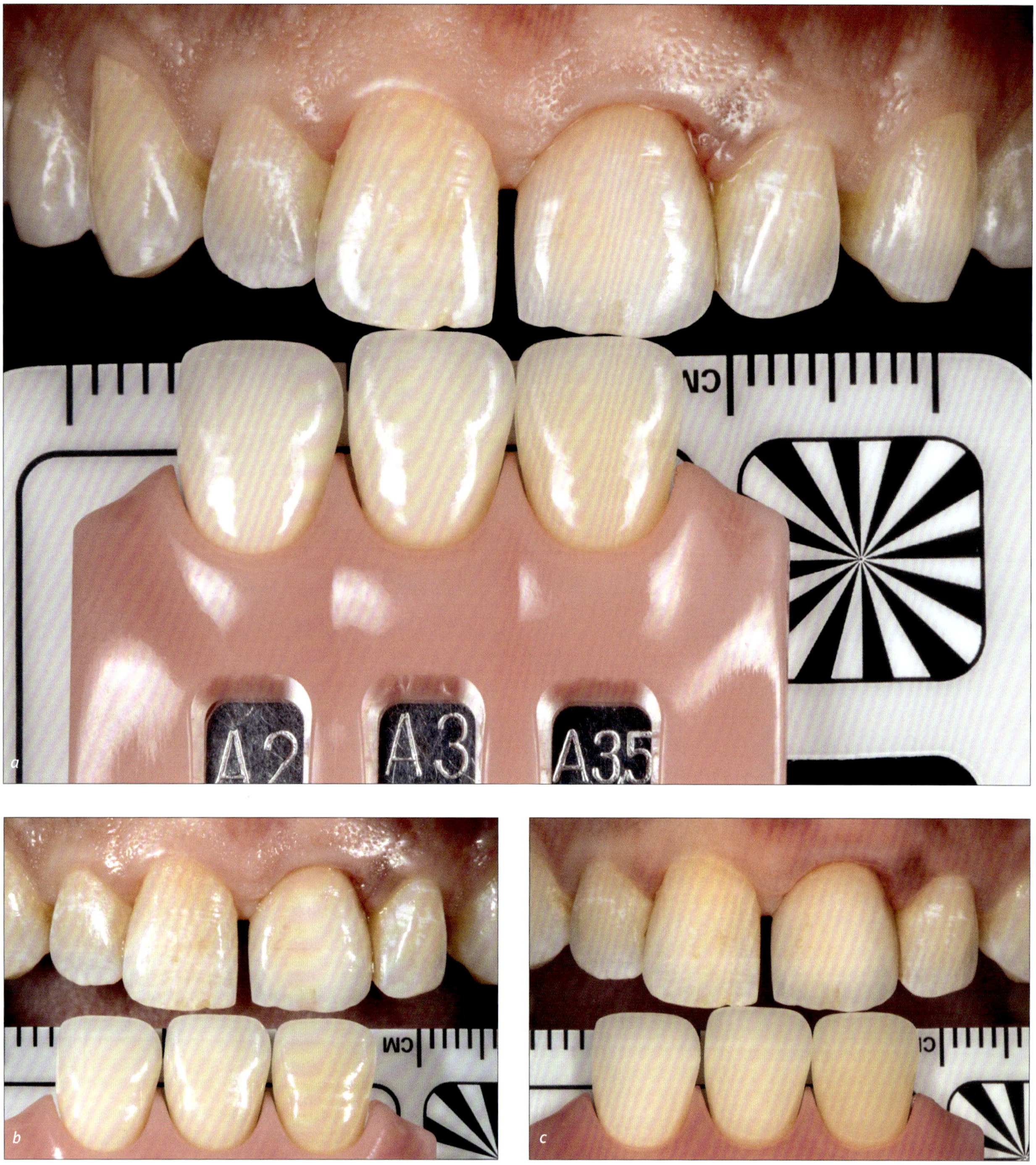

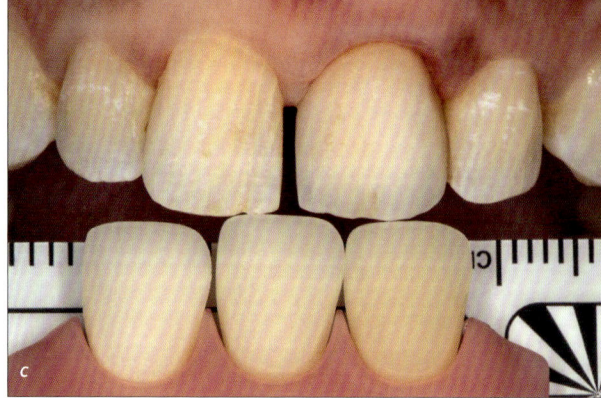

Figs 15a-c Digital photographs used at the try-in appointment to communicate required changes to the shade and contours of the restoration (a-b). including cross-polarized digital photographs (c).

During the try-in, the occlusion was assessed to maintain a slight shimstock clearance in maximum intercuspation and no excursive contacts. A periapical radiograph ensured adequate seating of the abutment on the implant. Digital photographs were used to communicate the required changes to the contours and shade of the restoration to the dental technician (Figs 15a-c).

At the delivery of the definitive crown (Fig 16a-d), the abutment screw was tightened to 35 Ncm; PTFE was used to protect the abutment screw, and composite resin was used to close the screw access hole.

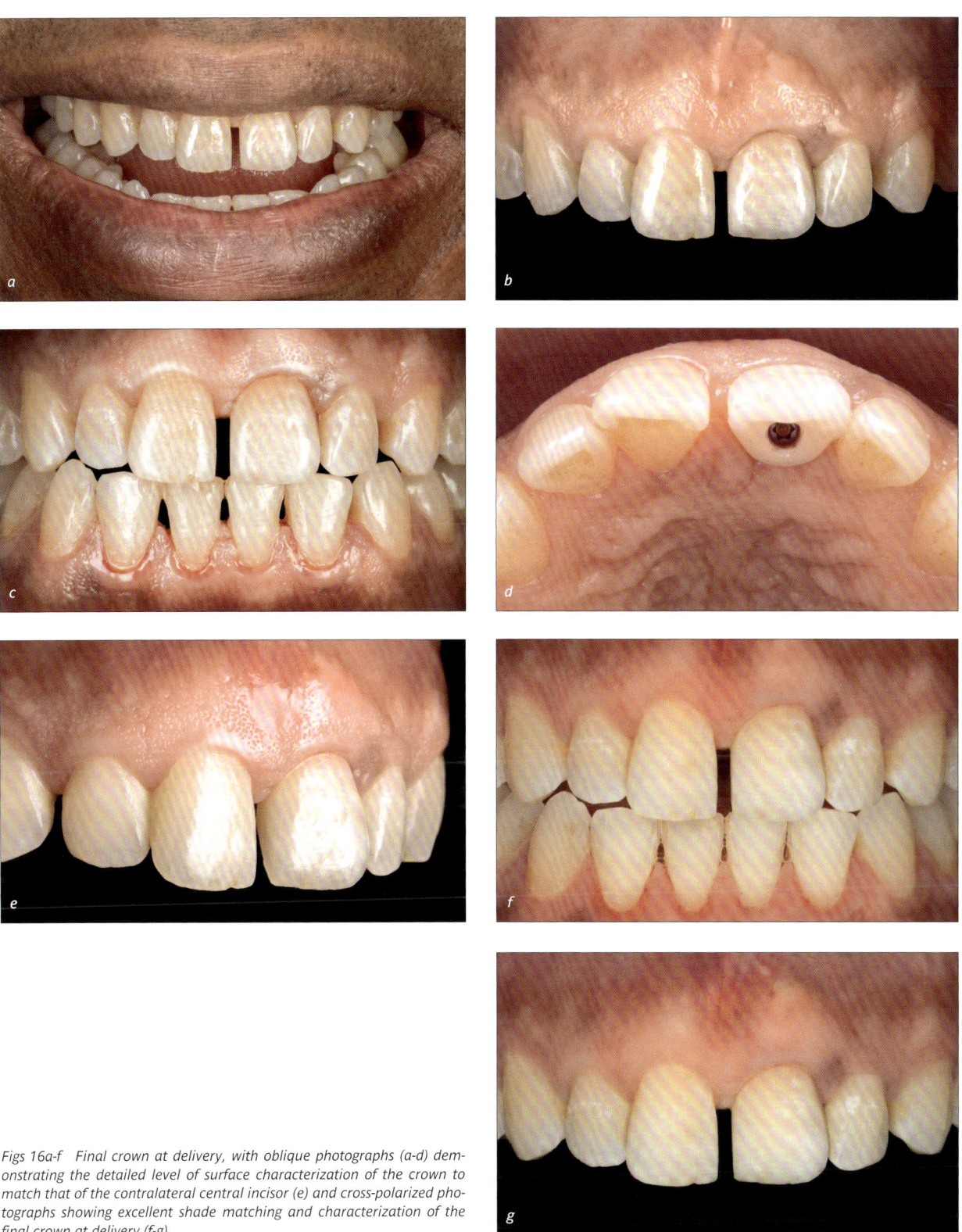

Figs 16a-f   Final crown at delivery, with oblique photographs (a-d) demonstrating the detailed level of surface characterization of the crown to match that of the contralateral central incisor (e) and cross-polarized photographs showing excellent shade matching and characterization of the final crown at delivery (f-g).

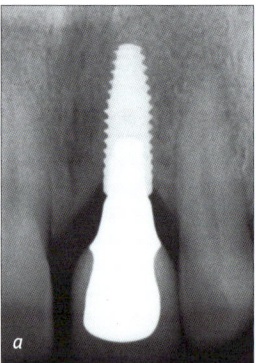

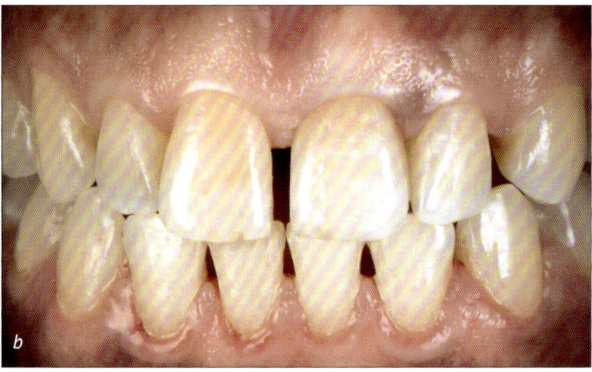

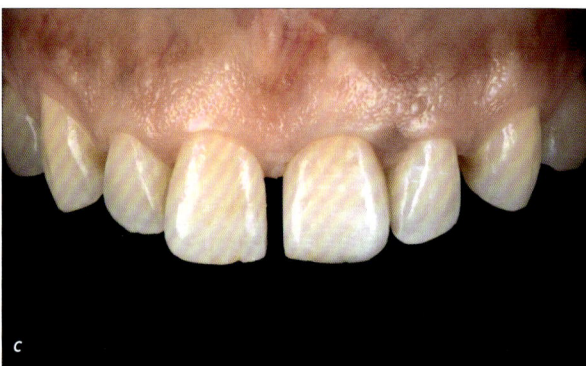

Figs 17a-c   Twelve-month follow-up radiograph and photographs showing excellent esthetics and soft-tissue health, with minor bone remodeling at the implant crest.

At the one-year follow-up, the periapical radiograph confirmed stable interproximal bone levels (Fig 17a). The peri-implant mucosa was healthy, with no signs of bleeding on probing or inflammation (Figs 17b-c). The patient was very happy with the esthetic and functional outcome. Oral hygiene reinforcement and instructions were given, and the patient will continue to be seen every twelve months for evaluation of his peri-implant health.

This case report demonstrates the successful application of digital technology combined with scientific principles and clinical techniques to provide an optimal esthetic and functional outcome for replacing a single missing maxillary central incisor. Virtual implant planning and guided implant surgery were a valuable adjunct to the treatment provided and permitted the use of a digitally prefabricated provisional restoration, delivered at the time of implant placement.

Acknowledgment

Laboratory procedures
Yasu Kawabe – Oral Design Boston, Boston, MA, USA

13.5 Replacing Four Upper Incisors with a Screw-Retained Bridge on Two Implants

K. Chmielewski, B. Roland

A 22-year-old female patient was referred to our office for implant therapy following an accident in which the patient lost the upper left central incisor (tooth 21) (Fig 1). The adjacent teeth had also been damaged; the right central incisor (11) and both lateral incisors (12, 22) showed grade II mobility. Immediately after the accident the first dental intervention involved repositioning of the mobile teeth and rigid splinting (Fig 2).

The patient presented three days after the trauma. A detailed examination was performed, including a cone-beam computed tomography (CBCT) examination (Fig 3). The patient was in good general health and was a non-smoker. Intraoral examination revealed local inflammation of the soft tissues, mobility of teeth 12, 11, and 22, and pain on occlusion with the opposing teeth. A laceration in the lower lip had been sutured. The cross-sectional views of the CBCT revealed fractures in the facial alveolar plate at sites 12, 11, and 22 (Fig 4).

An esthetic risk assessment (ERA; Martin and coworkers 2006) confirmed the clinical situation as being in the high-risk category.

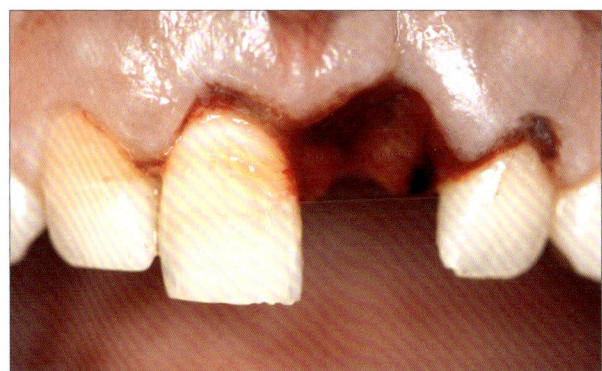

Fig 1   Clinical situation with missing tooth 21. Replacement of four upper incisors with a screw-retained bridge on two implants.

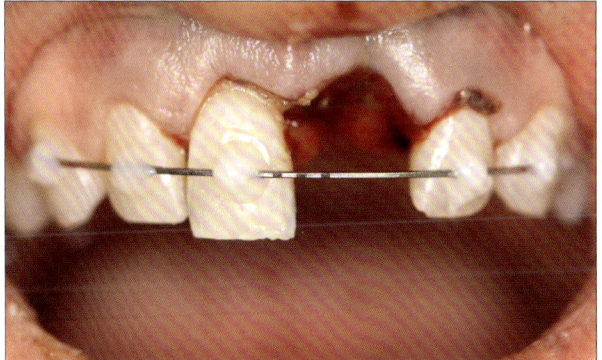

Fig 2   Splinting of mobile teeth.

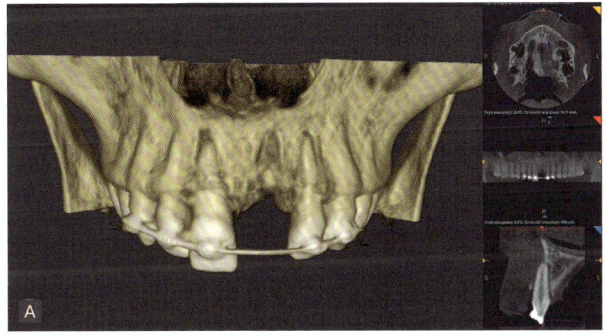

Fig 3   Reconstructed CBCT.

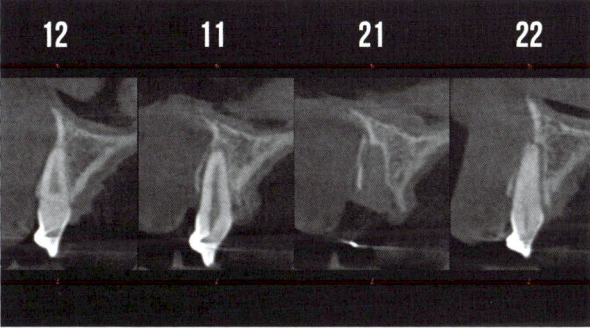

Fig 4   Cross-sectional views showing fractures of the facial plate at sites 11, 12, and 22.

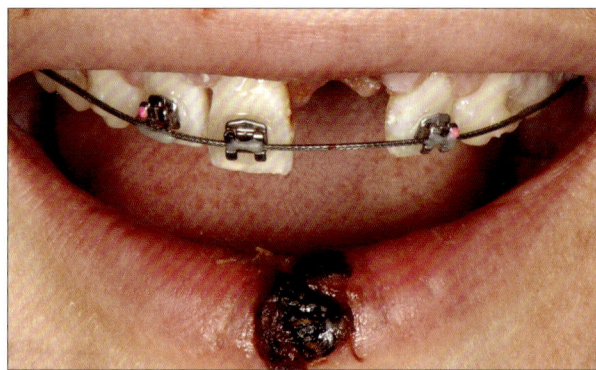

Fig 5   Elastic splinting.

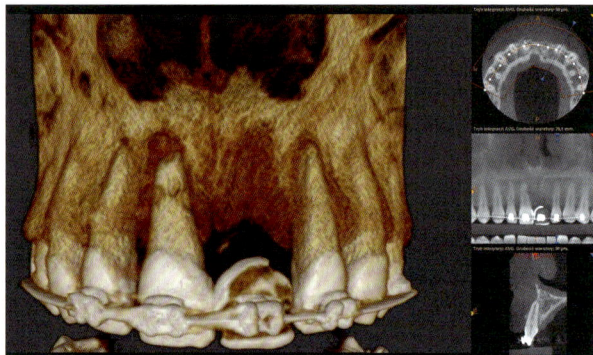

Fig 6   Overview showing bone destruction and tooth resorption.

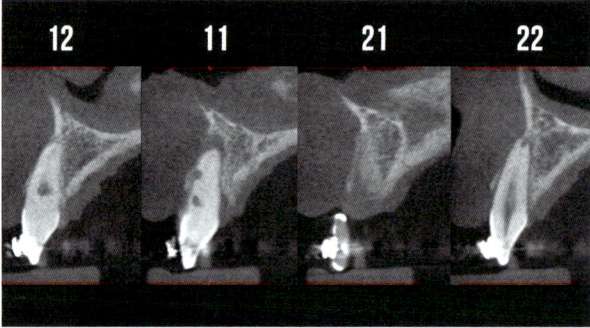

Fig 7   CBCT images detailing bone destruction and tooth resorption.

An orthodontist replaced the rigid splint with a fixed appliance for better tooth alignment (Fig 5), to be worn for three months to allow complete bone healing.

56 days after the trauma, the patient presented with pain in the region of tooth 11. Intraoral examination revealed a draining fistula above the apex of tooth 11.

Further CBCT scans demonstrated bone loss in the region of the previous injury, with additional root resorption of teeth 12, 11, and 22 (Figs 6 and 7).

Consequently, the remaining upper incisors had to be removed, resulting in an extended edentulous space. A surgical and esthetic risk assessment of the case resulted in a classification of "complex," with a low anatomic risk but a high risk of esthetic complications. The complexity of the case was classified as advanced.

After discussing the situation with the patient and her parents, a treatment plan was accepted that included guided surgery, immediate insertion of Straumann implants (Institut Straumann AG, Basel, Switzerland) with simultaneous bone regeneration, and immediate loading with a temporary restoration.

Following acceptance of the treatment plan, the following steps were planned:
- Extraction of teeth 11, 12 and 22
- Immediate implantation using computer-guided surgery at sites 12 and 22
- Guided bone regeneration (GBR) of the defect in the region of the missing tooth 21 and within the post-extraction sockets (teeth 12, 11, 22)
- Immediate non-functional loading of the implants with definitive hybrid abutments and a cemented temporary bridge
- Assessment of implant integration and soft-tissue contours after 4 to 5 months of loading
- Final restoration with a four-unit ceramic bridge at 6 months

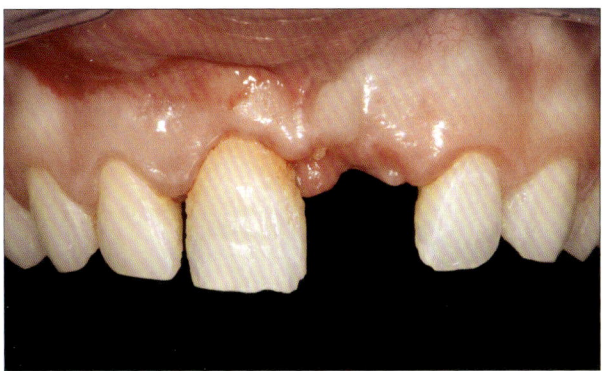

Fig 8   After bracket removal.

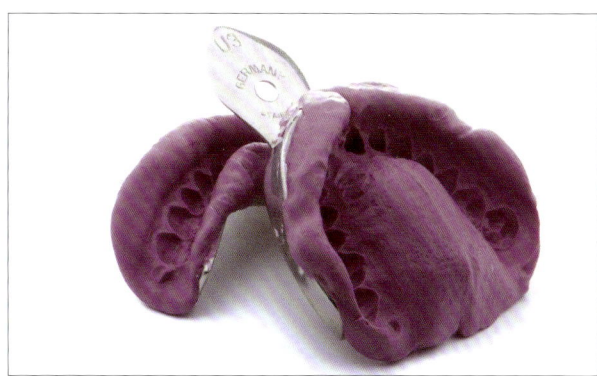

Fig 9   Alginate impressions for the casts.

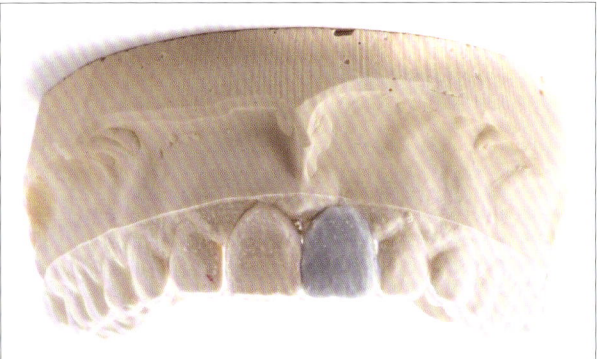

Fig 10   Wax-up of the missing tooth 21.

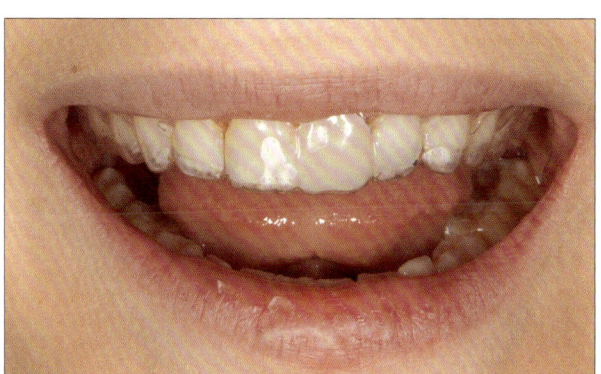

Fig 11   Provisional crown 21.

The surgical protocol agreed with the concept of immediate implant placement (Type 1) and immediate loading; however, a backup plan was also developed in case of the primary stability of the implant turned out to be insufficient at the time of placement.

Backup plan:
- Immediate implant placement using GBR
- Temporary denture for the 3 months of initial healing
- Temporary implant bridge for soft-tissue modeling
- Definitive restoration after 4 to 6 months

Actual treatment

The orthodontic appliance, including the brackets, was removed (Fig 8). Upper and lower alginate impressions were taken for conventional stone casts (Fig 9).

A basic wax-up of the missing tooth 21 allowed the fabrication of a vacuum-formed retainer (Fig 10), which, after filling the edentulous space with acrylic, served as an immediate temporary restoration for a few days (Fig 11).

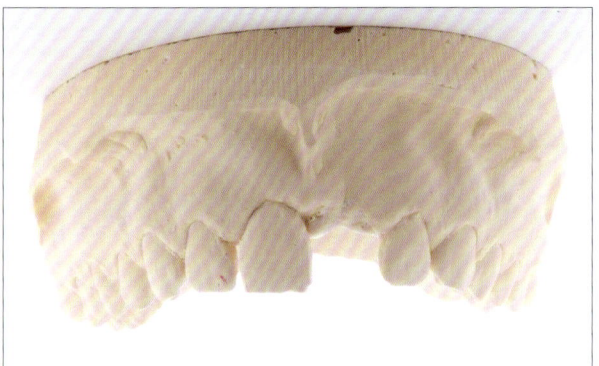

Fig 12   Cast ready for scanning.

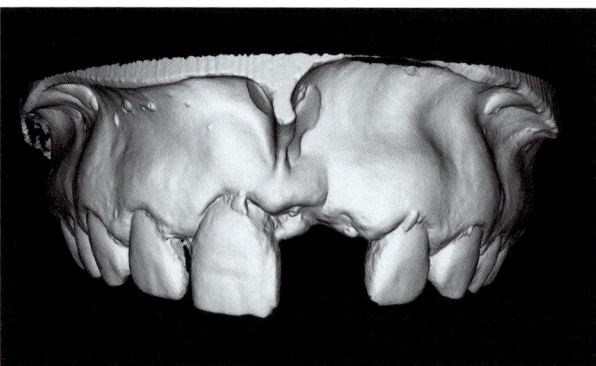

Fig 13   Representation of the STL file data of the maxilla.

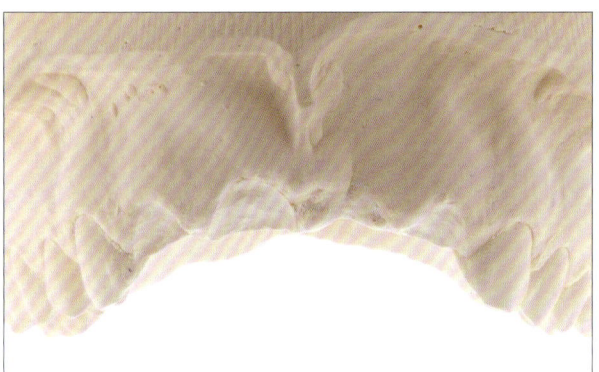

Fig 14   Re-scanned jaw after removing teeth 12, 11, and 22.

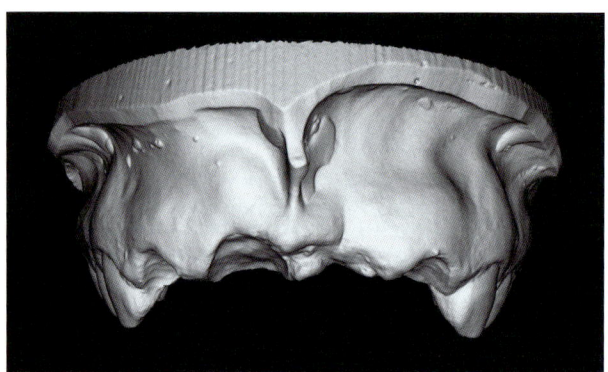

Fig 15   Resulting representation of the STL file data.

The maxillary and mandibular casts (Fig 12) were digitized with a desktop laboratory scanner, producing STL files (Fig 13). To optimize the planning and to design the surgical guide for Straumann Guided Surgery, teeth 12, 11, and 22 were removed and the upper model was re-scanned to produce an additional STL file (Fig 14).

Planning implant positions and designing the surgical guide

The implant positions and a surgical guide were planned with coDiagnostiX (Dental Wings, Montreal, Quebec, Canada). After importing the uncompressed DICOM files from the CBCT examination, planning proceeded as follows:

Step 1. Segmenting the data to create the 3D digital model of the maxilla representing the bone and teeth. For a better overview and better differentiation of structures, different colors are used for each segmentation layer (Fig 16)

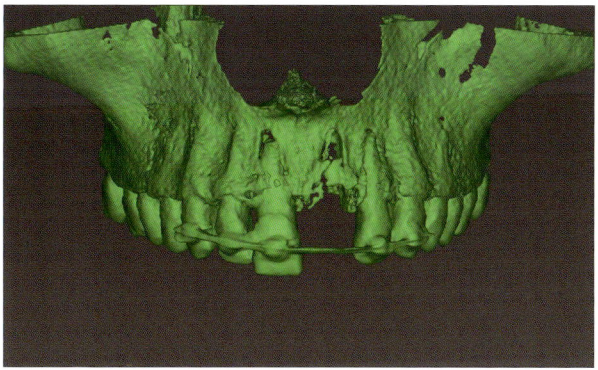

Fig 16   3D digital model of the maxilla.

Step 2. Merging the segmented DICOM data (green) with the STL data of the soft tissues and teeth (blue) (Fig 17).

Step 3. Further superimposition of the second set of STL data (of the maxilla) but with the teeth removed (Fig 18).

Step 4. Planning implants 12 (Fig 19) and 22 (Fig 20) to match the best prosthetically-driven 3D position. The availability of the STL soft-tissue information allows positioning the prosthetic platform of the implants according to the soft-tissue level (Fig 21).

To promote optimal osseointegration, the SLActive implant surface was preferred (Institut Straumann AG, Basel, Switzerland). Consequently, the planned implants were:

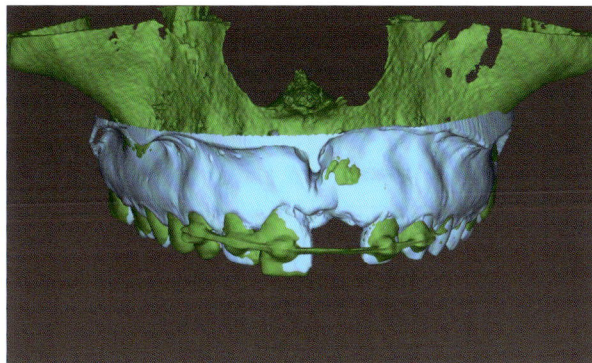

Fig 17   Superimposition of the DICOM model of the maxilla (green) with the STL data (blue).

- Implant 12: Straumann NC BLT SLActive Roxolid, diameter 3.3 mm, length 12 mm
- Implant 22: Straumann NC BLT SLActive Roxolid, diameter 3.3 mm, length 14 mm

Step 5. Planning the drilling sleeves. Sleeves 5 mm in diameter and 4 mm in height were selected (Fig 22).

Step 6. The surgical guide design was based on the STL data (Fig 23) using additional data to achieve the correct spatial orientation of the implant (Fig 24).

Step 7. Using the WeTransfer file transfer function within the coDiagnostiX software, the planning was sent to the dental laboratory together with the STL files of the scanned physical casts.

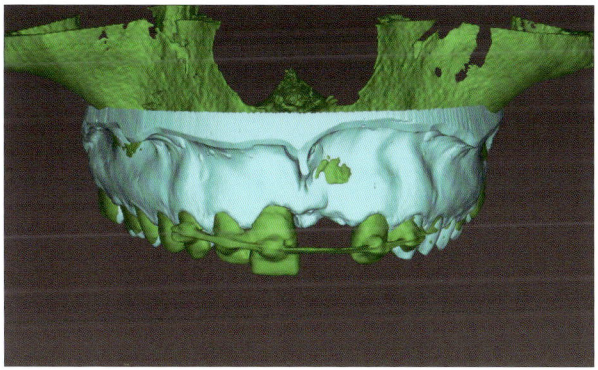

Fig 18   Superimposition of the DICOM model of the maxilla (green) with the STL data (blue) without teeth.

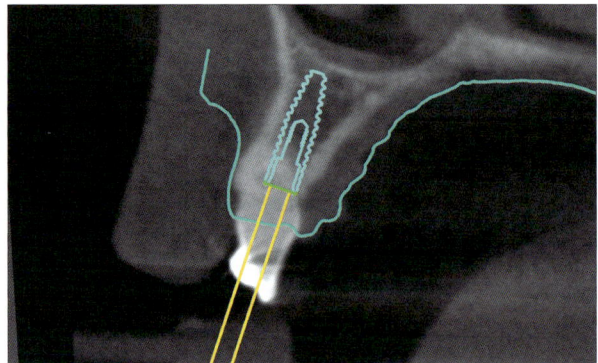

Fig 19   Planning of implant 12.

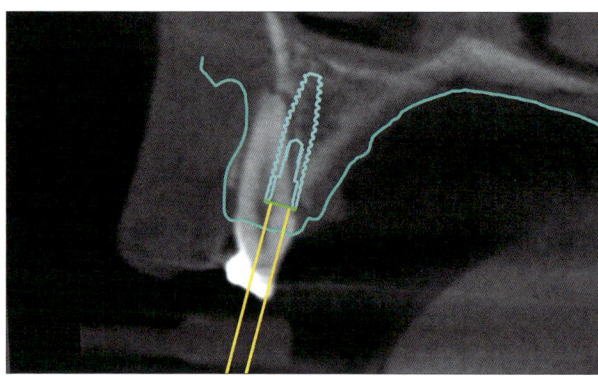

Fig 20   Planning of implant 22.

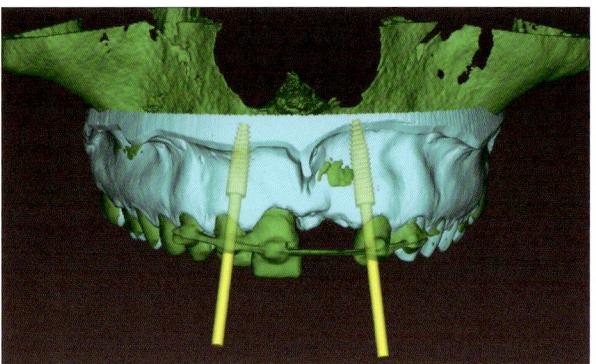

Fig 21   Checking the position of the prosthetic platform of the implants at the soft-tissue level.

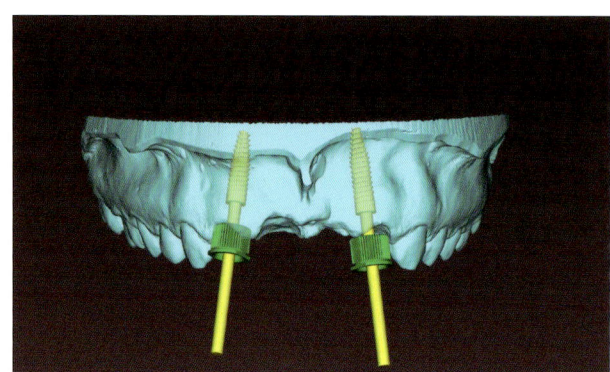

Fig 22   Planning of drilling sleeves (dark green).

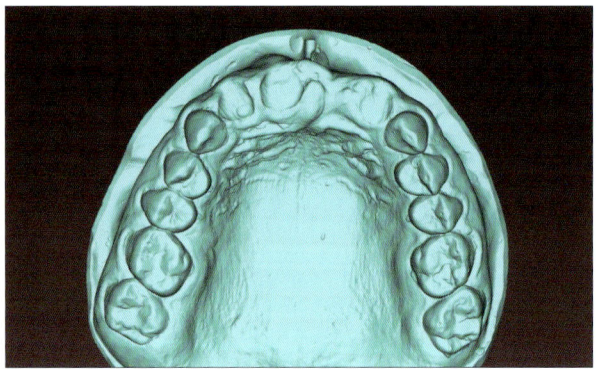

Fig 23   The guide design is based on the STL file of the maxillary model.

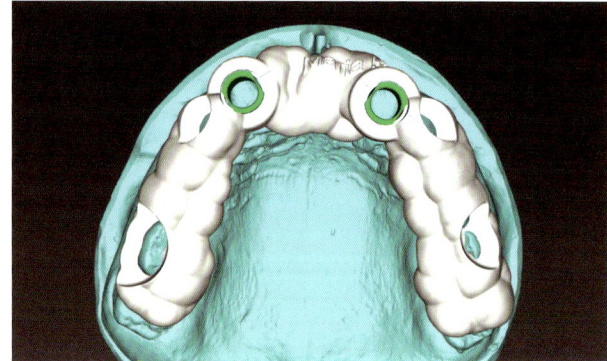

Fig 24   Design of the surgical guide.

Printing the surgical guide

Using the production version of coDiagnostiX, the dentist or dental technician can export the STL file of the designed surgical guide (Fig 25) for production using either 3D printing (additive) or milling (subtractive). In this case, the guide was printed using a Formlabs Form 2 SLA printer (Formlabs, Somerville, MA, USA) (Fig 26) and clear medical resin.

The guide was then rinsed in fresh isopropanol and fully post-cured to optimize its mechanical properties. Following insertion of the selected metal guide sleeves, the surgical template was ready for sterilization prior to intraoperative use. For additional visual reference, index lines were added with a black marker (Fig 27).

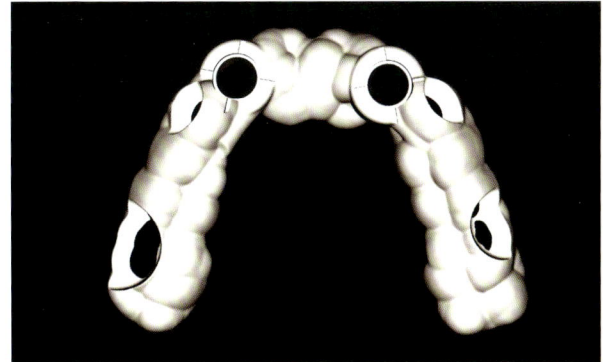

Fig 25 STL file data for the surgical guide.

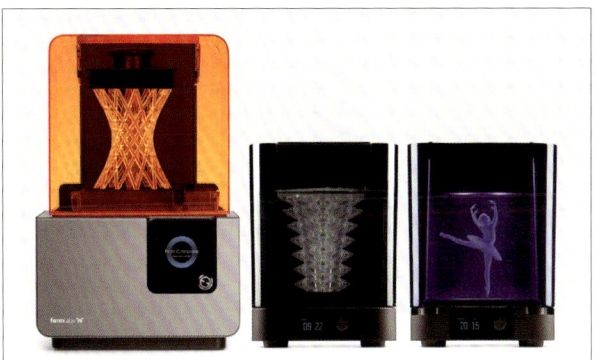

Fig 26 The Formlabs Form 2 SLA printer was used to print the guide.

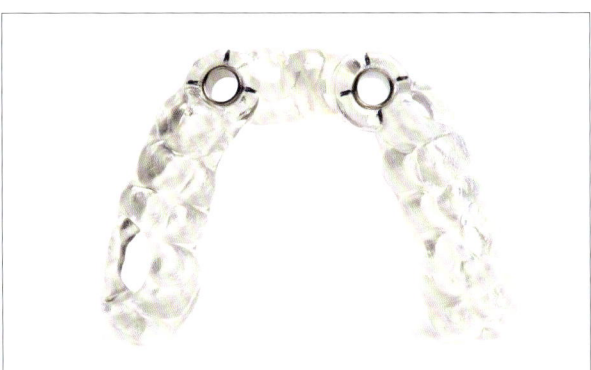

Fig 27 Index markings in black.

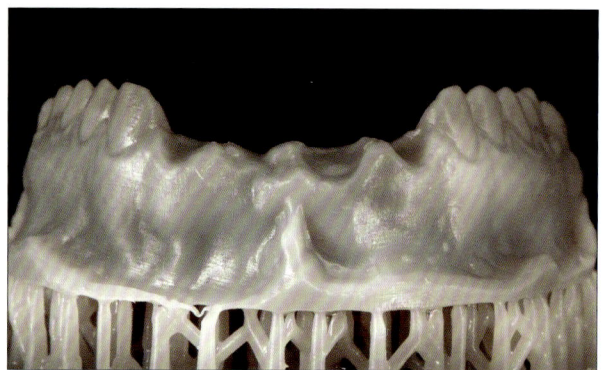

Fig 28   Printed model of the maxilla.

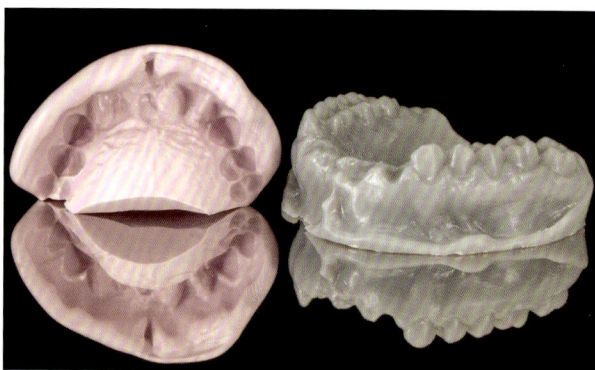

Fig 29   Silicone impression for the gingival mask.

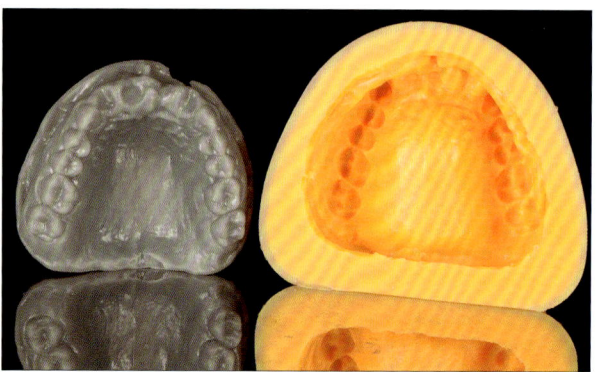

Fig 30   Duplicating the model using polyvinyl siloxane.

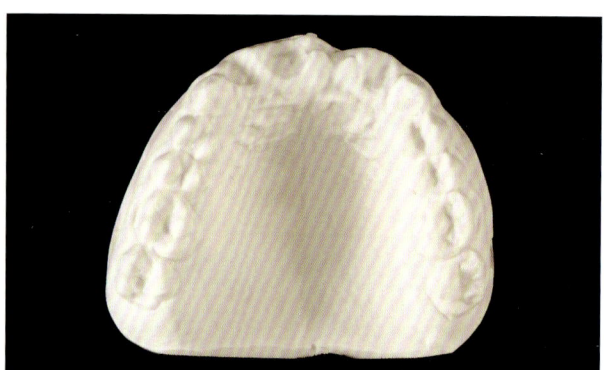

Fig 31   Duplicated stone model

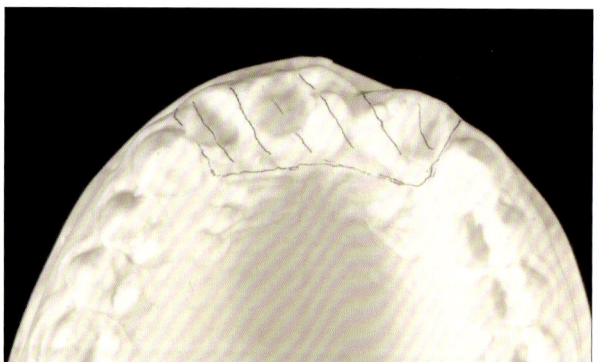

Fig 32   Anterior region marked up with a pencil.

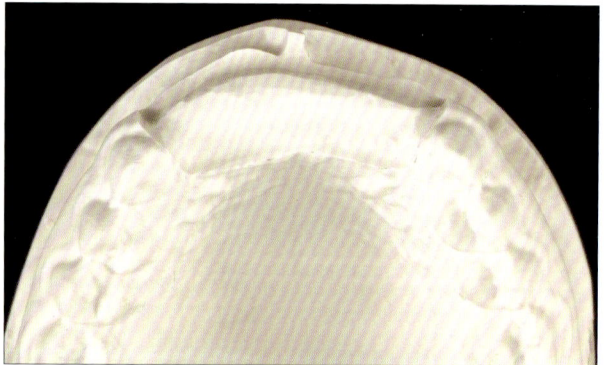

Fig 33   Plaster cast, reduced by 2 – 3 mm for the gingival mask in the anterior region.

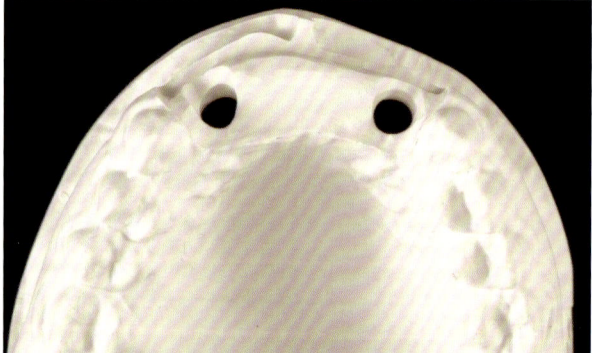

Fig 34   Implant position holes.

Preparing the abutments and the temporary bridge

Step 1. Using the Formlabs Form 2 SLA printer, models of the maxilla and mandible were printed in standard gray resin (Fig 28).

Step 2. To create a gingival mask, a silicone index (TS 5000; Merz Dental, Lütjenburg, Germany) was made (Fig 29).

Step 3. The 3D-printed gray model was duplicated in silicone (Elite Double 22 Fast; Zhermack, Badia, Italy) (Fig 30) to create a plaster cast (Quadro Rock white; Picodent, Wipperfürth, Germany) (Fig 31).

Step 4. The anterior region of the stone cast was marked up with a pencil (Fig 32) and reduced approximately 2 to 3 mm (Fig 33) to create space for the gingival mask.

Step 5. Based on the future implant positions, two holes were drilled in the model (Fig 34), where implant analogs were mounted in the correct position using the printed surgical guide (Fig 35). These analogs must not contact the walls of the plaster cast; they were secured in place with a resin material (TriadGel; Dentsply, York PA, USA) (Fig 36).

Step 6. Using the silicone index (from step 2), a gingival mask was made (Majesthetik Gingiimplant; Picodent, Wipperfürth, Germany) (Figs 37 and 38).

Step 7. Customized abutments were created from NC Vario Base crown abutments (Institut Straumann AG) and zirconia (Katana HT 12; Kuraray Noritake Dental, Tokyo, Japan) usitn opaque cement (Panavia V5; Kuraray Noritake) (Figs 39 and 40).

Step 8. The temporary bridge was designed using an STL file produced by scanning the abutment positions on the cast and importing the scan data into the CAD software (Exocad; Exocad, Darmstadt, Germany). The bridge was milled from a composite blank (Bredent Bio HIPC, shade A2; Bredent, Senden, Germany), cut back, and veneered using VisioLign material (Bredent) (Figs 41 and 42).

Step 9. The dental laboratory delivered the surgical guide, two individual hybrid abutments, the temporary bridge, and the printed models (Fig 43).

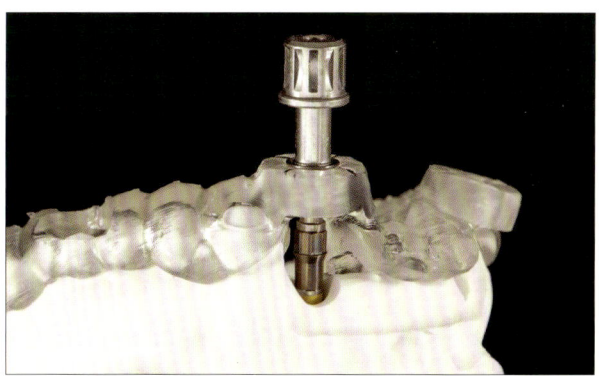

Fig 35   Implant analogs in the correct position thanks to the surgical guide.

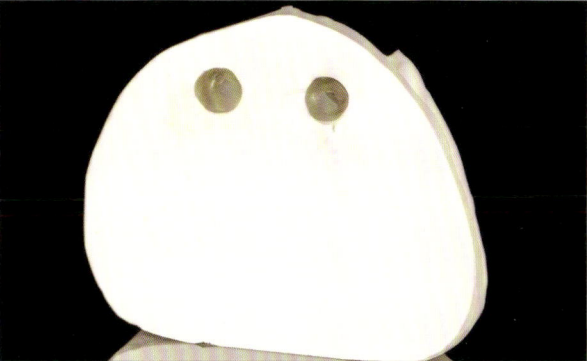

Fig 36   Implant analogs attached to the cast with resin.

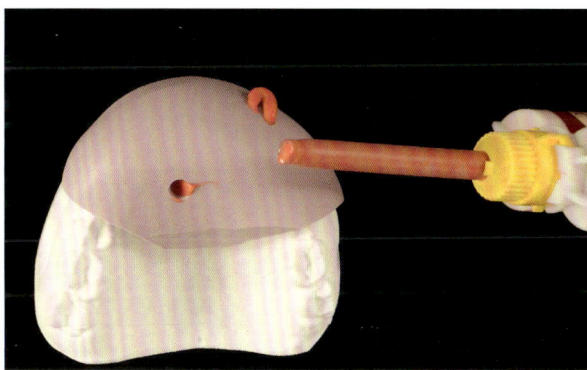

Fig 37   Silicone index used to produce the gingival mask.

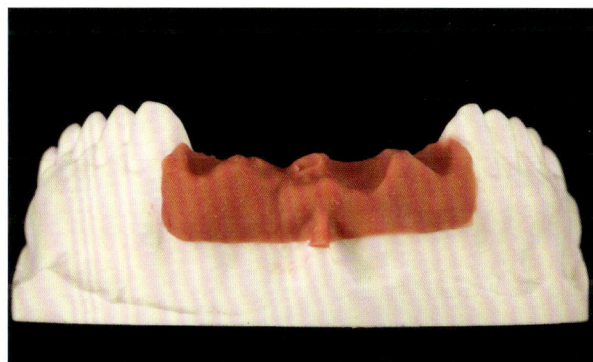

Fig 38   The gingival mask.

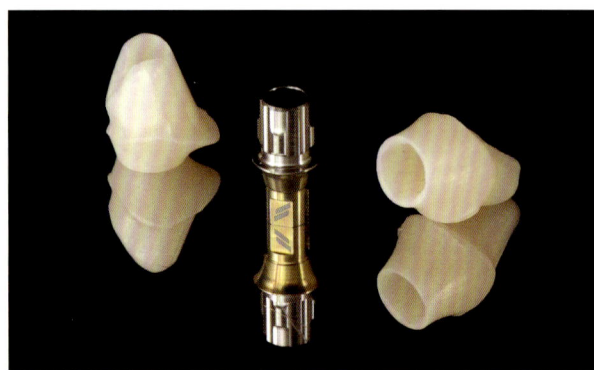

Fig 39   Custom abutments (Variobase + zirconia).

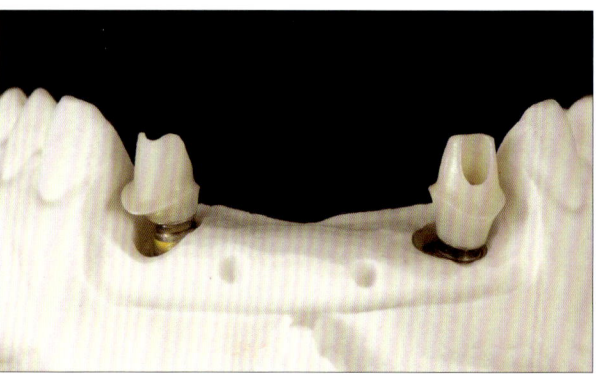

Fig 40   Custom zirconia abutments.

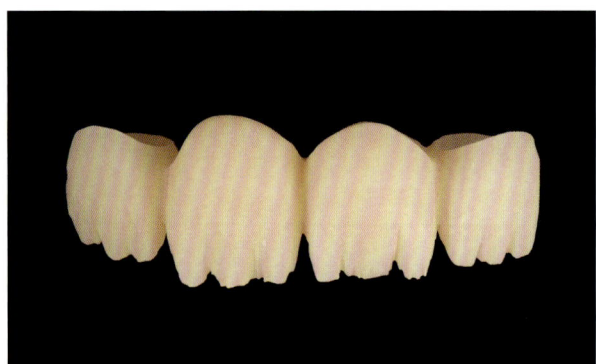

Fig 41   Temporary bridge after the cut-back.

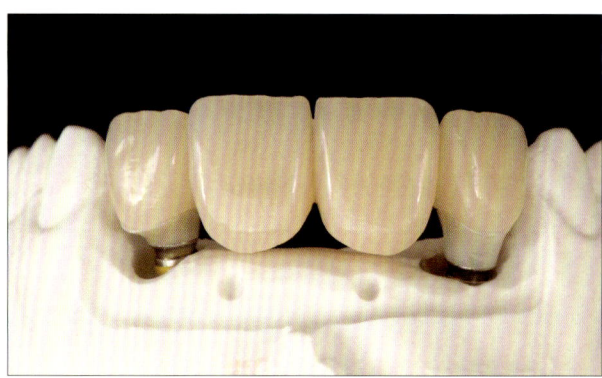

Fig 42   Completed temporary bridge.

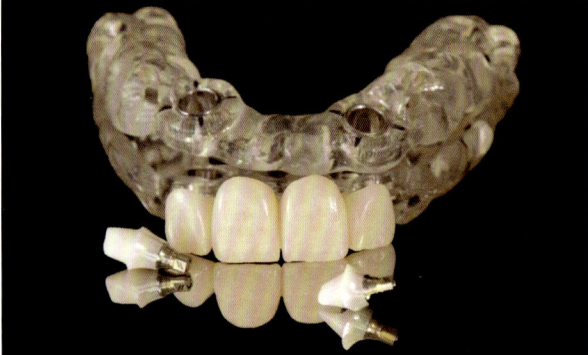

Fig 43   The surgical guide, two individual hybrid abutments, and the temporary bridge.

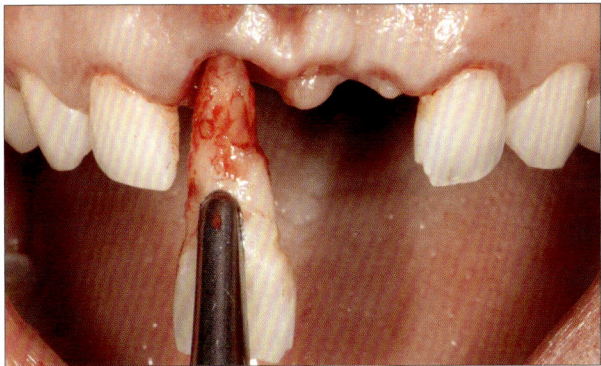

Fig 44   Extraction of tooth 11.

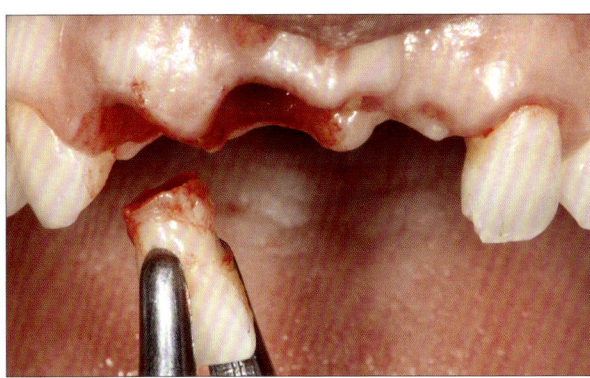

Fig 45   Removal of the fractured tooth 12.

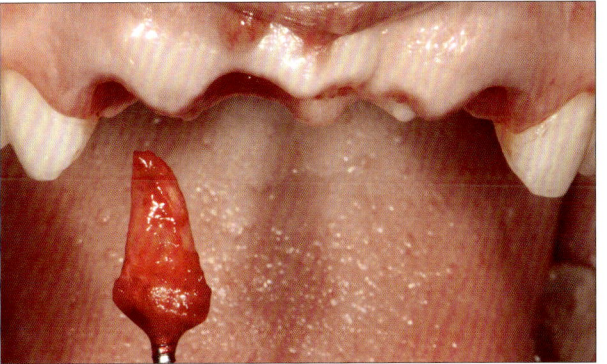

Fig 46   Removal of the apex of the fractured tooth 12 using the Benex extraction system.

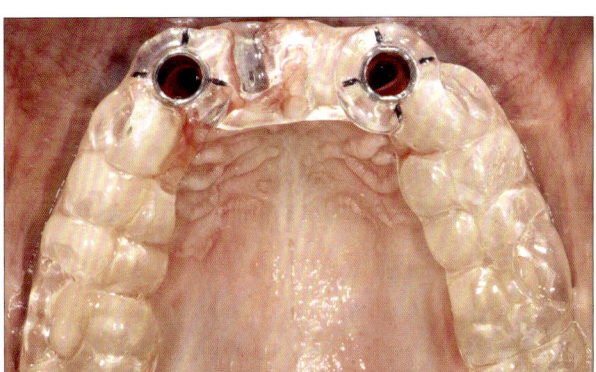

Fig 47   Checking the fit of the surgical guide.

Surgical procedures

Clindamycin (2 × 600 mg p.o.) was given 24 hours prior to surgery as prophylactic cover.

After achieving adequate local anesthesia (Ubistesin Forte; 4% articaine with 1 : 100,000 adrenaline), the remaining incisors were removed (Figs 44 and 45). The fractured root of tooth 12 was removed using the Benex extraction system (Zepf Medizintechnik, Seitingen, Germany) (Fig 46). The fit of the printed surgical guide was checked immediately after extraction (Fig 47).

The procedure was initiated with a trapezoidal flap using a full-thickness midcrestal incision and the split-papilla technique in the edentulous area and two vertical releasing incisions at the mesial line angles of teeth 13 and 23 (Fig 48). After elevating a full-thickness flap, the full extent of the local bone defect became apparent.

The osteotomy was performed with Straumann Guided Surgery instruments (Fig 49) following the surgical protocol derived from the coDiagnostiX software (Fig 50).

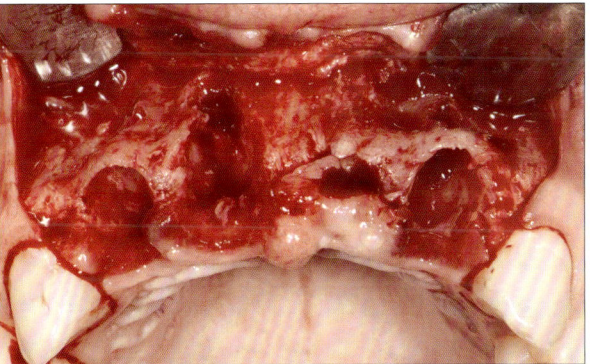

Fig 48   Flap design.

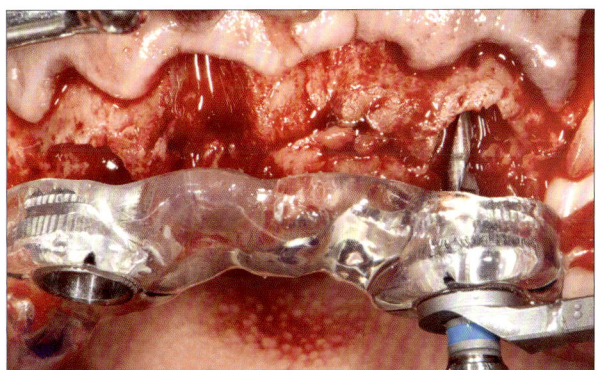

Fig 49   Osteotomy.

coDiagnostiX™	Patient data							
Version 9.6 Licensed to: 100002601 Kris Chmielewski,	Name: Date of birth: Patient ID: 685892669712297...							

Maxilla (Final [Date N/A]; Locked globally)		**Surgical protocol**					FDI notation (World Dental Federation)	
		Straumann® GuidedSurgery sleeve						
Color code	**Position**	**Implant art. no.**	**Implant**	**Sleeve**	**Sleeve position**	**Guided drill**	**Drill handle**	**Milling cutter**
🔵🟡 ⚫	12	021.3312	Bone Level Tapered Roxolid® SLActive® (NC) Ø 3.3 mm 12 mm	H: 5 mm Ø: 5 mm	H4	☰ extra long	●●● +3 mm	2.8 mm
🔵🟡 ⚫	22	021.3314	Bone Level Tapered Roxolid® SLActive® (NC) Ø 3.3 mm 14 mm	H: 5 mm Ø: 5 mm	H4	☰ extra long	● +1 mm	2.8 mm

Fig 50   Surgical protocol obtained from the coDiagnostiX software.

To minimize any deviation during insertion, the implants were placed through the guide (Fig 51). The depth of insertion was indicated by the H4 depth stop (Fig 52); the internal implant index position is attained by aligning the dots of the implant transfer with the black reference index printed on the guide (Fig 53).

After removing the guide together with the implant transfers, the planned implant platform position became visible. A 2-mm distance of the implant from the facial bone plate ensures the correct volume for stable space maintenance after augmentation with biomaterials (Fig 54).

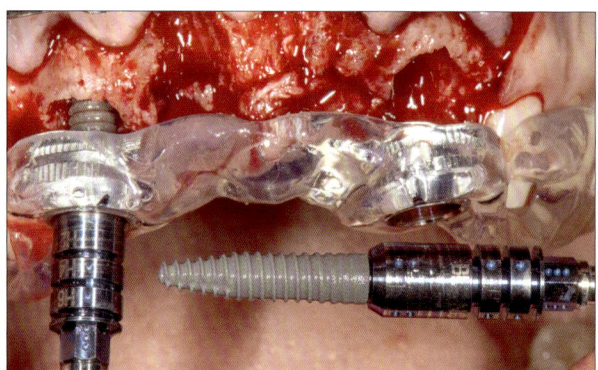

Fig 51   Insertion of Bone Level Tapered Roxolid SLActive (NC) implants.

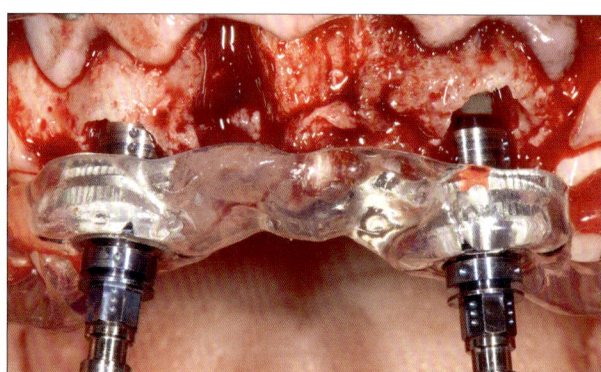

Fig 52   The depth of the insertion is indicated by an H4 depth stop.

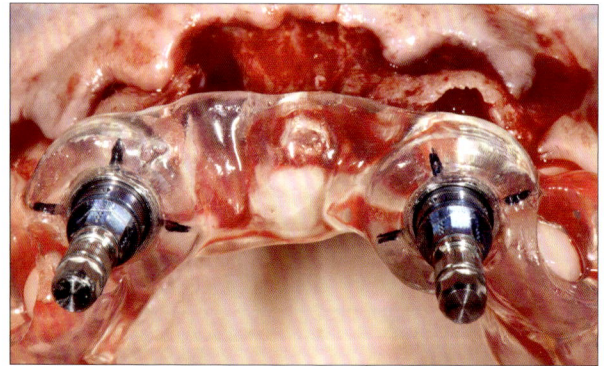

Fig 53   The index position has been achieved.

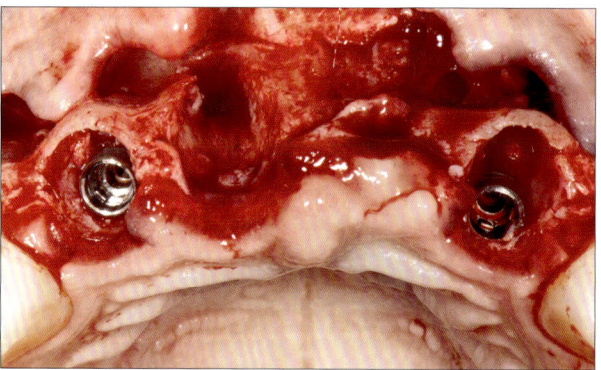

Fig 54   Implants placed in the optimum position with 2 mm of distance between the implants and the vestibular plates.

The correct fit of the abutments and temporary bridge was checked prior to introducing the augmentation materials (Fig 55). The offset (the gap for cementation) of the bridge has to be enlarged to compensate for the tolerance of fit immediately after delivery. The dental technician must design a cementation space that allows compensation for any misalignment between the implants and the restoration.

Guided bone regeneration was performed using 50% xenograft (Cerabone small particles; Botiss Biomaterials, Berlin, Germany) and 50% allograft (Maxgraft cortico-cancellous granules; Botiss Biomaterials). To promote soft-tissue healing and angioneogenesis, two platelet-rich fibrin membranes (APRF protocol) were cut into small pieces and mixed with the biomaterials (Figs 56 and 57). The augmented site was covered with additional APRF membranes and a pericardial collagen membrane (Jason membrane; Botiss Biomaterials).

The abutments were placed and the screw channels were closed with the PTFE tape. A non-resorbable polypropylene monofilament 5-0 suture material was used for tension-free wound closure achieved with periosteal releasing incisions (Fig 58). Immediately postoperatively, the temporary bridge was cemented with temporary cement (Temp-Bond NE; Kerr, Orange, CA, USA) (Fig 59).

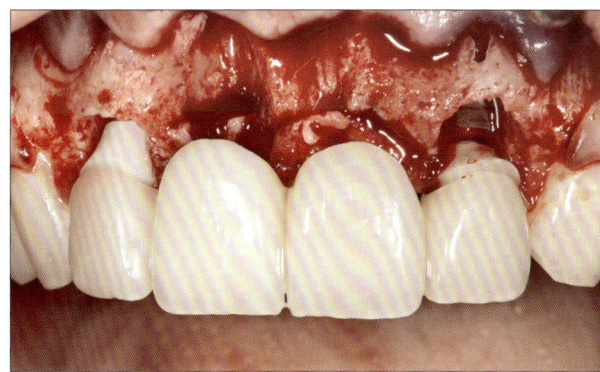

Fig 55   Checking the fit of the temporary bridge.

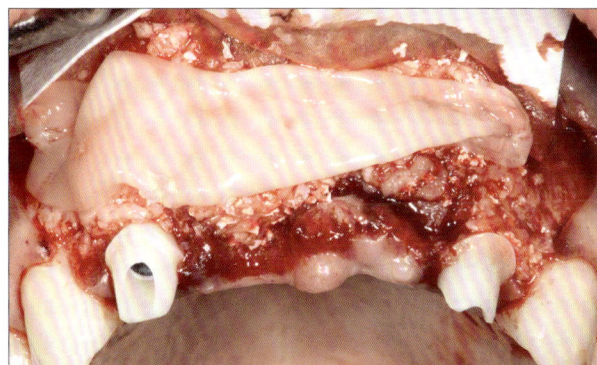

Fig 56   Augmented site covered with Jason membrane (Botiss Biomaterials).

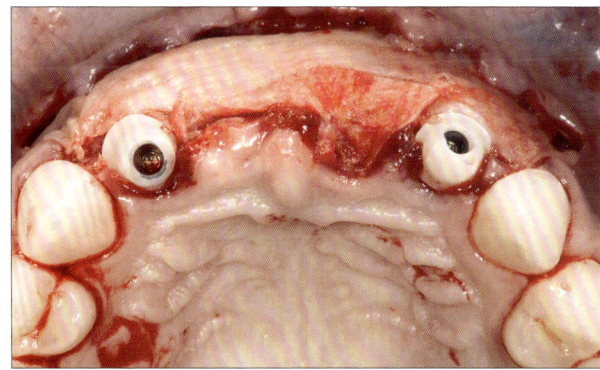

Fig 57   Augmented site with membrane in place.

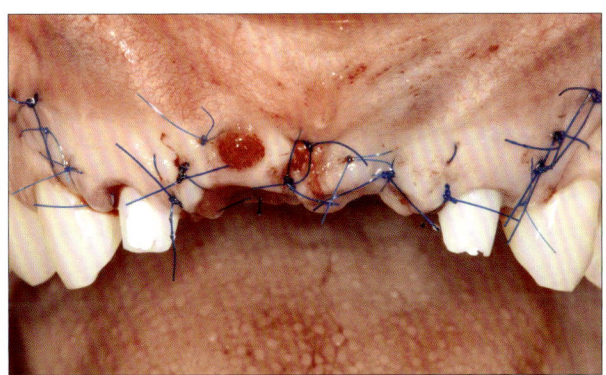

Fig 58   Sutures in place.

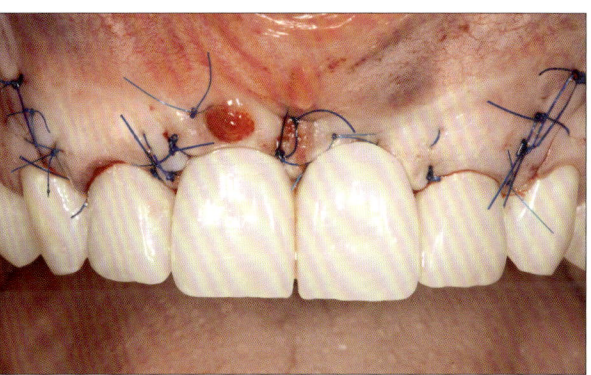

Fig 59   Cemented temporary bridge.

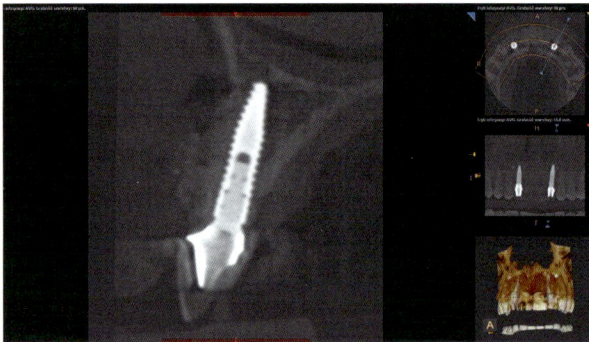

Fig 60   CBCT after the insertion of implant 22.

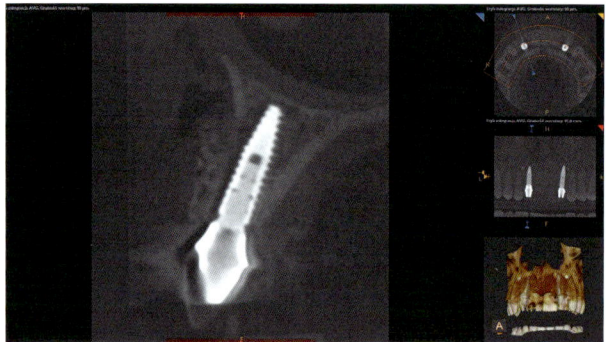

Fig 61   CBCT after the insertion of implant 12.

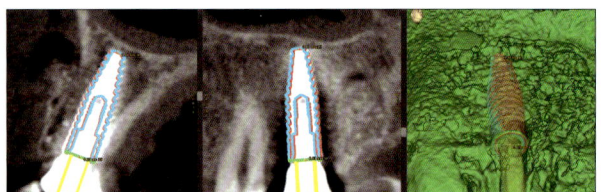

Fig 62   The blue and red implant outlines represent the planned and final implant positions, respectively.

Evaluating the position of the implants

Postoperative CBCT examination permitted the verification of the 3D implant positioning (Figs 60 and 61) in the cross-sectional views, with the additional vestibular volume of the augmentation material.

coDiagnostiX has a software tool for the scientific evaluation of implant positions compared to the initial planning, allowing to check for offsets or misfits following the guided procedure. The blue and red outlines of the implant shape represent the initial plan and final position of the implant, respectively. In this case, the 3D offset was −0.19 mm at site 12 and −0.04 mm at site 22 (Fig 62).

Healing

The sutures were removed two weeks after surgery (Fig 63). Within four months of surgery, the soft tissue had adapted well to the outline of the temporary prosthesis. However, the mesial surface of the hybrid abutment 12 started to become visible (Fig 64). After another three months of healing, a slight improvement of the soft tissue was noted (Fig 65).

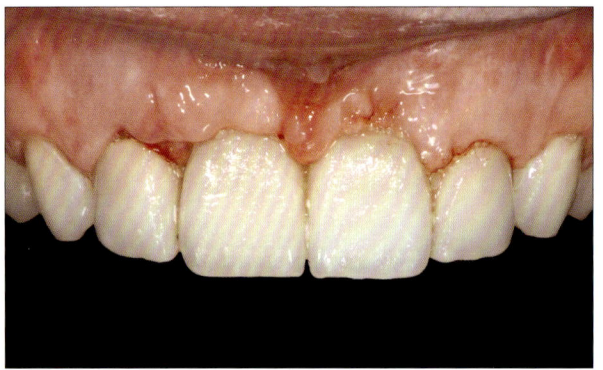

Fig 63   Two weeks after surgery, with sutures removed.

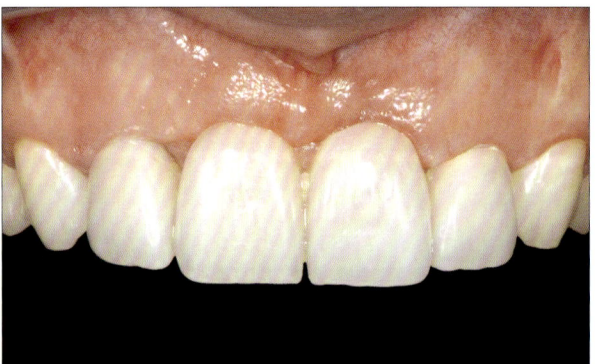

Fig 64   Implant 12 with mesial hybrid abutment margin visible four months after surgery.

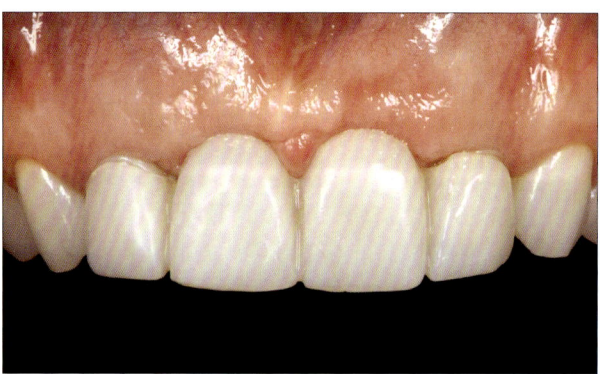

Fig 65   Seven months after surgery.

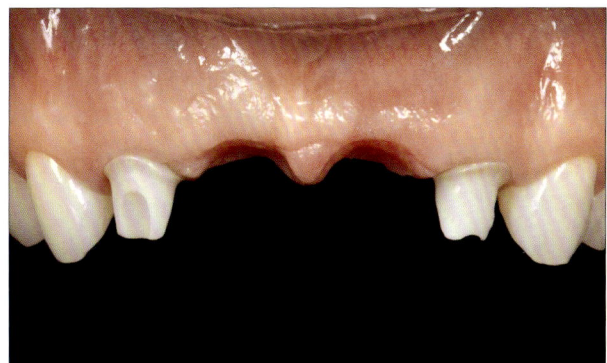

Fig 66 Soft tissue after nineteen months of healing.

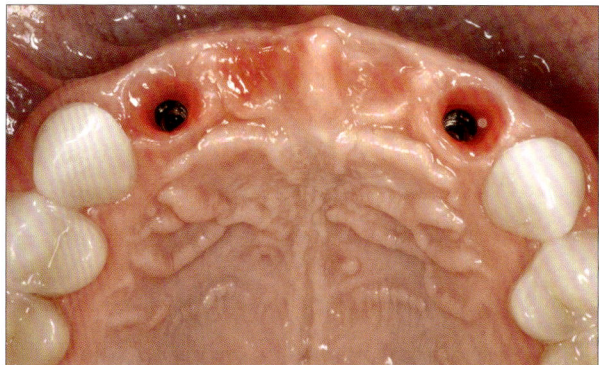

Fig 67 Healthy soft-tissue situation.

Definitive restoration

After nineteen months of healing and function from immediate implantation and loading, the volume, shape, and quality of the mature soft tissue appeared to be stable (Fig 66).

The initial concept of using the initial abutments for the final prosthesis had to be revised. It was decided that new abutments would be needed for the definitive screw-retained bridge. On removal of the hybrid abutments, the soft tissues appeared healthy and presented with enough volume for the final restoration (Fig 67).

Impression copings for a closed-tray impression were placed on the implants (Fig 68) and a silicone impression was taken. Implant analogs were inserted into the impression, which was then sent to the laboratory (Fig 69).

Additional clinical photographs were taken with shade tabs in both reflected and cross-polarized light (Figs 70 and 71) for shade matching.

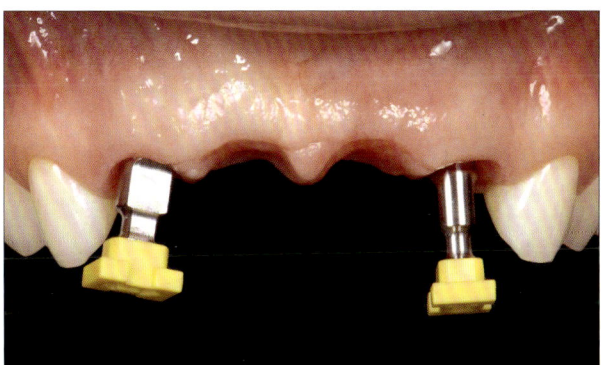

Fig 68 Closed-tray impression analogs.

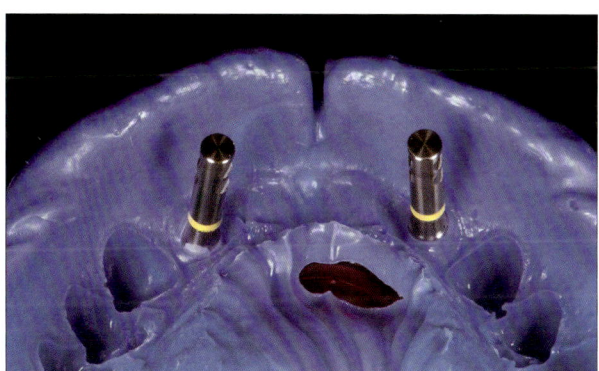

Fig 69 Impression.

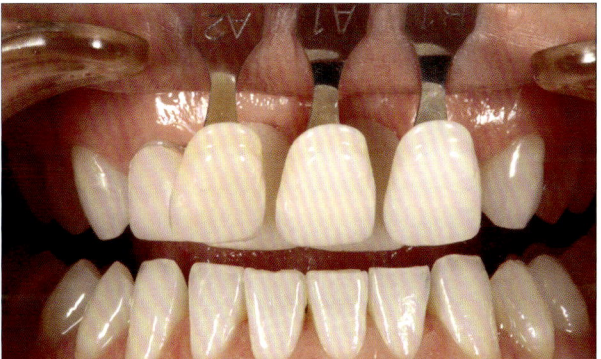

Fig 70 Photograph with shade tabs.

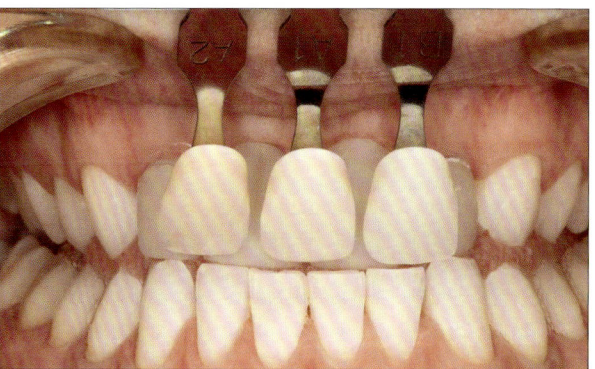

Fig 71 Photograph with shade tabs in cross-polarized light.

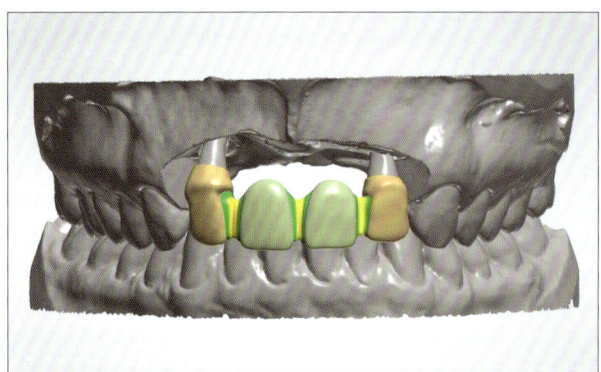

Fig 72   Planning the definitive framework.

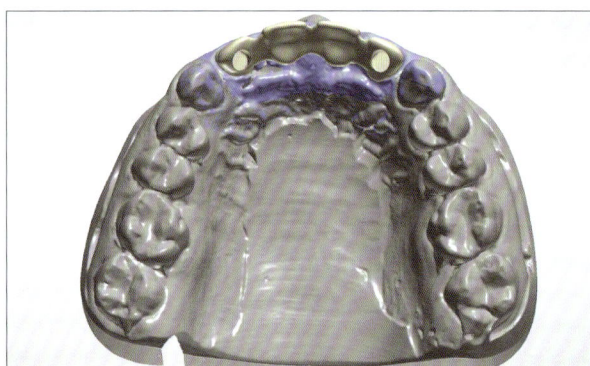

Fig 73   Planning the definitive framework.

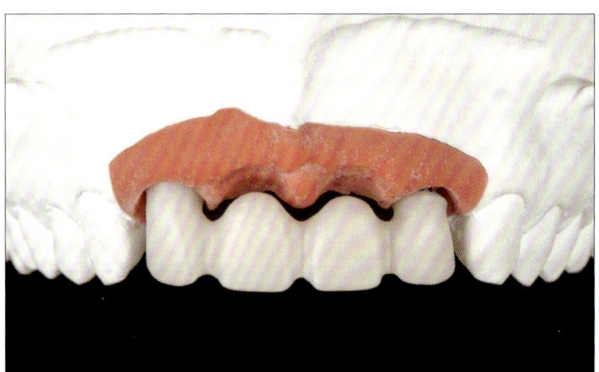

Fig 74   Checking passive fit of the framework before veneering.

The Exocad planning software was used to design and produce the elements of the definitive restoration. The shape of the zirconia framework was planned and sent for milling (Figs 72 and 73). Thanks to the angulated system of the Variobase abutments employed, palatal screw access is available with up to 25 degrees of angular discrepancy from the ideal implant position, giving more esthetic options with screw-retained restorations on angled implants.

The prosthetic framework was milled from a zirconia blank (Katana HT 12; Kuraray Noritake) and sintered (Austromat 664i furnace; Dekema, Freilassing, Germany) at 1,500°C for 120 minutes, according to the manufacturer's instructions. The passive framework fit was checked on the cast prior to veneering (Fig 74).

The framework was then veneered with ceramics (CZR, shade A1; Kuraray Noritake) and fired accordingly (Austrat 624; Dekema). Two ceramic veneers were fabricated from the same material on refractory die material for the adjacent canines (13 and 23) (Fig 75).

After the final firing, the framework was bonded to the Variobase abutments (Panavia V5 opaque cement; Kuraray Noritake) and checked on the cast (Figs 76 and 77). Palatal access to the Variobase abutments requires the use of dedicated screws and screwdrivers (Fig 78). Figures 79 and 80 show the clinical situation and the prosthesis immediately prior to delivery.

The screws were covered with PTFE tape (Fig 81) and sealed with composite resin (Genial Flo; GC, Tokyo, Japan) (Fig 82).

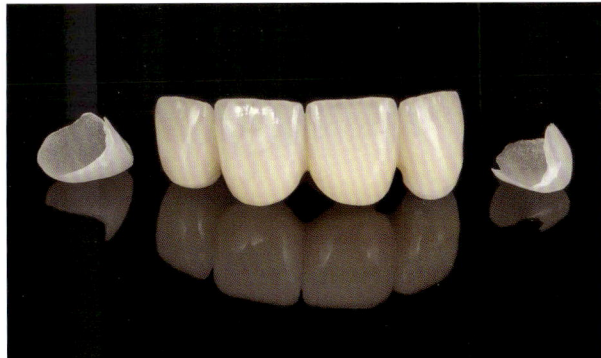

Fig 75 Definitive restorations.

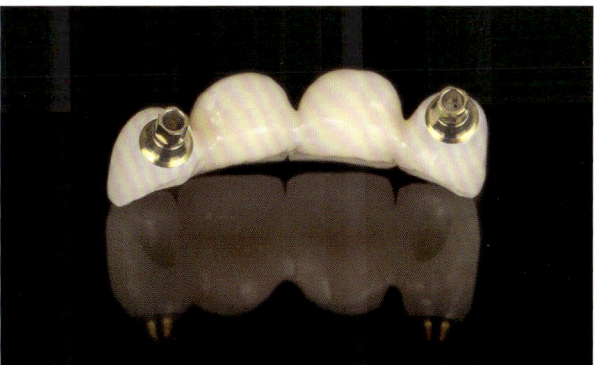

Fig 76 Variobase abutments adhesively connected to the framework.

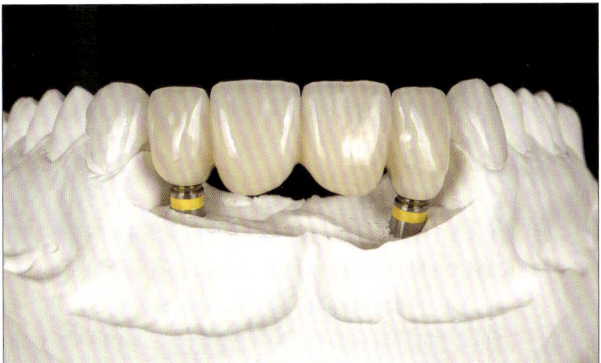

Fig 77 Checking the restoration on the cast.

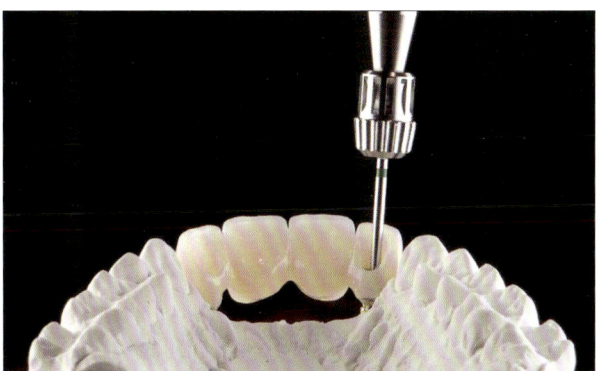

Fig 78 Palatal access to the AS abutment.

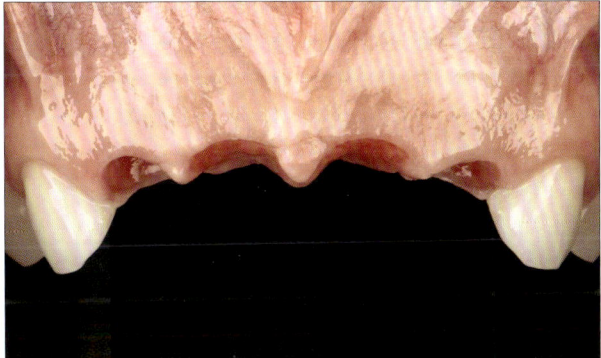

Fig 79 Soft-tissue situation before delivery (facial view).

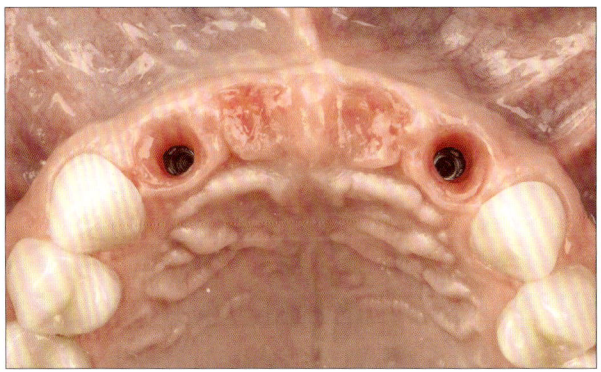

Fig 80 Soft-tissue situation before delivery (occlusal view).

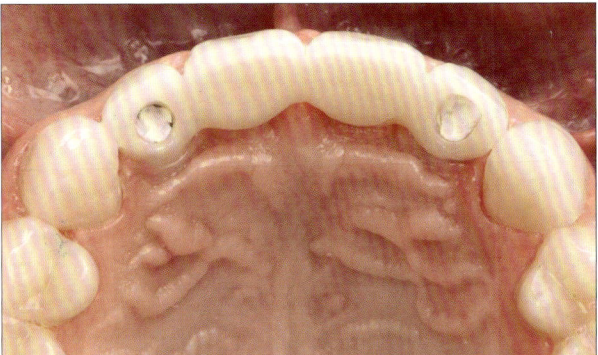

Fig 81 PTFE tape in the screw holes.

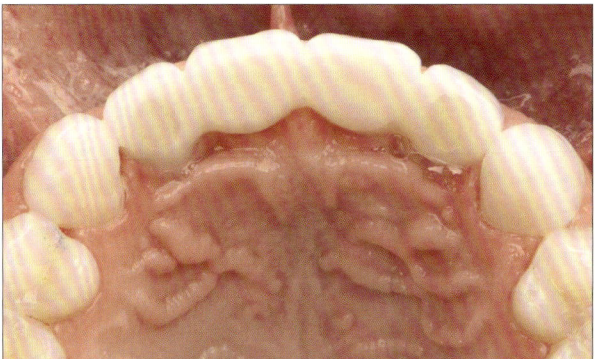

Fig 82 Screw holes closed with composite resin.

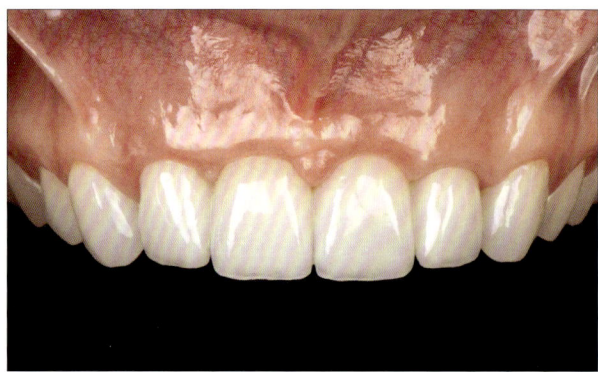

Fig 83   Final result, maxilla (facial view).

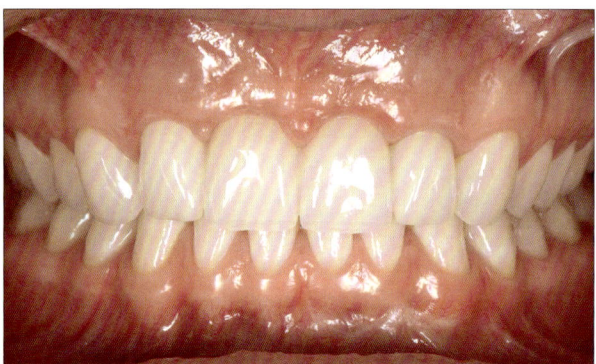

Fig 84   Final result (facial view).

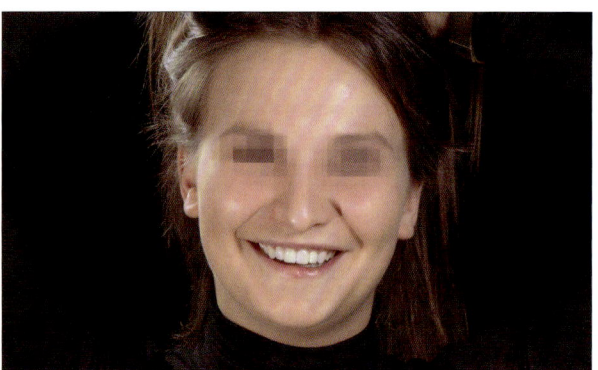

Fig 85   The patient is happy with her new smile.

The final esthetic appearance of the restoration and soft tissues was excellent (Figs 83 to 85).

Periapical x-rays demonstrated stable bone levels 2 years after immediate loading of the implants (Figs 86 and 87).

Discussion

The treatment of the present case yielded a pleasing esthetic outcome—even though the initial clinical situation had been very challenging. The treatment plan in this patient included the extraction of three additional teeth, as they were past further restorative efforts. The resulting edentulous space, extending over four teeth, was managed by placing only two implants.

This approach avoids the risks of adjacent implants in the esthetic zone and gives better control over the shape of the soft tissues in the pontic area where "papilla"-like tissue is higher than between implants. Horizontal contour augmentation at the pontic site provided an opportunity to optimize the esthetic outcome. A single surgical procedure with immediate placement and bone augmentation at the time of extraction significantly reduced the treatment time and morbidity for the patient. However, bone remodeling around the implant after immediate placement may yet affect the final outcome.

Clinicians should understand that this may be a direct result of a "trendy" initial surgical intervention and possible limitations in treatment outcomes, something that may be associated with "doing everything at once."

Acknowledgments

Laboratory procedures
Björn Roland – Klein-Winternheim, Germany

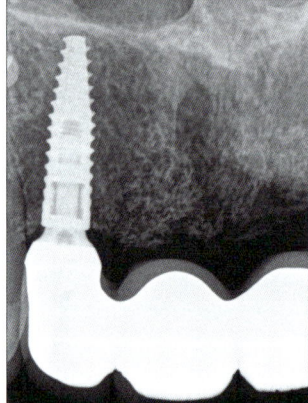

Fig 86   Stable bone situation 2 years after loading implant 12.

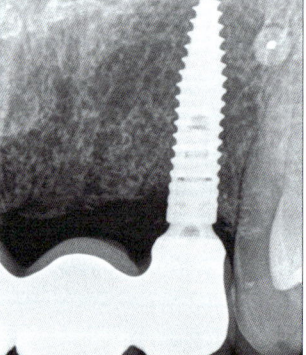

Fig 87   Bone situation 2 years after implant loading with indications of bone loss on the mesial aspect. The mesial probing pocket depth (PPD; implant 22) was 6 mm, up from 4 mm earlier.

13.6 Replacing Three Mandibular Posterior Teeth with an Immediately Loaded Fixed Dental Prosthesis

W. D. C. Derksen

A 60-year-old healthy male patient presented with problems involving a fixed dental prosthesis (FDP) in the lower left quadrant (Figs 1a-b). The bridge had de-cemented from abutment teeth 33 and 35; tooth 33 was decayed, and tooth 35 had little structure remaining. Since removing the FDP spanning sites 33 to 38 would have compromised function and raised esthetic concerns, the possibility of immediate implant placement and provisionalization was investigated.

Preoperative surgical planning

A cone-beam computed tomography (CBCT) scan and an intraoral scan (IOS) were taken (3M True Definition scanner; 3M, St. Paul, MN, USA). Both scans were uploaded to guided-surgery software (coDiagnostiX; Dental Wings, Montreal, Quebec, Canada). To combine the assessment of the surgical and prosthetic information, the scans were aligned in the same geometrical position using the so-called "best-fit" alignment with the teeth as reference points (Fig 2). Since the posterior teeth had already been restored with metal-based and zirconia restorations, this alignment could only be accurate if it included the anterior teeth.

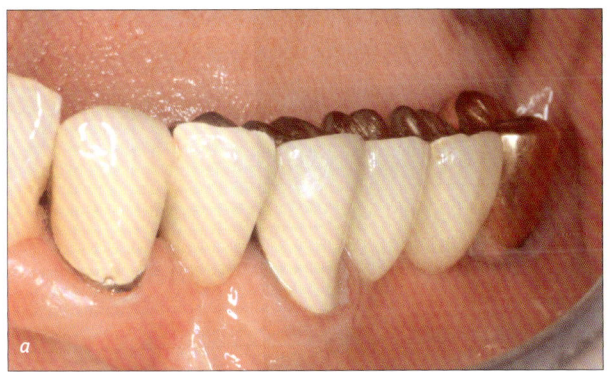
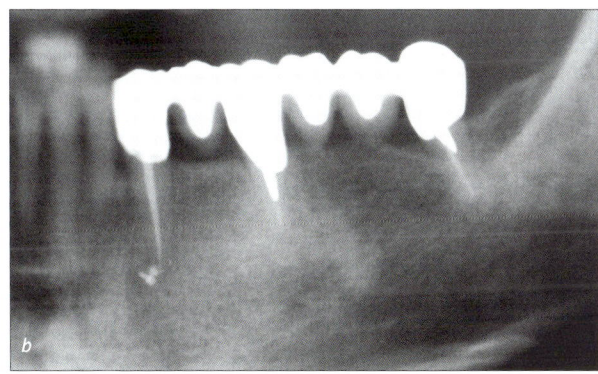

Figs 1a-b   Preoperative clinical (a) and radiological (b) situation.

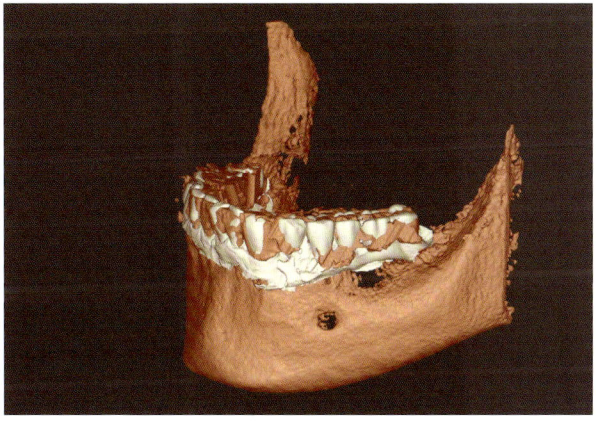

Fig 2   Matching CBCT (brown) and IOS (white) in the guided-surgery software (coDiagnostiX; Dental Wings).

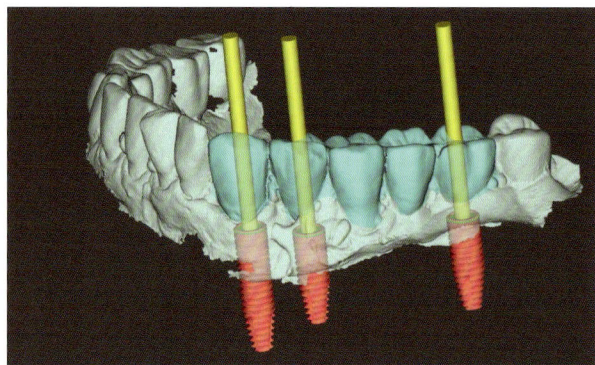

Fig 3   Implant positioning based on existing prosthetic set-up.

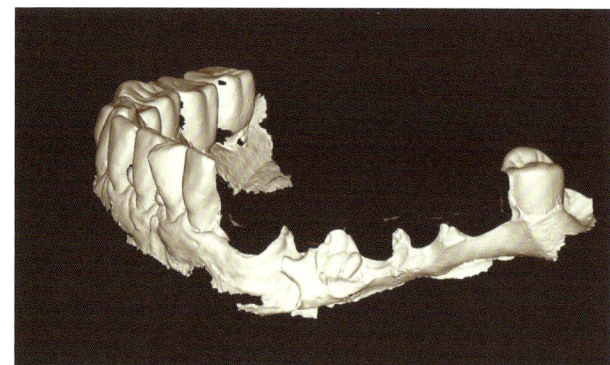

Fig 4   Selected teeth were digitally erased from the intraoral scan.

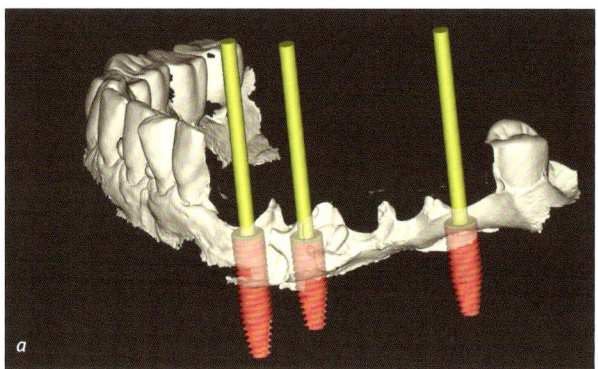

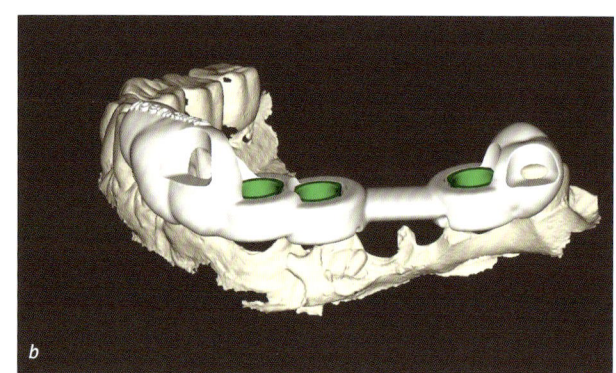

Figs 5a-b   Design of the surgical guide.

After evaluating the available bone volume, it was decided that immediate placement would be possible in this particular case. As the existing restorations were of acceptable shape and position, no separate prosthetic design was required, and the implants could be planned based on the existing prosthesis (Fig 3). The software allowed the selection of appropriate implant types, sizes, and positions. As the treatment plan called for immediate placement and possibly for immediate restoration, an implant with a tapered design (allowing underpreparation of the osteotomy) was selected in order to achieve high primary stability (Bone Level Tapered RC; Institut Straumann AG, Basel, Switzerland).

Because computer-guided placement using a tooth-supported surgical guide was planned but the existing FDP was to be removed in the same session, teeth 33 to 37 were removed from the intraoral scan digitally in the CAD/CAM software (DWOS; Dental Wings). A new STL file was created and imported into the guided-surgery software (Fig 4).

This STL file was aligned to the same geometrical position as the other scans. A surgical guide was designed based on the planned implant positions, to be supported by the remaining teeth (Figs 5a-b). To provide extra support for the surgical guide and to retain posterior stability and proprioception, it was decided to leave tooth 38 and its crown in place.

The failing FDP was sectioned mesially of tooth 38. The surgical guide was milled from a transparent PMMA blank, and the required titanium guide sleeves were manually inserted at the designated positions.

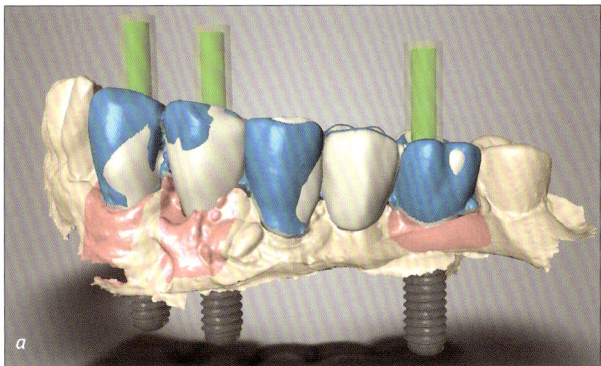

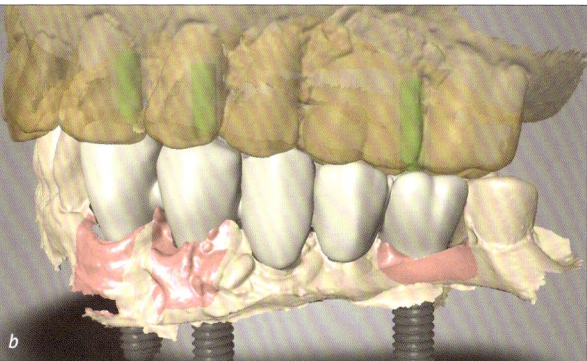

Figs 6a-c   Preoperative prosthetic design in CAD/CAM software (Dental Wings). The blue image is the scan of the old prosthesis, which functions as a virtual wax-up.

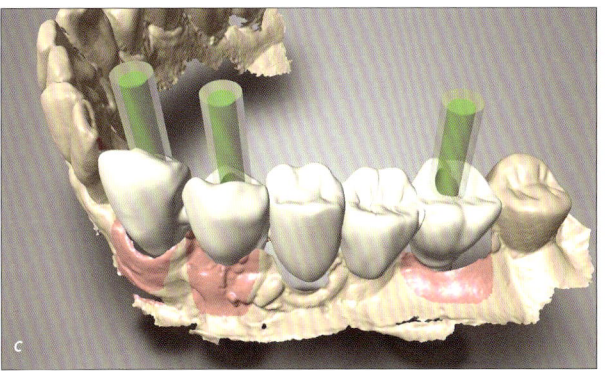

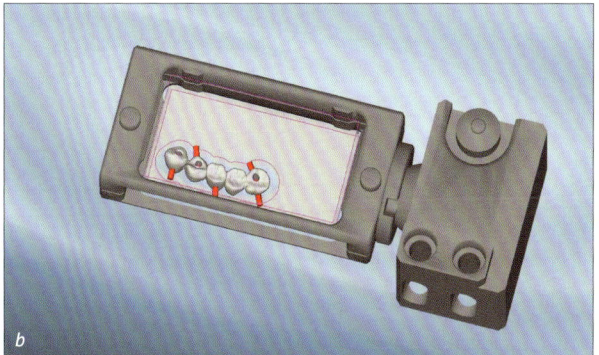

Fig 7   Designing the temporary bridge in the CAD/CAM software.

Preoperative prosthetic planning

The planned implant positions were exported from the guided-surgery software to the CAD/CAM software (Dental Wings) for the presurgical prosthetic design of the immediate temporary restorations. The intraoral scan with the old FDP in situ was used as a virtual wax-up for rapid transformation into a design for an implant-supported temporary fixed bridge (Figs 6a-c). This prosthetic information significantly reduced the time it took to complete the design.

The temporary FDP was milled from a PMMA blank (Fig 7). A CAD/CAM restoration produced prior to implant surgery can be used for immediate provisionalization if implants can be placed in the planned positions and sufficient primary stability can be achieved (Schrott and coworkers 2014). Guided surgery is not absolutely accurate; minor deviations between the planned and actual implant positions can occur (Tahmaseb and coworkers 2014). These potential inaccuracies require the cementing space between the planned abutments and the temporary PMMA bridge to be enlarged somewhat to ensure a passive fit between the bridge and the abutments after implant insertion.

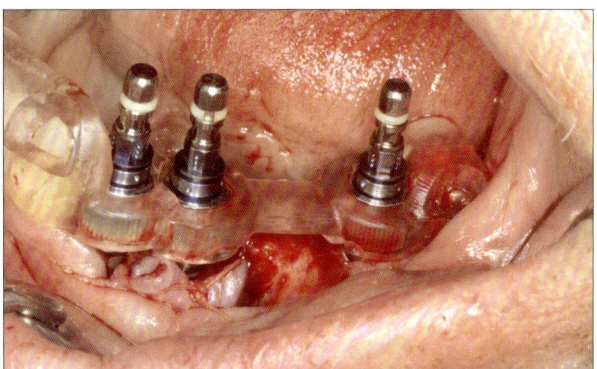

Fig 8   Guided implant placement.

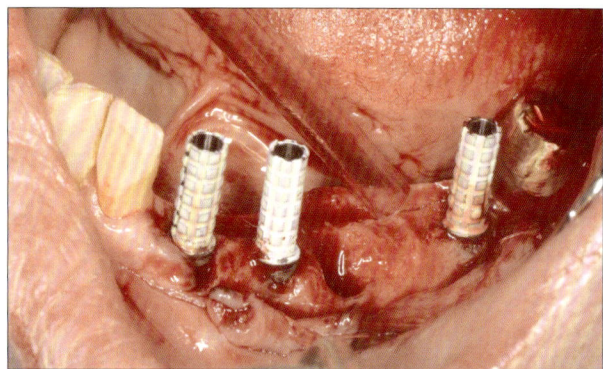

Fig 9   Temporary abutments connected to the implants.

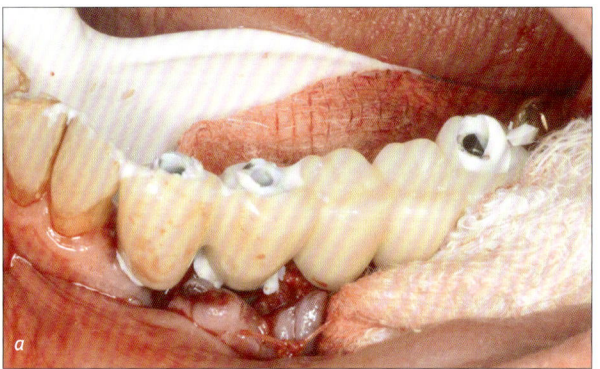

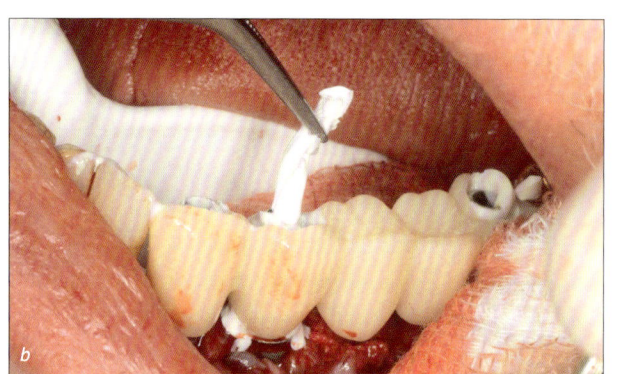

Figs 10a-b   Relining the PMMA FDP on the temporary abutments.

Surgical phase

After sectioning the FDP mesially of tooth 38 and removing it, the remaining roots of teeth 33 and 35 were removed, and implants were inserted at sites 33, 34, and 37 using the surgical guide (Fig 8). Appropriate primary stability (> 35 Ncm) was achieved. Temporary non-engaging abutments were inserted after applying a resin opaque extraorally (Fig 9). Prior to wound closure, the temporary bridge was tried in to confirm its passive fit and relined on the temporary abutments using a dual-cure opaque composite resin. After curing, the PTFE tape sealing the screw access channels was removed

and the bridge—now connected to the abutments—was unscrewed (Figs 10a-b). Excess cement attached to the bridge and abutments was removed.

While the surgeon performed guided bone regeneration in the socket defects and closed the soft tissues, the prosthodontist adapted and finished the temporary bridge extraorally (Figs 11a-c). Excess cement was removed, voids were filled with flowable composite resin, and the bridge was polished, cleaned ultrasonically, and disinfected.

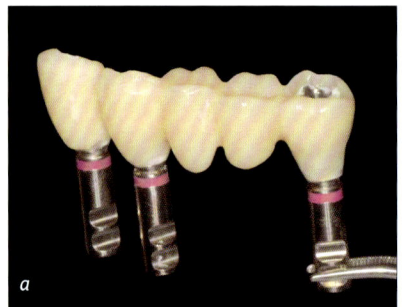

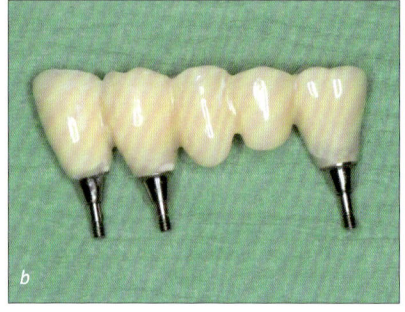

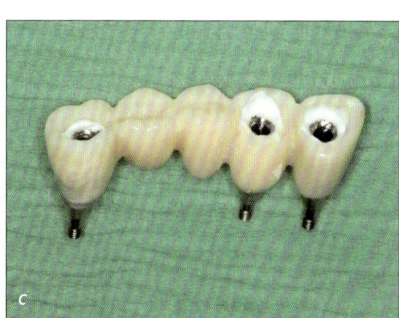

Figs 11a-c   Extraoral finishing of the PMMA FDP.

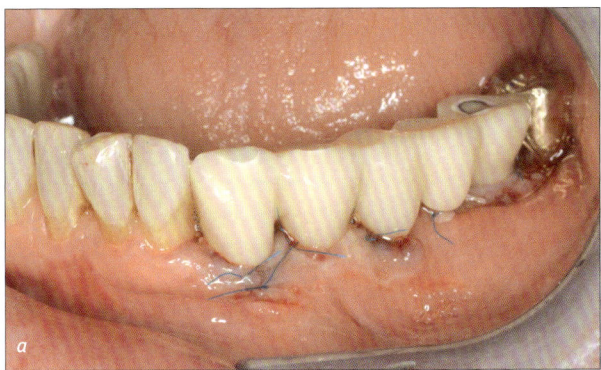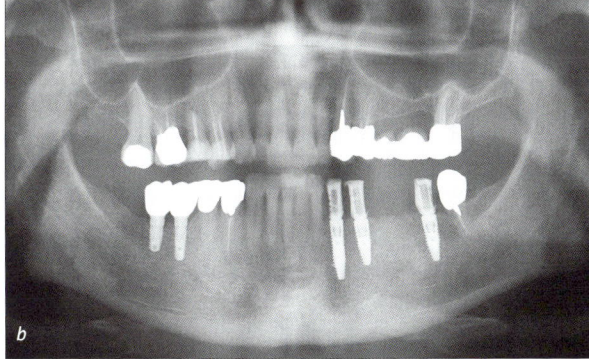

Figs 12a-b   Clinical (a) and radiological (b) situation after implant placement and temporary restoration.

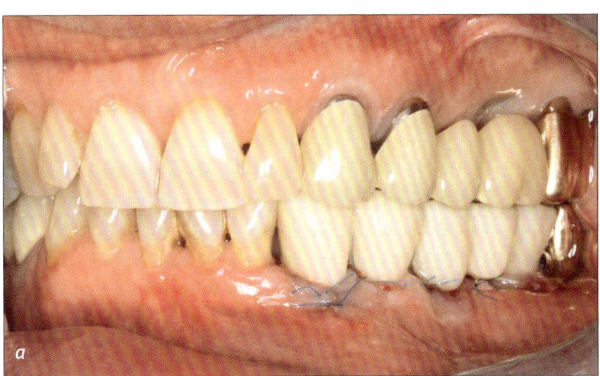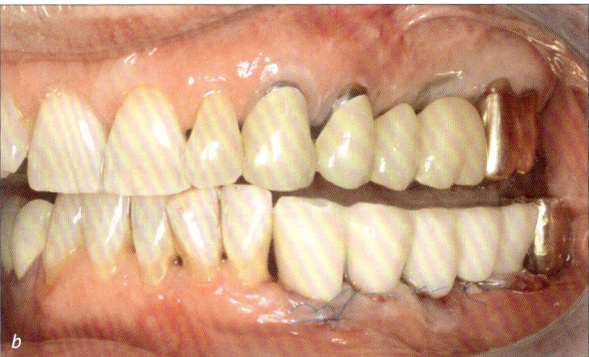

Figs 13a-b   Confirmation of the desired occlusion and freedom in lateral excursions.

Immediate restoration

After suturing, the screw-retained temporary implant bridge was connected to the implants (with max. 20 Ncm to prevent rotation). The occlusal screw access holes were sealed with Teflon and composite resin (Figs 12a-b). The bridge was designed to be in occlusion but protected from lateral occlusal forces, which was confirmed intraorally (Figs 13a-b). The patient was satisfied with the appearance of his temporary restoration (Fig 14).

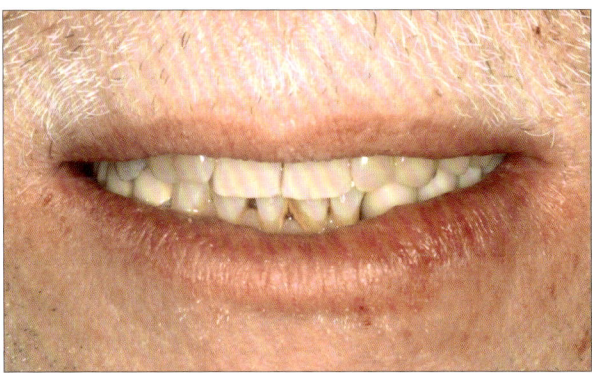

Fig 14   Extraoral view directly after implant placement and restoration

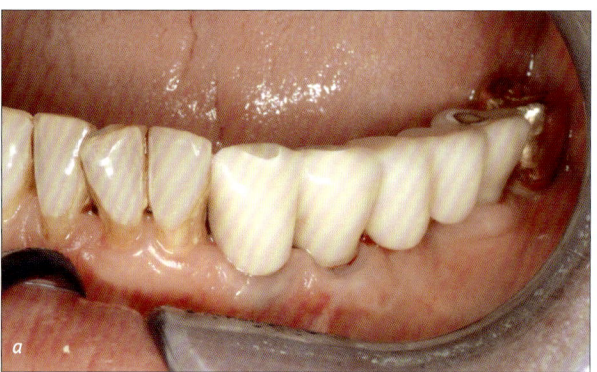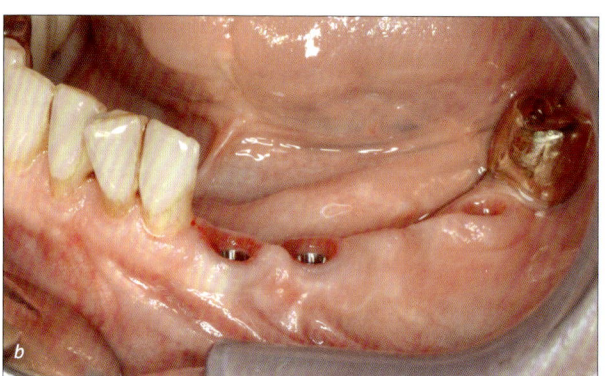

Figs 15a-b   Healing status after 3 months.

Final restoration

Healing was uneventful. Three months after implant insertion, the provisional bridge was unscrewed (Figs 15a-b). A digital impression (True Definition Scanner; 3M) of the implant locations was obtained using scan bodies (RC Mono; Institut Straumann AG) (Fig 16).

A monolithic zirconia FDP was designed using CAD technology (Fig 17). To provide the dental technician with a working cast, a stereolithographic model was made that included three specially designed repositionable analogs (Fig 18). The monolithic screw-retained zirconia bridge was adhesively connected to three titanium abutments (Variobase RC; Institut Straumann AG). Since the guided implant placement resulted in completely parallel implant axes, engaging abutments could be used (Fig 19).

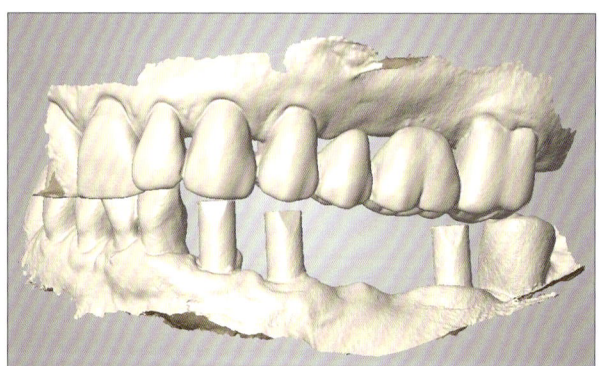

Fig 16   STL file with scanbodies, obtained using a 3M True Definition scanner.

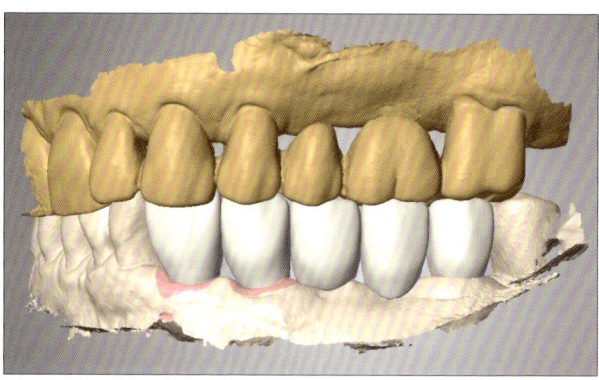

Fig 17   CAD/CAM design of definitive FDP using Dental Wings software.

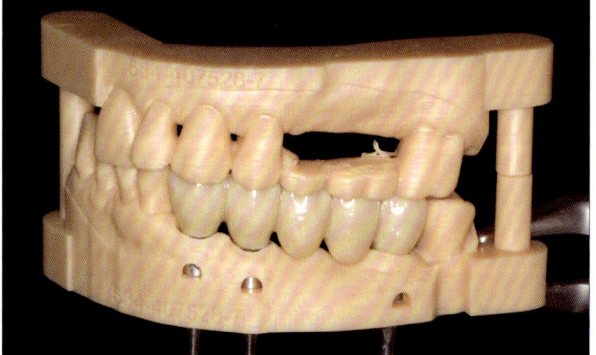

Fig 18   Definitive monolithic zirconia FDP on a stereolithographic model.

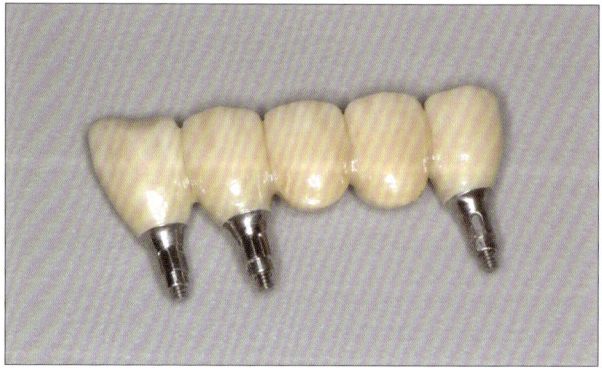

Fig 19   Screw-retained FDP adhesively connected to titanium abutments.

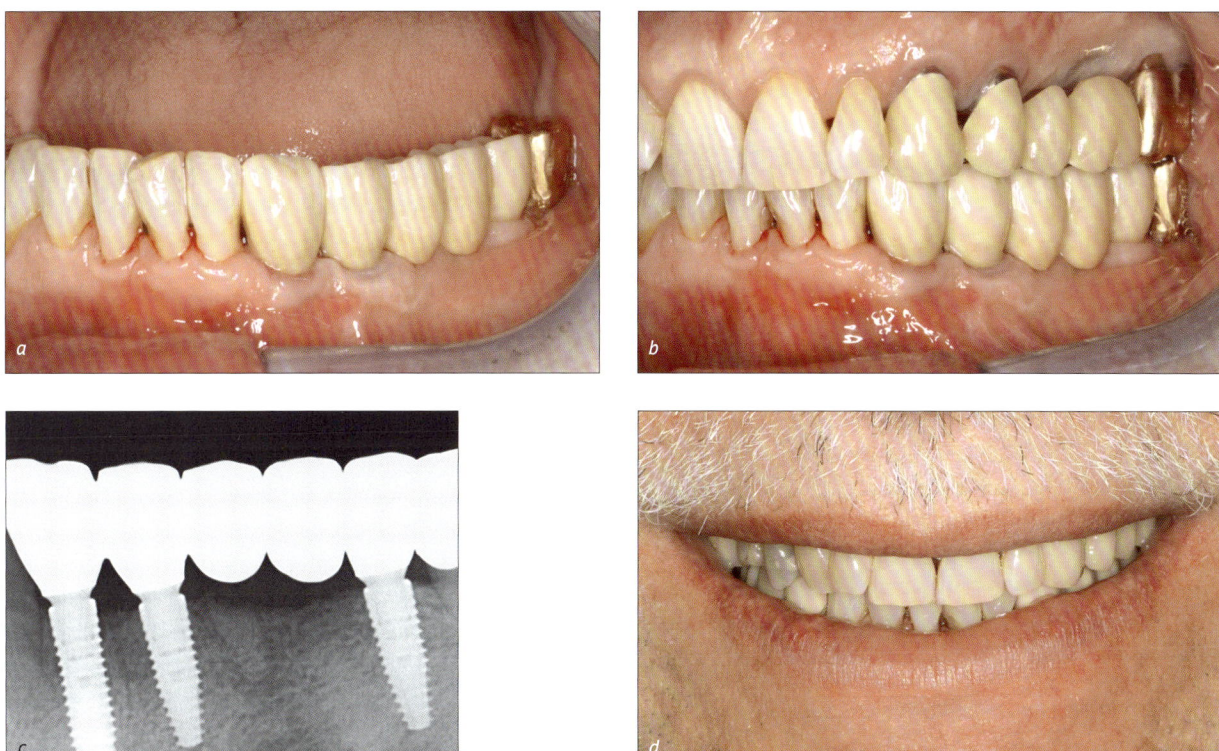

Figs 20a-d   Intraoral (a and b), radiological (c), and extraoral (d) views directly after the placement of the definitive FDP.

Apart for some bone loss distally of implant 33, the implants appeared to be well integrated, with adequate keratinized tissue (Figs 20a-d). It was decided to retain tooth 38 and its gold crown, as it was still in good condition and in function and gave the patient a pleasant feeling due to the proprioception it provided.

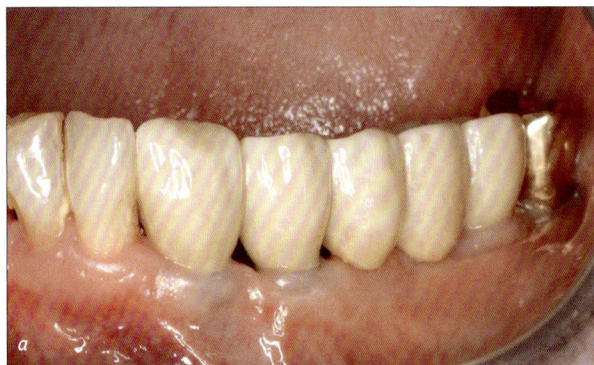

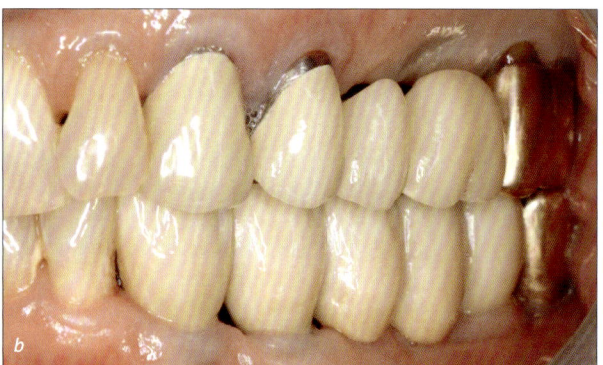

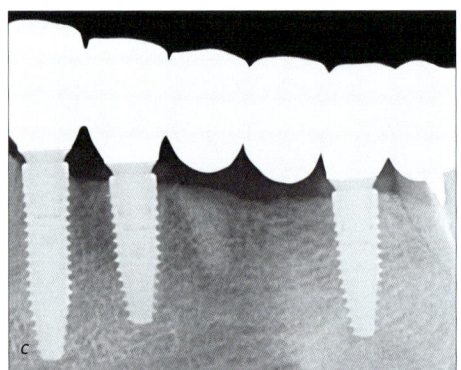

Figs 21a-c   Clinical and radiological situation at the two-year recall.

Follow-up

The patient was recalled at one and two years after delivery of the definitive restoration. The periapical radiograph showed some additional remodeling of the bone surrounding implant 34; however, all peri-implant tissue had a healthy appearance, with no inflammation, suppuration, or deep pockets (Figs 21a-c).

Acknowledgments

Clinical procedures

W. D. C. Derksen – Arnhem, Netherlands
H. B. Derksen – Arnhem, Netherlands

13.7 Replacing a Mandibular Denture with a Full-Arch Implant-Supported Mandibular Fixed Dental Prosthesis

P. Papaspyridakos

A 68-year-old male patient with a mandibular complete denture opposing a full-arch maxillary provisional fixed dental prosthesis (FDP) presented for an implant consultation (Figs 1 and 2). His medical history was non-contributory, and there was no contraindication to dental implant treatment.

The patient's chief complaint was dissatisfaction with the stability of his denture while chewing and a desire for a fixed mandibular prosthesis. The patient had already had two dental implants (Certain; Biomet 3i, West Palm Beach, FL, USA) placed seven years before, and the existing mandibular denture had been relined on healing abutments. Clinical examination revealed that the quality of the mandibular denture was acceptable in terms of phonetics, esthetics, vertical dimension of occlusion, and tooth position. One of the two existing implants was considered hopeless due to advanced bone loss, while the second implant was considered restorable. Following a comprehensive diagnostic mock-up and the presentation of various treatment options, the patient consented to a complete implant-supported mandibular fixed rehabilitation.

A duplicate of the mandibular denture was used as a radiographic template for the cone-beam computed tomography (CBCT) scan using the dual-scan technique. This technique (Nobel Guide; Nobel Biocare, Yorba Linda, CA, USA) is required in the edentulous jaw; one scan is obtained of the patient wearing the radiographic template, and a second scan is made of the radiographic template alone (Papaspyridakos and coworkers 2017). Radiopaque fiducial markers were incorporated into the template and used to merge the two scans in the virtual planning software.

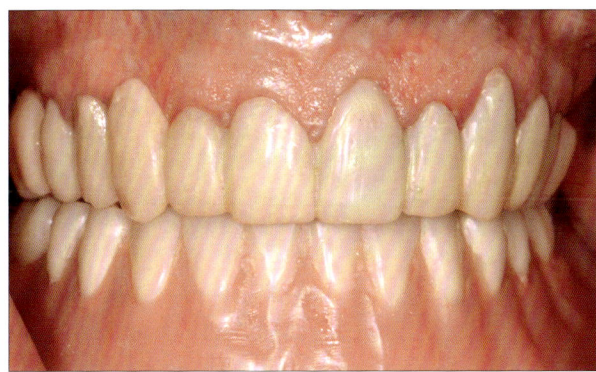

Fig 1   Initial situation.

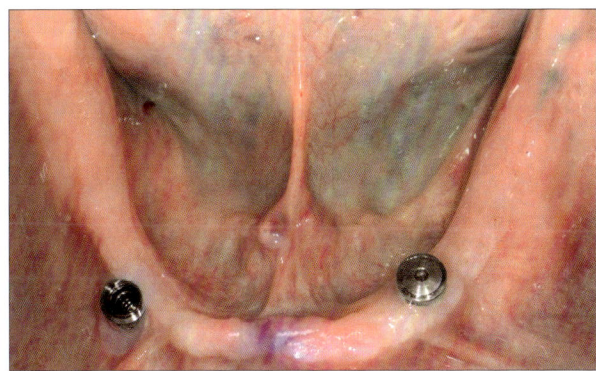

Fig 2   Occlusal view of the edentulous mandible.

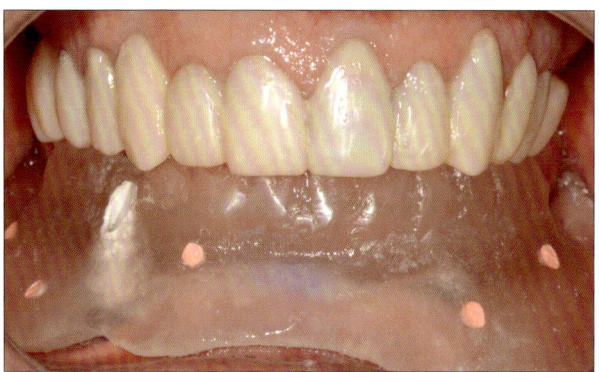

Fig 3   Radiographic template, screw-retained on one existing implant and relined on the healing abutment of the second implant. A dual-scan technique is necessary for the edentulous jaw—one of the patient wearing the radiographic template and a second one with the template itself. The fiducial markers of gutta-percha were used to merge the two scans in the CAD software for virtual planning.

The radiographic template was screw-retained on one of the existing implants and relined on the healing abutment of the second implant (Fig 3) to provide additional stability of the template during the CBCT scan, given the resiliency of the soft tissues in the edentulous jaw. The DICOM file generated from the CBCT examination was imported into virtual computer-assisted design (CAD) software (Nobel Clinician; Nobel Biocare, Zürich, Switzerland). After the virtual plan was completed, the file was emailed to a computer-assisted manufacturing (CAM) facility for production of the guided surgery template using stereolithography (Fig 4). On receipt of the completed stereolithographic surgical template, it was tried in and verified. A bite registration was taken to facilitate the positioning of the template (Fig 5).

Four bone-level type implants were placed (NobelReplace Conical Connection; Nobel Biocare) in the mandible using computer-guided surgery and a guided placement procedure (Figs 6 and 7). As a primary stability of more than 35 Ncm had been achieved, it was decided to employ an immediate-loading protocol.

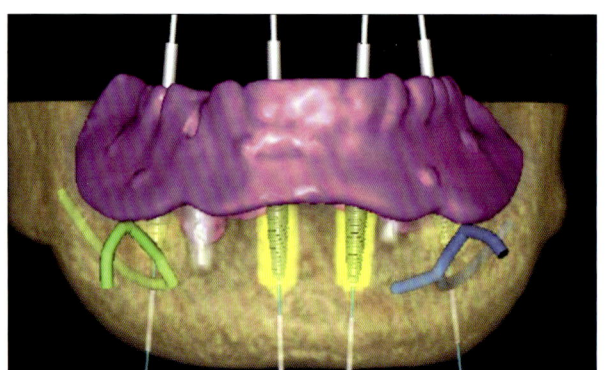

Fig 4   Prosthetically driven digital implant planning using CAD software.

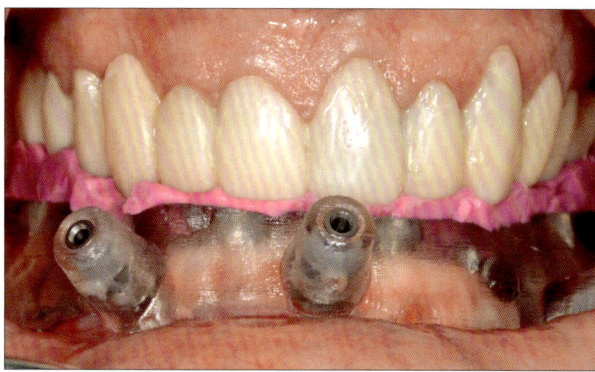

Fig 5   The stereolithographic surgical template stabilized with a bite index and anchor pins inserted into the bone.

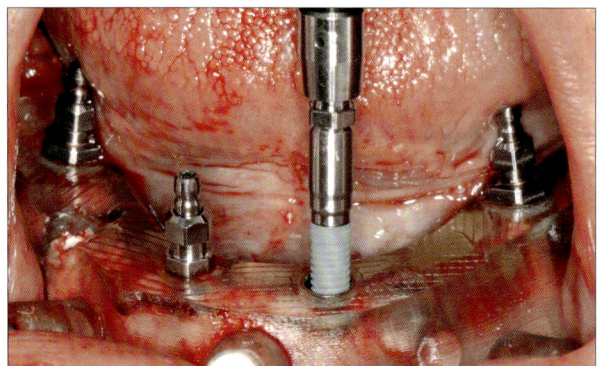

Fig 6   Guided implant placement through the template. The preparation of the implant site had been guided with drilling sleeves that fit the stereolithographic template.

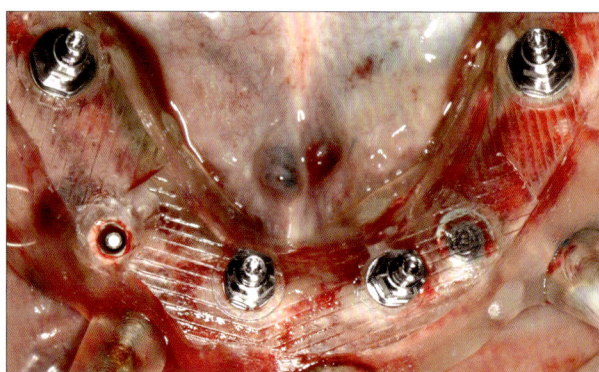

Fig 7   All implants inserted through the template.

Consequently, straight multi-unit abutments were connected to the implants at a torque of 35 Ncm. Temporary abutments were connected to the multi-unit abutments and the mandibular denture was relieved to accommodate the temporary abutments (Fig 8). Rubber dam was used to isolate the underlying soft tissue. The temporary multi-unit abutments were hand-tightened on the implants, and a panoramic radiograph was taken (Fig 9). The temporary abutments were connected to the mandibular denture with acrylic resin and picked up with the conversion prosthesis technique, which involves relieving the existing denture to accommodate temporary abutments connected to the implants. Acrylic resin was injected around the temporary abutments, and the denture was picked up. While the conversion prosthesis was being trimmed and contoured in the laboratory, the failing implant was explanted. The screw-retained conversion prosthesis was then delivered (Fig 10), and the screw access channels were sealed with PTFE tape and composite resin.

After a two-month uneventful healing period, the conversion prosthesis was removed and implant osseointegration was confirmed after torque-testing the implants at 35 Ncm. The conversion prosthesis was assessed for esthetics, phonetics, and vertical dimension of occlusion over the healing period. The patient expressed his satisfaction with the fixed prosthesis. The prosthodontic procedures were completed during four clinical appointments using the following digital workflow (Papaspyridakos and coworkers 2017):

1st clinical appointment. A final abutment-level implant impression was taken using an open-tray splinted technique and the working cast was fabricated using the double-pour technique. A verification jig was also made intraorally to verify the accuracy of the working cast.

2nd clinical appointment. The occlusion of the maxillary provisional FDP against the mandibular conversion prosthesis was registered with a centric relation record, and the conversion prosthesis was screwed in place on the working cast. The casts were then mounted in a semi-adjustable articulator using a facebow transfer. Subsequently, dual digital scanning of the conversion prosthesis and the respective working cast was performed using a high-precision laboratory scanner (Activity 880 scanner; Smart Optics, Bochum, Germany). The conversion prosthesis was then returned to the patient.

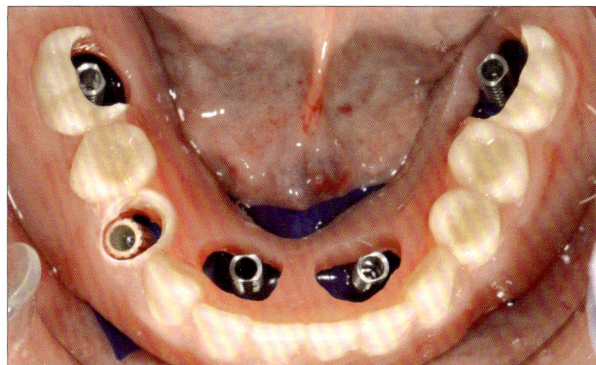

Fig 8   Denture conversion technique. The mandibular denture is relieved, and the temporary abutment ready for pick-up with acrylic resin.

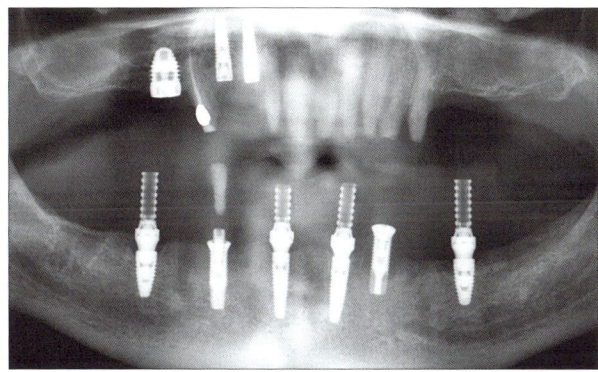

Fig 9   Post-placement panoramic radiograph. Multi-unit abutments and temporary abutments were placed prior to the procedures for the conversion prosthesis.

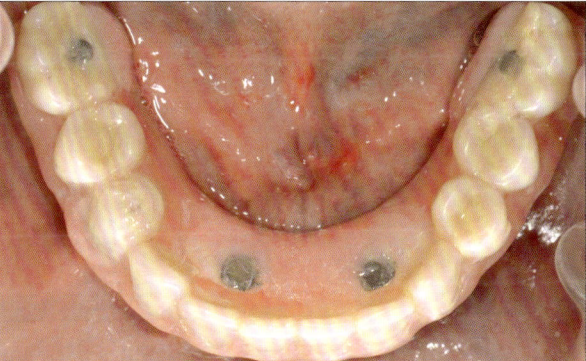

Fig 10   The immediately loaded conversion prosthesis in situ, after explantation of the failing left implant.

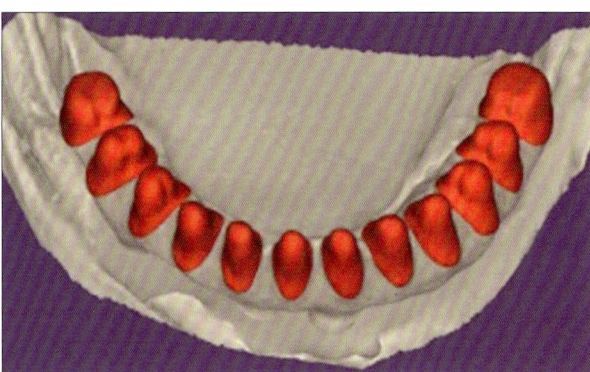

Fig 11   STL data after digital scanning of the physical pattern of the framework, imported into CAD software. The conversion prosthesis had previously been digitally scanned and a duplicate prototype milled in PMMA, followed by a conventional manual cutback to create a physical pattern of the framework.

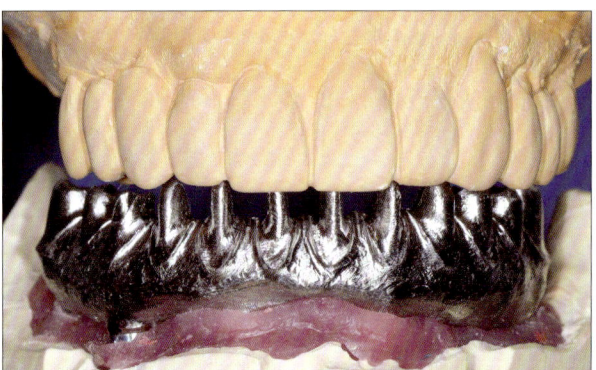

Fig 12   Milled CAD/CAM titanium framework mounted in the articulator.

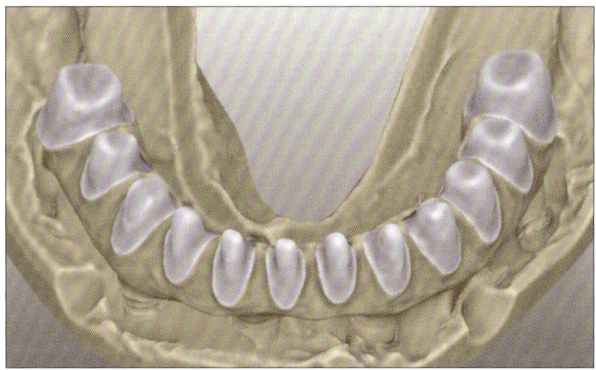

Fig 13   STL data after re-scanning of the CAD/CAM titanium framework with abutment preparations, imported into CAD software.

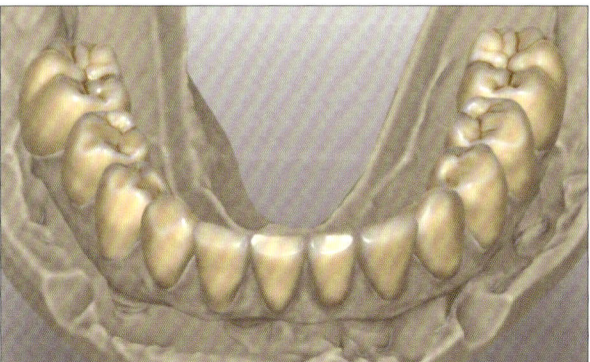

Fig 14   STL data after re-scanning of the CAD/CAM titanium framework with abutment preparations, imported into CAD software.

In the laboratory, the standard tessellation language (STL) files generated by the scanner were merged and imported into a CAD software package (Exocad DentalCAD; exocad, Darmstadt, Germany) linked to a CAM milling unit (Tizian Cut plus; Schütz, Rosbach, Germany). A duplicate prototype of the conversion prosthesis was milled from prefabricated polymethyl methacrylate (PMMA) blocks (ZCAD Temp-Fix 98; Harvest Dental, Brea, CA, USA). The PMMA prototype was then manually cut back to design a framework with custom abutment preparations. The custom abutment preparations were to serve as abutments for all-ceramic single crowns. The PMMA framework prototype was re-scanned with the same laboratory scanner (Fig 11). The generated STL data were sent to a CAM facility (NobelProcera, Nobel Biocare) to mill a titanium framework.

3rd clinical appointment. The milled titanium framework was tried in and the accuracy of its fit confirmed clinically and radiographically. The framework was seated on the articulator and re-scanned with the laboratory scanner (Figs 12 and 13). Single crowns were designed with the CAD software (Exocad) and milled in lithium disilicate (Katana EMAX; Kuraray Noritake, Tokyo, Japan) (Fig 14). The prescribed occlusal scheme was for a mutually protected occlusion with anterior guidance.

A bisque try-in was performed, at which minor esthetic adjustments were made. An occlusal assessment was performed using red articulating paper (AccuFilm II; Parkell, Edgewood, NY, USA) and Hanel shimstock foil (Coltene Whaledent; Langenau, Ulm, Germany).

At the laboratory, all but three lithium disilicate single crowns were cemented to the titanium framework as follows (Fig 15):

The internal surfaces of the crowns were sandblasted and etched with 4.9% hydrofluoric acid for 20 seconds, rinsed with water for 1 minute, and air-dried with oil-free air.

Next, a 10-methacryloyloxydecyl dihydrogen phosphate (MDP)-containing bonding/silane coupling agent mixture (Clearfil Ceramic Primer; Kuraray Noritake, Tokyo, Japan) was applied on both the crowns and the titanium frameworks for 60 seconds, then cemented with a self-adhesive resin cement (Clearfil SA; Kuraray Noritake, Tokyo, Japan). The remaining three crowns were not cemented extraorally because the screw access channels interfered with the crowns, so these were planned to be cemented intraorally.

4th clinical appointment. The screw-retained abutment-level titanium framework was torqued to 15 Ncm and the screw access holes filled with PTFE tape and composite resin. The remaining three crowns were also cemented, using the aforementioned technique (Figs 16 and 17). The patient was given oral-hygiene and prosthesis-cleaning instructions.

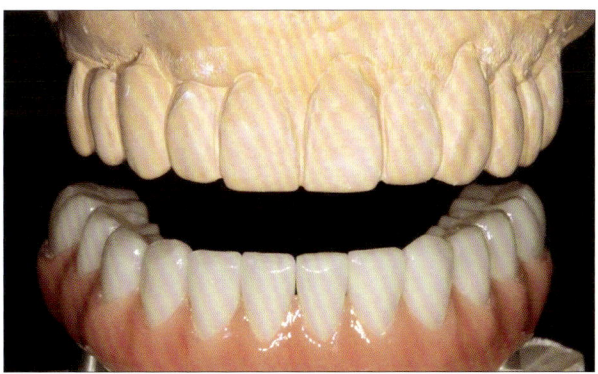

Fig 15   CAD/CAM milled lithium disilicate crowns cemented on the CAD/CAM titanium framework at the laboratory, except for three crowns that were cemented intraorally.

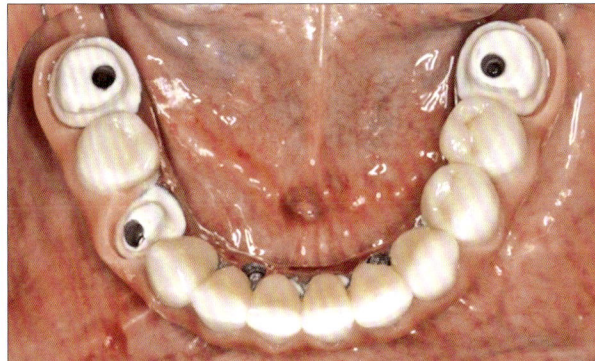

Fig 16   CAD/CAM titanium framework prior to intraoral cementation of the remaining three CAD/CAM milled lithium disilicate crowns.

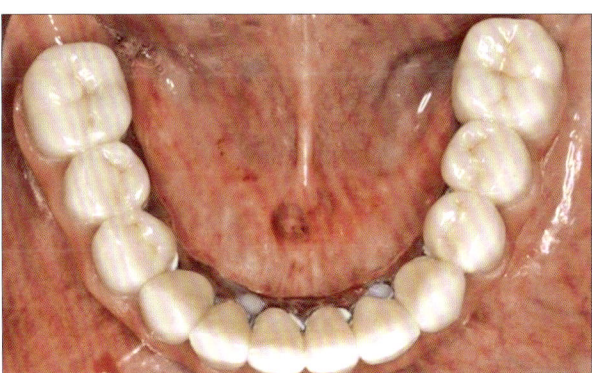

Fig 17   Post-insertion occlusal view of the CAD/CAM titanium framework with CAD/CAM milled lithium disilicate crowns.

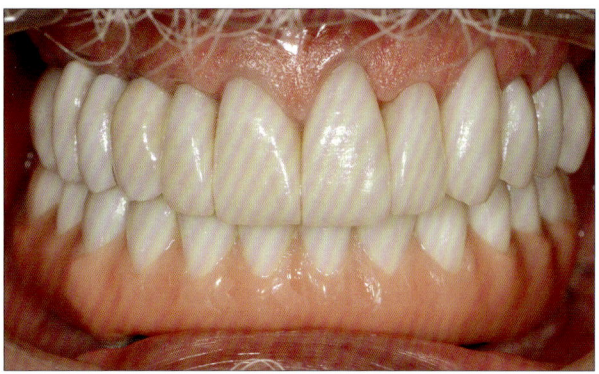

Fig 18 Post-insertion frontal view of the inserted maxillary and mandibular prostheses.

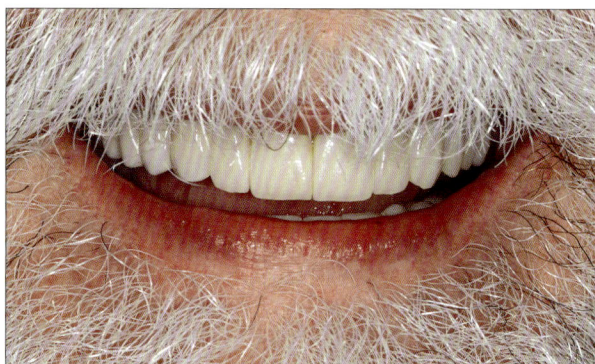

Fig 19 Post-insertion smile.

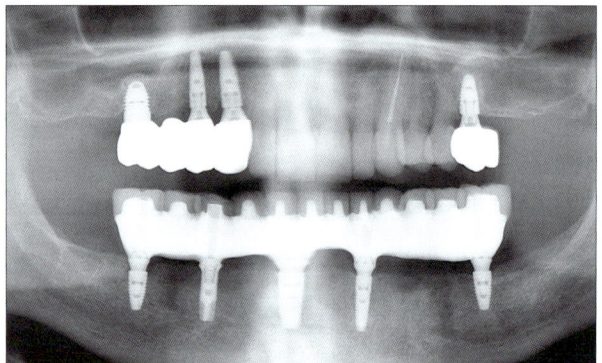

Fig 20 Panoramic radiograph after 1 year in clinical function.

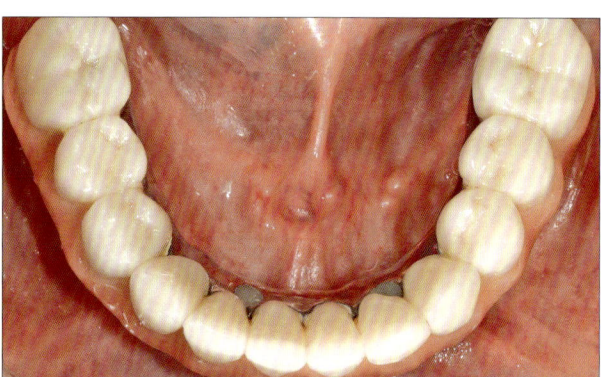

Fig 21 Occlusal view of mandibular prosthesis after 1 year in clinical function.

One month later, the segmented maxillary reconstruction using a combination of tooth- and implant-supported single crowns and FDPs was delivered. The patient expressed his complete satisfaction with the esthetics and function of his rehabilitation (Figs 18 and 19). A nightguard was delivered to protect the prostheses from ceramic chipping and parafunctional challenges.

At the one-year follow-up, a clinical and radiographic examination revealed a stable outcome (Figs 20 to 22). At the two-year follow-up, patient satisfaction remained high, with no biologic or technical complications (Fig 23). The final prosthesis was not removed at any point throughout the follow-up period, as per the clinic's protocol.

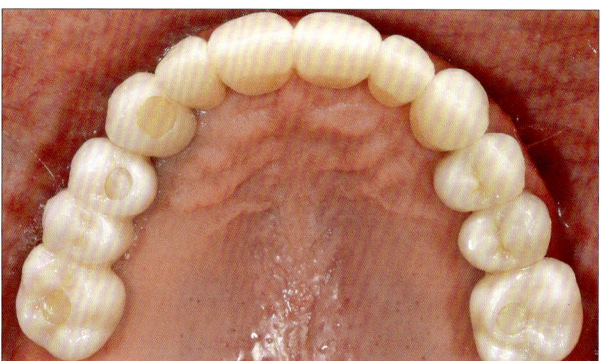

Fig 22 Occlusal view of maxillary prostheses after 1 year in clinical function.

Discussion

This clinical report describes the digital workflow for a full-arch implant-supported rehabilitation with a screw-retained titanium framework with a custom abutment preparation design and individually cemented lithium disilicate single crowns. A two-year follow-up confirmed the stability of the treatment outcome up to that time point. No signs of peri-implant bleeding or suppuration were evident.

The long-term prosthodontic results with 108 edentulous jaws restored with titanium frameworks with individually cemented single crowns have been reported to be favorable up to the 10-year clinical follow-up with the same prosthodontic design as in the present clinical report (Maló and coworkers 2012). However, little evidence on peri-implant parameters was reported on the aforementioned study.

The use of digital technology in all aspects of implant dentistry, from digital imaging and computer-guided implant placement to digital impressions and CAD/CAM prosthodontics is a reality (Papaspyridakos and coworkers 2017, 2018). This present clinical report illustrates a current clinical application of digital technology in implant dentistry for a fully edentulous patient and the integration of digital technology.

"Digital impressions" are in fact surface scans acquired by an intraoral scanner (IOS) to produce an STL file. They have several advantages over conventional impression techniques: they eliminate the need for tray selection, dispensing and setting of impression materials, disinfection, and impression shipping to the laboratory; greater patient comfort may be an additional advantage (Papaspyridakos and coworkers 2016). The STL file can be stored electronically, which eliminates storage management issues, supports the paper-free practice, and contributes to efficient record-keeping, while also serving as a patient education tool.

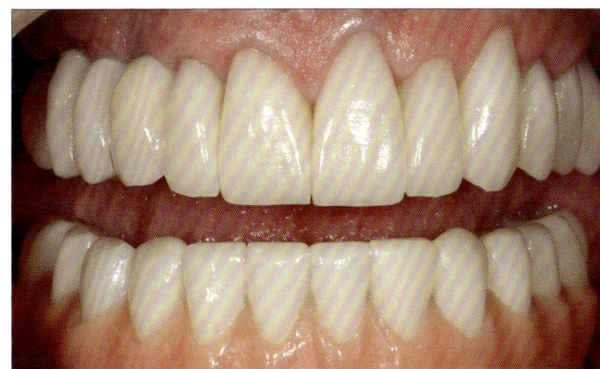

Fig 23   Frontal view after 2 years in clinical function. A stable and pleasant outcome.

The STL data are used to generate either a physical cast or a digital cast for a complete digital workflow. When the patient was treated in 2015, digital impressions using an IOS were not scientifically validated. Instead, a conventional impression was performed from which conventional stone casts were made; these were then digitized with a laboratory scanner. Digital technology is advancing with enormous speed, with recent advances showing promising results. Several recent studies suggest that full-arch digital impressions of implants (TRIOS; 3shape, Copenhagen, Denmark) may display the same accuracy as or greater accuracy than conventional impressions (Amin and coworkers 2017; Papaspyridakos and coworkers 2016).

The continuous progress of full-arch digital impressions may soon render complete digital workflows feasible, without the need for conventional impressions or digitized stone casts. The digital impressions can also be used to generate printed casts using 3D-printing technology.

More research is necessary regarding the accuracy of printed casts generated from full-arch digital impressions.

In regard to the CAD/CAM prosthodontic phase, the conversion prosthesis was digitally scanned and a PMMA prototype was copy-milled. Subsequently, the milled prototype was cut back conventionally to obtain a physical pattern of the framework with custom abutment preparations and then re-scanned. There is no longer any need for such a physical pattern today, since CAD software can now be used to perform a virtual cutback prior to milling the framework (Papaspyridakos and coworkers 2017). Hence, the STL data of the scanned conversion prosthesis can be used for the digital cutback and a framework can be milled within a complete digital workflow.

Prosthodontically, the main benefit was the reduced risk of material fracture, a frequently encountered complication with both metal-acrylic and metal-ceramic hybrid full-arch prostheses. Potential technical complications with the single crowns used in this approach can be managed by CAD/CAM milling of new crowns. This can reduce the cost of maintenance and repairs in the long term. However, the use of a titanium framework limits this approach to patients with adequate restorative space; more space may be required than for other types of ceramic hybrid prosthesis, which must be taken into consideration during the treatment planning phase.

When designing a full-arch implant-supported fixed prosthesis, a complete digital workflow currently remains unattainable. A combination of digital and conventional workflows is the current standard of care. Enormous progress continues to be made in the fields of virtual articulation, virtual facebow recordings, and printed-cast fabrication, which means that a complete digital workflow may be a reality for full-arch implant-supported rehabilitations in the near future.

Acknowledgments

Clinical procedures
Dr. Sarah Amin, BDS, MS – Cairo, Egypt

Laboratory procedures
Yukio Kudara, CDT, MDT – Boston, MA, USA
(definitive prostheses)

13.8 Rehabilitating an Edentulous Maxilla with Three Separate Bridges

G. Finelle

A 55-year-old woman was referred to our clinic for implant therapy. She was healthy and had stopped smoking two years previously. Ten years before, the patient had received extensive dental treatment in both jaws. The patient reported that her dental condition had deteriorated progressively since that time. At the time of presentation, the maxillary bridge was loose. The clinical and radiographic examinations revealed a highly compromised situation for all the teeth that supported the bridge and for other teeth (Figs 1 to 4).

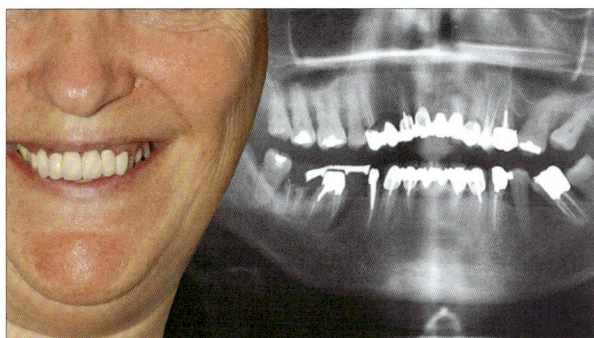

Fig 1   Patient smile and panoramic radiograph at baseline.

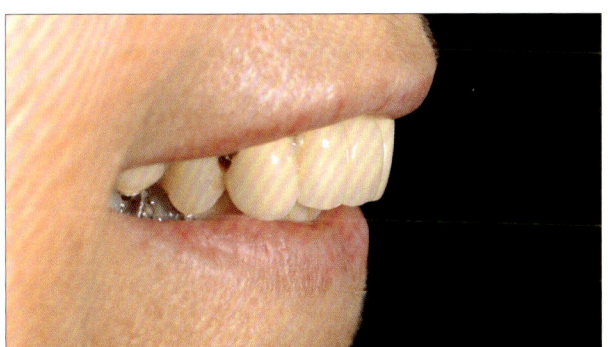

Fig 2   Profile view of the smile at baseline.

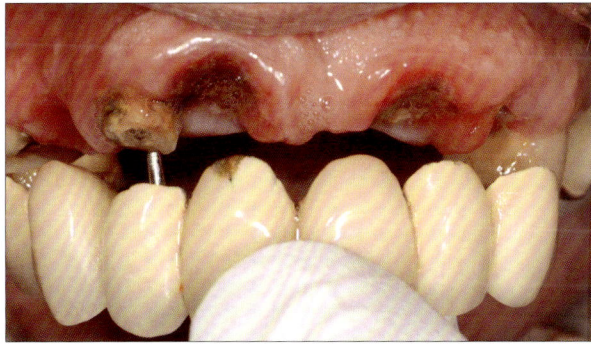

Fig 3   Intraoral baseline situation.

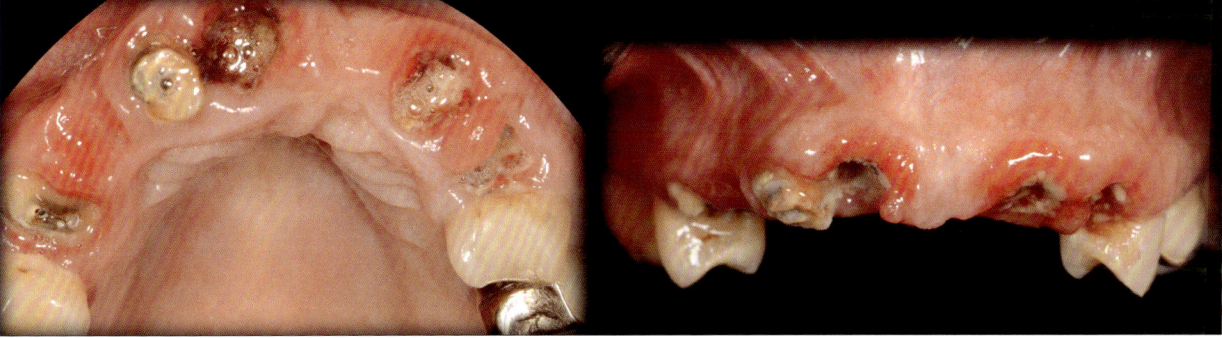

Fig 4   Intraoral situation after bridge removal (occlusal and frontal views).

Table 1 Esthetic Risk Assessment

Esthetic risk factors	Level of risk		
	Low	**Medium**	**High**
Medical status	Healthy, uneventful healing		Compromised healing
Smoking habit	Non-smoker	Light smoker (≤ 10 cigs/day)	Heavy smoker (> 10 cigs/day)
Gingival display at full smile	Low	Medium	High
Width of edentulous span	1 tooth (≥ 7 mm)[1] 1 tooth (≥ 6 mm)[2]	1 tooth (< 7 mm)[1] 1 tooth (< 6 mm)[2]	2 teeth or more
Shape of tooth crowns	Rectangular		Triangular
Restorative status of neighboring teeth	Virgin		Restored
Gingival phenotype	Low-scalloped, thick	Medium-scalloped, medium-thick	High-scalloped, thin
Infection at implant site	None	Chronic	Acute
Soft-tissue anatomy	Soft tissue intact		Soft-tissue defects
Bone level at adjacent teeth	≤ 5 mm to contact point	5.5 to 6.5 mm to contact point	≥ 7 mm to contact point
Facial bone-wall phenotype*	Thick-wall phenotype ≥ 1 mm thickness		Thin-wall phenotype < 1 mm thickness
Bone anatomy of alveolar crest	No bone deficiency	Horizontal bone deficiency	Vertical bone deficiency
Patient's esthetic expectations	Realistic expectations		Unrealistic expectations

* If three-dimensional imaging is available with the tooth in place
[1] Standard-diameter implant, regular connection
[2] Narrow-diameter implant, narrow connection

A detailed interdisciplinary clinical and radiographic examination was made to evaluate the prognosis of the teeth to establish a proper treatment plan. The analysis revealed chronic generalized moderate (and locally severe) periodontitis combined with numerous restoratively and endodontically compromised teeth in both jaws.

Panoramic and periapical radiographs confirmed the clinical findings, demonstrating severe restorative and periodontal damage in the entire maxilla, suggesting an implant-supported fixed full-arch rehabilitation. The treatment plan for the mandible was to retain the natural teeth, with the exception of the non-salvageable 46 and 47. Am implant-supported prosthetic rehabilitation was to be provided once periodontal health was established, with periodontal recalls every 4 to 6 months.

Based on the Esthetic Risk Analysis (ERA), the case was classified as "complex," with ten of the thirteen parameters examined falling into a risk category (Table 1).

After a thorough discussion of the situation with the patient, it was decided to pursue the following treatment plan:

1. Flapless extraction of teeth 15 to 25 and socket debridement
2. Delivery of an immediate removable partial denture
3. Generalized periodontal therapy

4. After three months of healing: 3D digital analysis, virtual planning of implant positions, and 3D-printed surgical-guide production
5. Placement of eight SLActive implants (Institut Straumann AG, Basel, Switzerland) using computer-generated surgical guides based on the combined tooth and mucosal support; simultaneous guided bone regeneration was to be provided
6. After another two months: Delivery of a full-arch screw-retained fixed provisional restoration milled from a PMMA block
7. After another two months: Final loading of the implants with definitive screw-retained segmented CAD/CAM bridges (three parts), with each framework milled from titanium and single monolithic lithium disilicate CAD/CAM crowns (e.max; Ivoclar Vivadent, Schaan, Liechtenstein) cemented to the framework at the laboratory

Initial debridement and periodontal therapy

Due to the presence of active infection and in order to obtain fully healed soft tissue at the time of implant placement, a delayed approach (twelve weeks) was chosen over immediate placement. Initial gingival and periodontal debridement was performed to reduce the intraoral bacterial load. Teeth 15 to 25 as well as 45 and 46 were extracted. A temporary removable partial denture was constructed based on a facially driven prosthetic set-up that included occlusal, functional, and esthetic considerations.

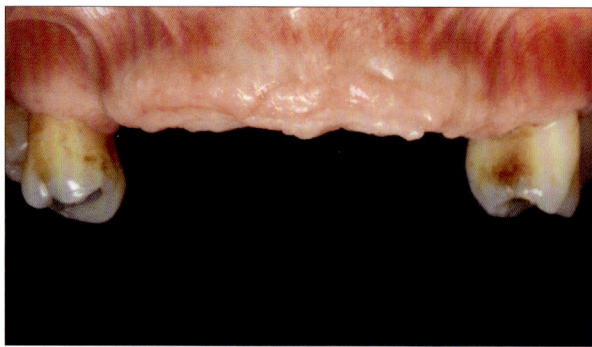

Fig 5   Healing of the maxillary ridge eight weeks after extraction.

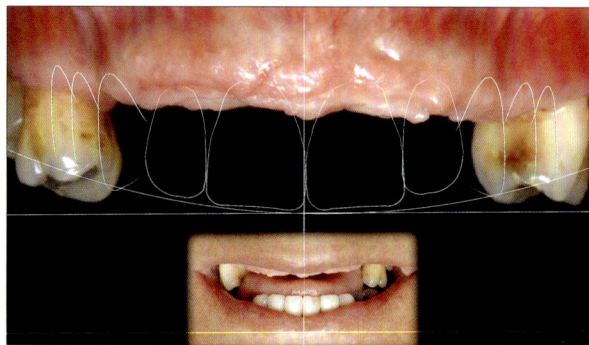

Fig 6   Digital Smile design (DSD) analysis.

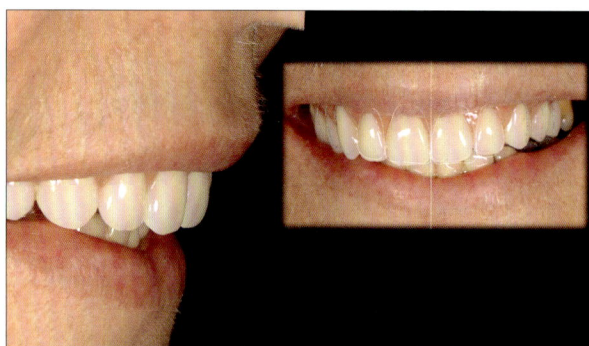

Fig 7   Delivery of the provisional removable restoration based on the DSD process.

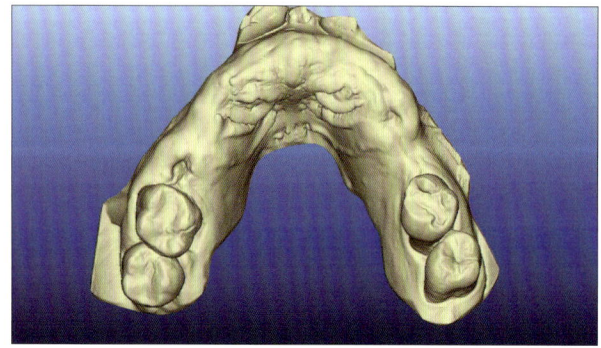

Fig 8   Surface scan of situation eight weeks after extraction.

Digital diagnosis and virtual implant planning

After eight weeks of healing (Fig 5), the clinical and esthetic analysis was reassessed to determine the patient's esthetic risk profile. At full smile, the patient presented a medium lip line displaying part of the existing gingiva in the edentulous anterior region. The patient's gingival biotype was thick, with sufficient keratinized gingiva. A digital analysis was performed to meet the following objectives:

- To confirm esthetic requirements using Digital Smile Design (DSD) analysis and a facially driven set-up (Figs 6 and 7) (Coachman 2016)
- To merge the prosthetic and esthetic (extra- and intraoral) information with the underlying bony structures using 3D planning software
- To determine the ideal 3D positions of the proposed implants in a prosthetically driven approach
- To design and fabricate a 3D-printed surgical guide based on the above-mentioned plan
- To ensure communication of the proposed treatment to all members of the dental team

Unlike a conventional diagnosis, 3D implant planning software packages (CoDiagnostiX; Dental Wings, Montreal, Quebec, Canada) allows different types of clinical information to be superimposed and merged on a common planning platform for an integrated diagnosis. This allows the dental team (prosthodontist, surgeon, laboratory technician) to concurrently visualize information regarding the hard and soft tissues, the planned prosthesis, the intended implant positions, and extraoral facial references.

In this specific case, the following information was recorded:

- The 3D bone volume, using cone-beam computed tomography (CBCT; output: DICOM files)
- The clinical situation showing the teeth and soft-tissue contours through digital intraoral surface scanning (output: STL files) (Fig 8)

The intended treatment outcome with the esthetic set-up based on the DSD analysis demonstrated the ideal prosthetic situation at the end of treatment through further intraoral surface scanning (output: STL files) (Fig 9)

The digital workflow for virtual 3D planning and fabrication of a surgical guide is as follows:

1. Import and segmentation of maxillary bony structure data (from CBCT)
2. Import of maxillary surface scan to assess the position and thickness of the soft tissues relative to the bone
3. Import of a digitized ideal set-up based on the DSD facial analysis
4. Prosthetically driven implant selection and 3D positioning (Figs 10 and 11)
5. Corresponding positioning of the drilling sleeves
6. Virtual design of the surgical guide (Figs 12 and 13)
7. Export of the surgical-guide design (STL file) and drilling protocol (PDF)
8. Surgical-guide fabrication by CAD/CAM additive manufacturing (3D printing) (Fig 14)

The superimposition of the CBCT data and several STL files allows the surgeon to plan the implant procedure with a global and multidisciplinary vision of the prosthetic requirements and the soft-tissue situation.

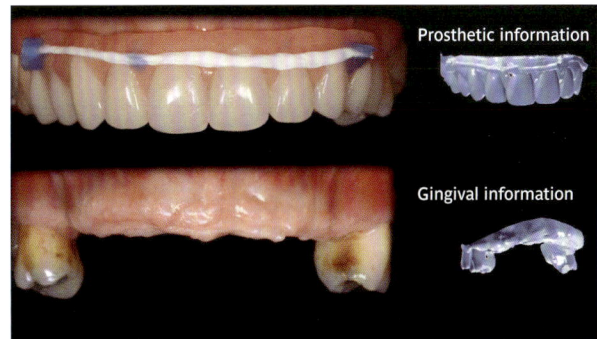

Fig 9   Digital information on the prosthetic position (esthetic set-up), position of lip line (PTFE cord), and soft-tissue position (intraoral situation).

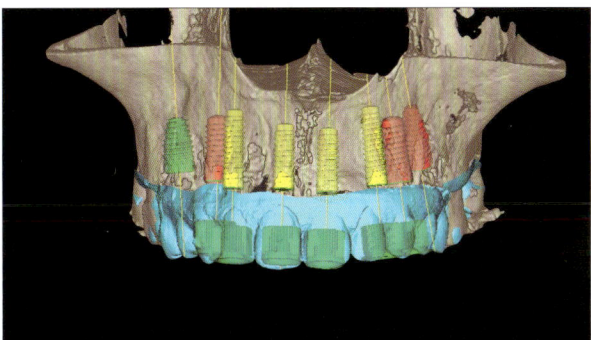

Fig 10   Prosthetically driven implant positions and the prosthetic design.

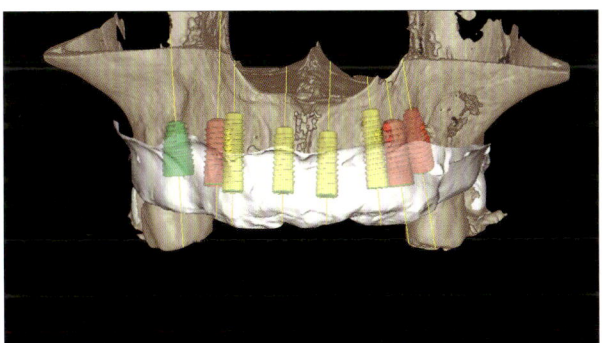

Fig 11   Implant position and the available soft tissue.

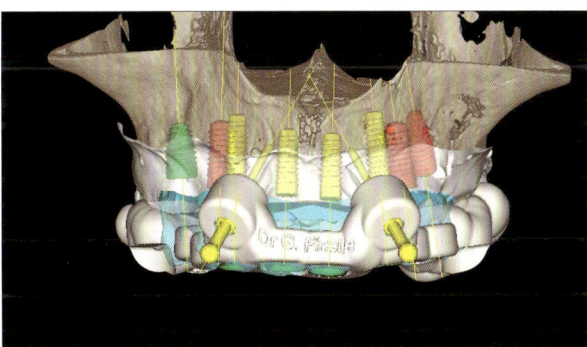

Fig 12   Design of the hybrid tooth- and mucosa-supported surgical guide.

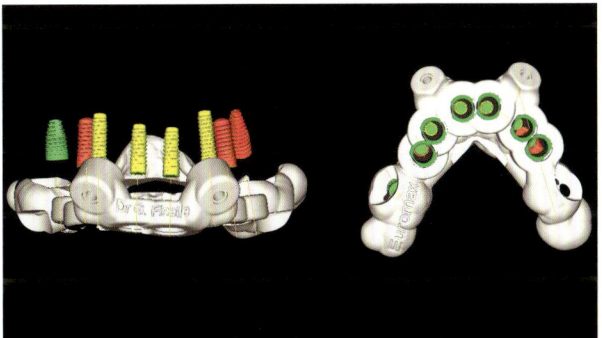

Fig 13   Surgical-guide design and the implant positions.

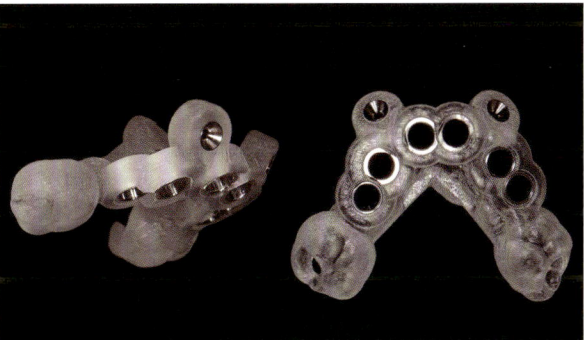

Fig 14   CAD/CAM-generated (3D printed) surgical guide.

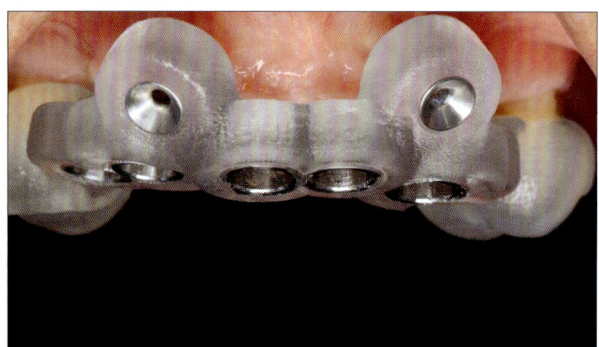

Fig 15   Seating of the surgical guide before surgery.

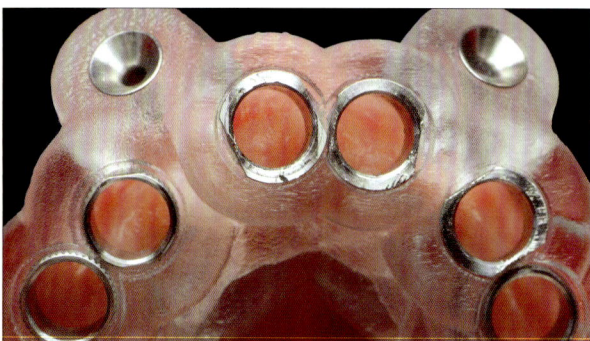

Fig 16   Occlusal view of the surgical guide in place.

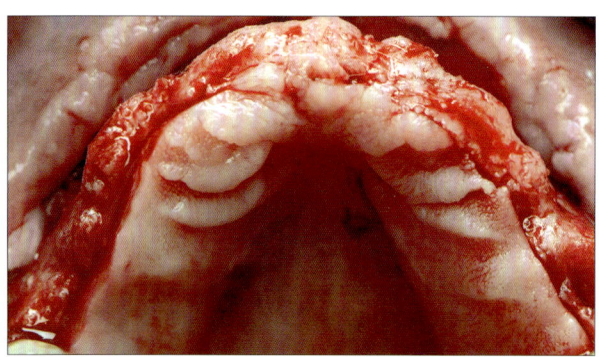

Fig 17   Palatal position of the crestal incision to optimize the supply of buccal keratinized tissue.

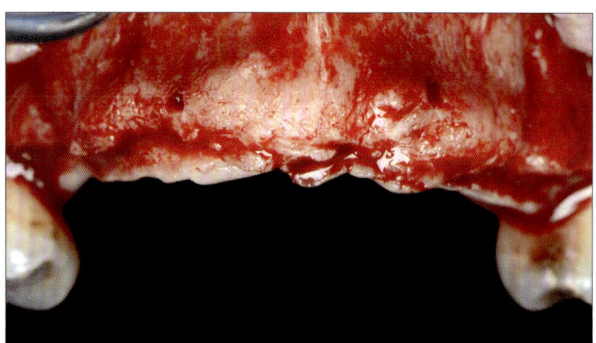

Fig 18   Flap elevation.

Computer-guided implant surgery

After twelve weeks of soft-tissue healing following the extractions (delayed implant placement protocol), the implants were placed with simultaneous contour augmentation using guided bone regeneration (GBR) based on the prosthetically driven digital planning.

As suggested by Gallucci and coworkers (2008), a segmented prosthetic design was selected for this case, with three separate bridges supported on implants (16–14, 13–11–21–23, 24–26).

Regarding implant placement at site 26, the patient was given a detailed explanation of the risks and benefits of sinus floor elevation versus a tilted implant. The patient chose the less invasive circumnavigation of the sinus by a tilted implant 26.

An initial hybrid surgical guide was supported by the palatal mucosa and by teeth 16, 17, 26, and 27. The stability and reproducibility of the position were checked (Figs 15 and 16). A palatal crestal incision was accompanied by flap elevation on the buccal side only, to allow for palatal seating. To improve the retention and stability of the guide during implant preparation, two stabilizing screws served as anchors at sites 12 and 22 (Figs 17 to 19).

Implant osteotomies were performed following the surgical protocol exported from the software (coDiagnostiX) and as recommended by the implant manufacturer for computer-guided surgery:

1. Milling cutter (Fig 20)
2. Successive guided drills matching the corresponding guide-sleeve handles of the corresponding diameter (Fig 21)
3. Guided profile drills

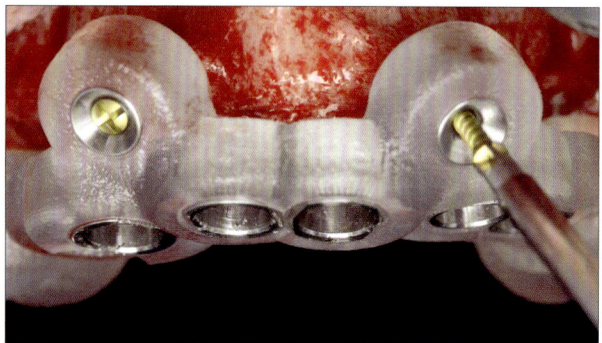

Fig 19   Insertion of a stabilizing screw before drilling through the guide.

Eight implants (Institut Straumann AG) (Table 1) with specific guided transfer abutments were placed under full surgical guidance, ensuring control of the axial position of the implant and its insertion depth (Figs 22 and 23).

Following the placement of the six anterior implants, teeth 16 and 25 were extracted and a second surgical template was utilized immediately to place implants into the interseptal bone of the sockets using a guided sequence similar to the one already described (Fig 24).

As expected from 3D planning, guided bone regeneration (GBR) using bone substitute with a low substitution rate (Cerabone; Botiss, Berlin, Germany) was required to increase the bone support on the buccal aspect of the anterior implants and to fill in the defects in the fresh extraction sockets. The grafts were covered with a non-crosslinked porcine resorbable collagen membrane (Jason membrane; Botiss) as a temporary barrier (Fig 25) during initial bone healing, in accordance with the principles of guided bone regeneration.

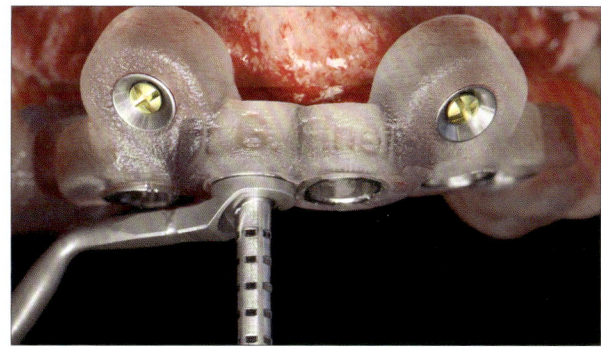

Fig 20   The first rotary instrument used for computer-guided surgery is the milling cutter (Institut Straumann AG).

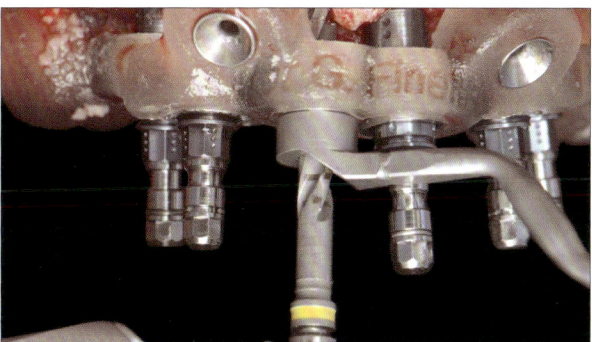

Fig 21   Implementation of the drilling sequence using surgical drills and a matching handle set.

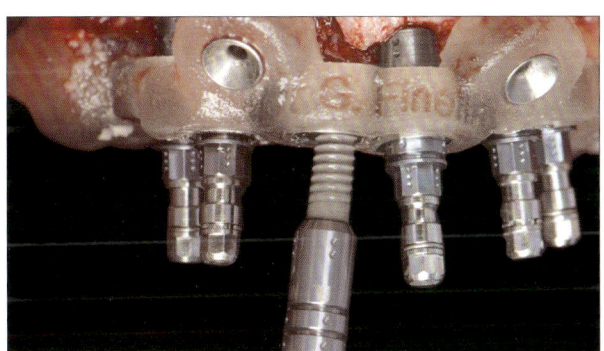

Fig 22   Guided insertion of the implant through the guide sleeves.

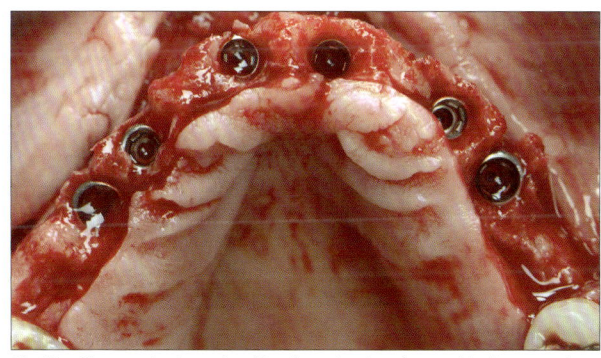

Fig 23   Six anterior bone-level implants in place (central incisors, canines, first premolars).

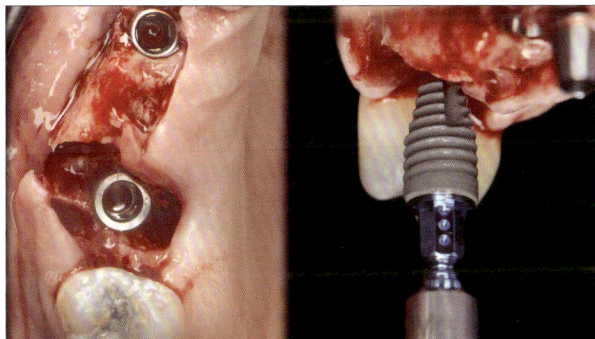

Fig 24   Immediate implant placement after the extraction of teeth 16 and 26.

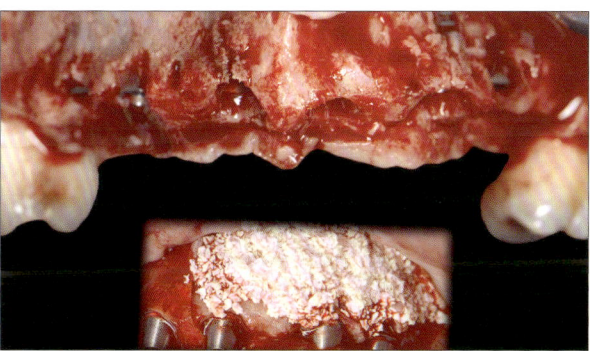

Fig 25   GBR procedure using a particulate xenograft bone substitute and a resorbable membrane.

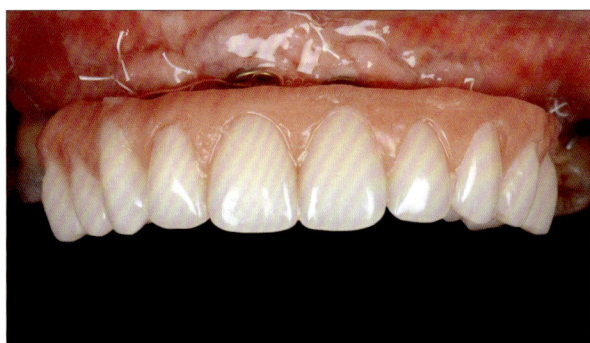

Fig 26   Interim removable prosthesis used during osseointegration.

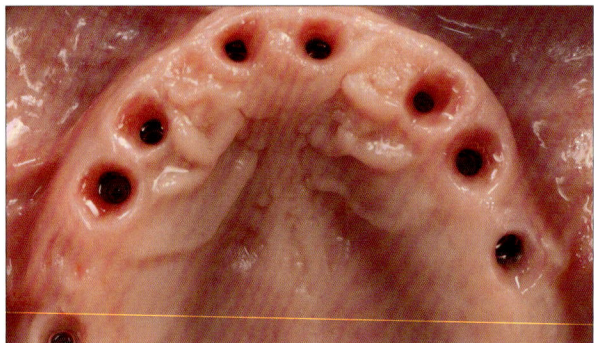

Fig 27   Clinical situation at eight weeks.

Table 1   List of implants placed

Site	Diameter (mm)	Length (mm)	Type	Surface
16	4.8	8	Regular CrossFit/ Bone Level Tapered	SLActive
14	4.1	10	Regular CrossFit/ Bone Level	SLActive
13	3.3	12	Narrow CrossFit/ Bone Level	SLActive
11	3.3	10	Narrow CrossFit/ Bone Level	SLActive
21	3.3	10	Narrow CrossFit/ Bone Level	SLActive
23	3.3	12	Narrow CrossFit/ Bone Level	SLActive
24	4.1	10	Regular CrossFit/ Bone Level	SLActive
26	4.1	10	Regular CrossFit/ Bone Level Tapered	SLActive
45	3.3	8	Regular Neck/ Standard Plus	SLActive
46	4.1	8	Regular Neck/ Standard Plus	SLActive

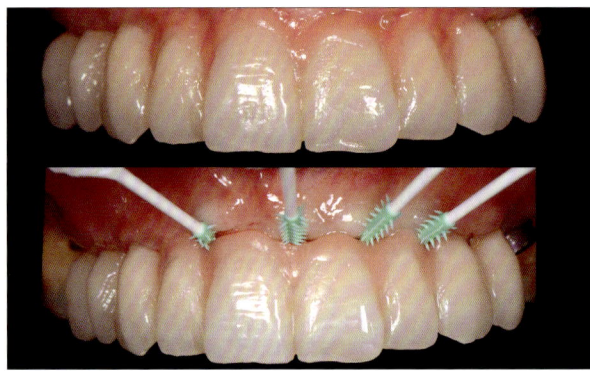

Fig 28   Screw-retained provisional: One-piece full-arch fixed restoration, designed with adequate access for plaque control.

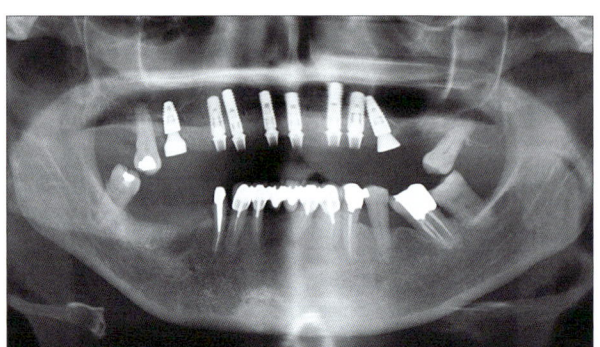

Fig 29   Panoramic radiograph after implant placement.

The flap was advanced using periosteal releasing incisions and the wound was closed with non-resorbable 5-0 suture material (Gore-Tex suture; Gore Medical, Flagstaff, AZ, USA). Teeth 17 and 27 were not extracted at the time, for the following reasons:

- To provide stable tooth support for the surgical guides
- To maintain the vertical dimension of occlusion (VDO) during the entire treatment up to the delivery of the final prosthesis)
- To help stabilize the provisional removable partial denture during implant osseointegration (six weeks) (Fig 26)

Provisionalization
Eight weeks postoperatively, the soft-tissue situation was healthy, and the contour of the of the arch was favorable (Fig 27). A conventional closed-tray impression was taken and a one-piece CAD/CAM (PMMA) screw-retained fixed provisional restoration was made in the laboratory following the initial diagnostic set-up (from the Digital Smile Design) (Figs 28 and 29).

Definitive rehabilitation

After a complication-free temporary phase, the final rehabilitation was planned to include three segmented bridges to allow for easier revision in case of technical complications, to offer improved options for cleaning, and to simplify laboratory procedures.

To minimize the distortion of the full-arch implant-level impression, a conventional open tray technique was performed using a polyvinyl siloxane (PVS) impression material, with the impression copings splinted together intraorally with rigid resin material (DuraLay; Reliance, Alsip, IL, USA) (Fig 30). A facebow recording was made at the same visit (Fig 31). The intermaxillary relationship was recorded using an implant-supported maxillary resin-based rim (DuraLay; Reliance) on which bite-registration material was positioned. The VDO was controlled by teeth 17, 27, which had been retained for this purpose.

In order to aid the CAD/CAM design of the definitive prosthetic framework, a polyvinyl siloxane impression of the provisional restoration was taken. A conventional stone master model with implant analogs was then poured from the impressions.

To validate the precision and trueness of the master cast and ensure a predictable passive fit of the future restoration, three stone verification indices (corresponding to the segmented design selected) were inserted into the implant connections. No fractures of these indices occurred, confirming a satisfactory passive fit (Fig 32).

Both models were mounted in an articulator (Artex; Amann Girrbach, Koblach, Austria) in the correct intermaxillary relationship and digitized (Dental Wings) (Fig 33). Prior to scanning the models, digital scanbodies were inserted into each implant analog. The mounted maxillary and mandibular casts and the model of the provisional restoration were sent to an external milling facility (Createch Medical, Pabellón, Spain) to assist in the digital workflow of model scanning and the design and milling of a titanium framework.

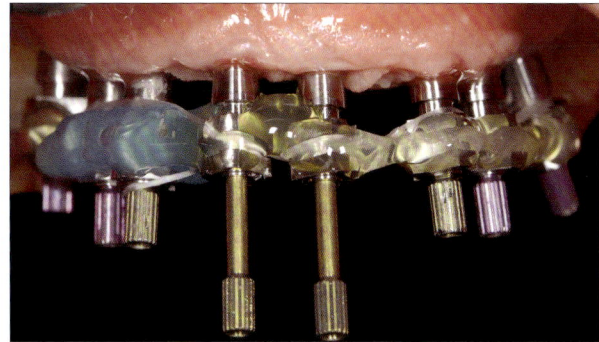

Fig 30   Final conventional open tray impression with splinted impression posts.

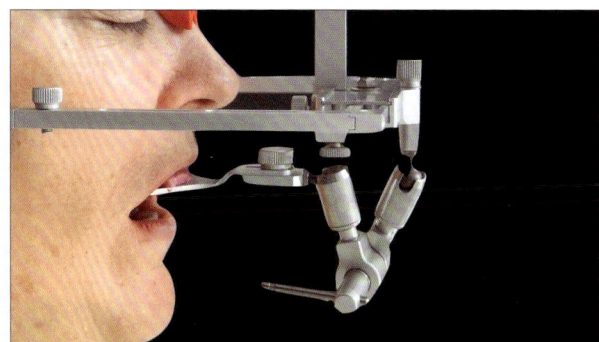

Fig 31   Facebow registration.

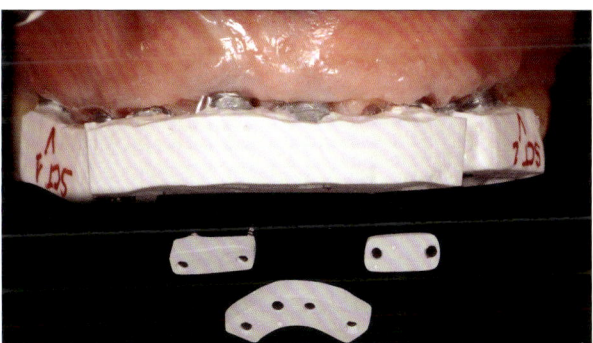

Fig 32   Validation of the accuracy of the working model with segmented stone indices.

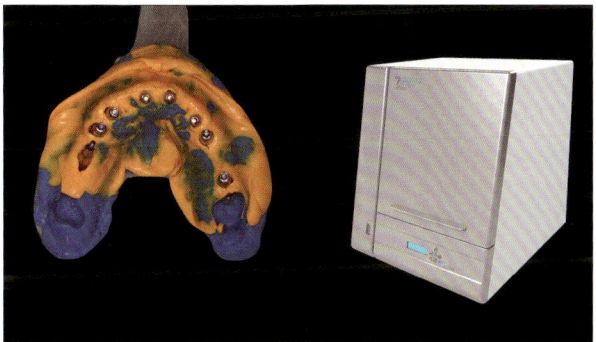

Fig 33   The impression is poured out and the model scanned.

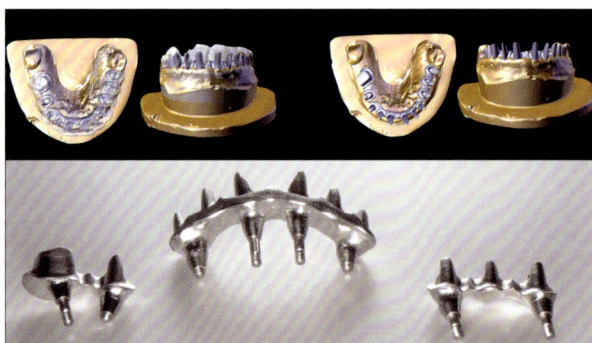

Fig 34   Design of three reduced titanium frameworks.

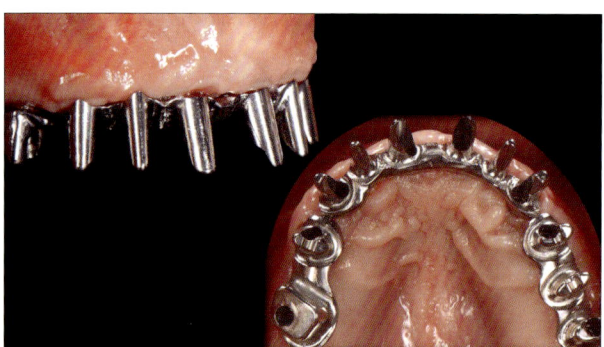

Fig 35   Framework try-in.

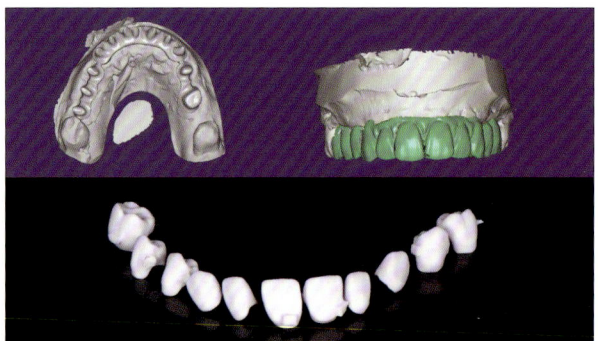

Fig 36   Design and fabrication of twelve individually milled monolithic CAD/CAM ceramic crowns (e.max CAD; Ivoclar Vivadent; lithium disilicate).

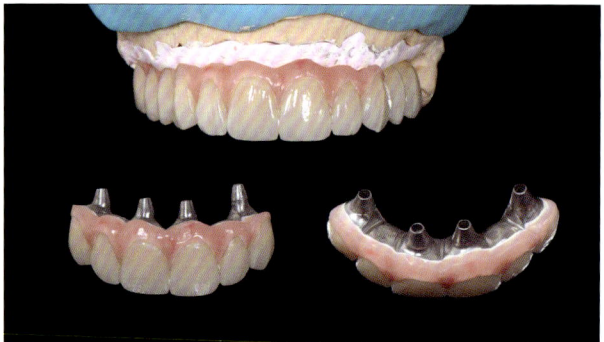

Fig 37   Final bridge ready for delivery after staining and cementation of the individual crowns onto the framework.

The design of the titanium framework was carried out by the laboratory (Laboratoire Nouvelle Technologie, Paris, France) in collaboration with the milling company (Createch Medical). Three titanium frameworks were constructed using non-indexed implant connections. The gingival framework was veneered with gingiva-colored ceramics. Individual monolithic crowns were constructed and cemented onto the framework (Figs 34 and 35). A passive fit with adequate occlusal space was confirmed at the clinical try-in.

Gingiva-colored ceramic material was layered and sintered onto the titanium framework at the laboratory. Sixteen custom CAD/CAM crowns were designed (Dental Wings) and milled in lithium disilicate (IPS e.max CAD; Ivoclar Vivadent). After staining and sintering, the crowns were individually cemented (glass-ionomer cement) onto the framework. Crowns located at implant positions were designed to allow screw access (Figs 36 and 37).

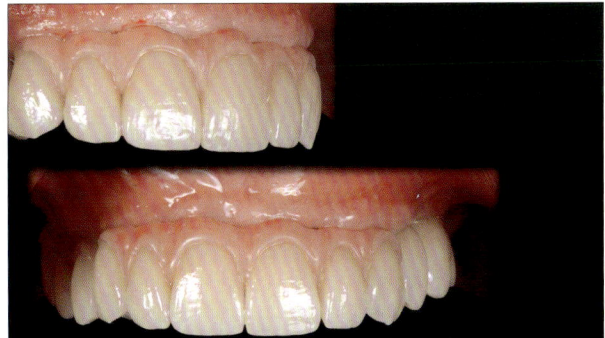

Fig 38   Final delivery of the bridge.

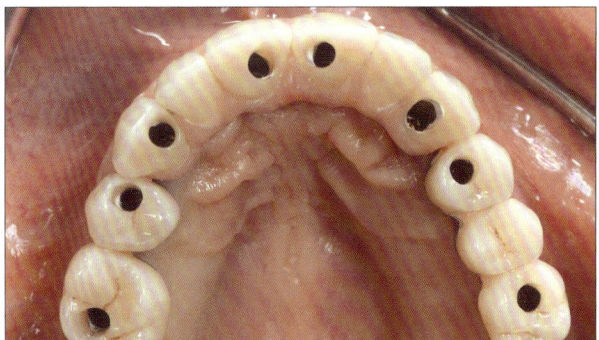

Fig 39   Occlusal view showing the screw-retained design.

The three segmented bridges (16 – 14, 13 – 11 – 21 – 23, 24 – 26) were screwed onto the respective implants at a torque of 35 Ncm. The screw access holes were sealed with PTFE rubber and composite (Gænial A02; GC, Tokyo, Japan) (Figs 38 and 39). At the 18-month follow-up, the peri-implant soft tissues showed no signs of inflammation and no significant bone resorption, and panoramic radiographs confirmed the correct insertion of the prosthesis. The patient felt comfortable and was satisfied with the esthetics, phonetics, and function of the restoration (Figs 40 to 42).

The lower arch was reconstructed using conventional restorative techniques, with a combination of conventional ceramic crowns and bridge restorations on the retained teeth (e.max Press; Ivoclar) and implant-supported crowns bonded onto Variobase abutments (Institut Straumann AG).

Follow-up visits including professional oral hygiene were scheduled every six months to ensure proper maintenance and check the efficacy of the patient's own oral hygiene.

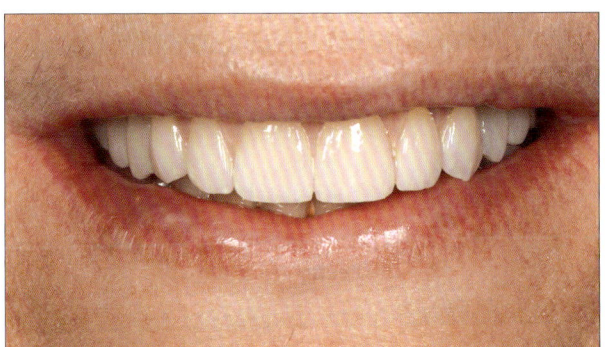

Fig 40   Patient smile after delivery.

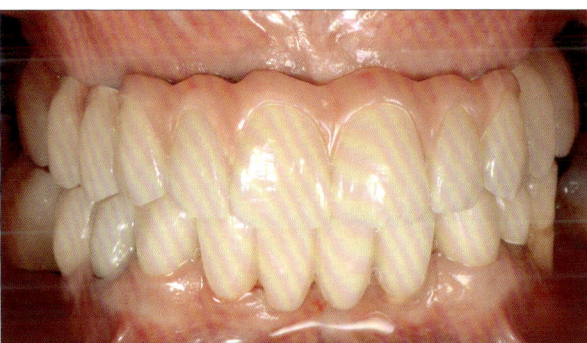

Fig 41   Intraoral view at the 18-month follow-up, including all definitive restorations.

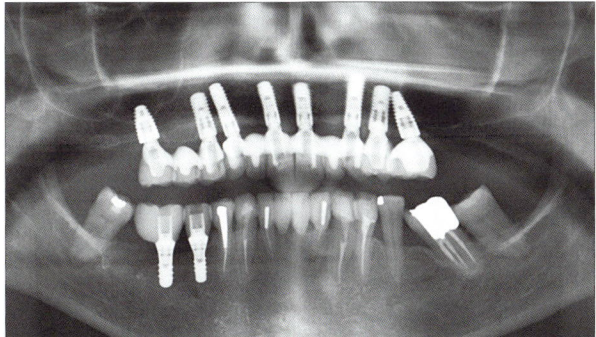

Fig 42   Panoramic X-ray at the 18-month follow-up.

13.9   Rehabilitating an Edentulous Maxilla with a Fixed Dental Prosthesis Following Provisional Immediate Loading

A. Lanis, O. Álvarez

A 54-year-old female patient in good general health was referred to the Advanced Prosthodontics and Digital Dentistry Clinic in Santiago, Chile for an evaluation. Her main complaint was the total absence of maxillary teeth and a failing removable upper complete acrylic prosthesis (Figs 1 to 4). She requested a fixed restoration based on osseointegrated implants. As part of the clinical examination, the SAC Assessment Tool was used, resulting in a surgical and restorative risk classification as "complex" (Figs 5 and 6). Preliminary diagnostic photographs were also taken.

The intraoral examination revealed three retained maxillary roots (teeth 13, 14, 23), which were deemed to be beyond further conventional treatment (Figs 7 to 9). The periodontal assessment revealed gingivitis (Figs 10 and 11).

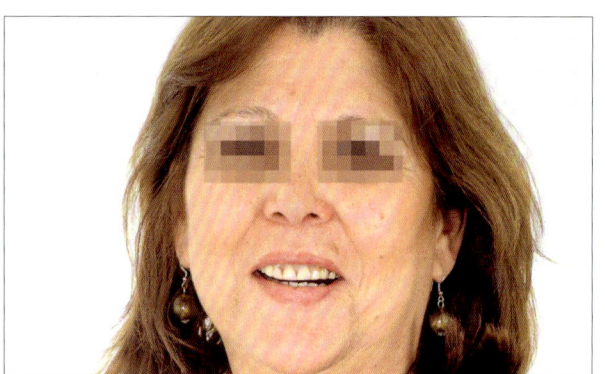

Fig 1   Initial situation. Patient with her removable maxillary prosthesis.

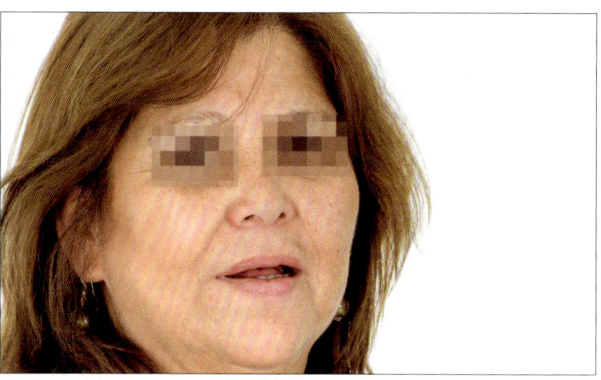

Fig 2   Initial situation. Patient without her removable maxillary prosthesis.

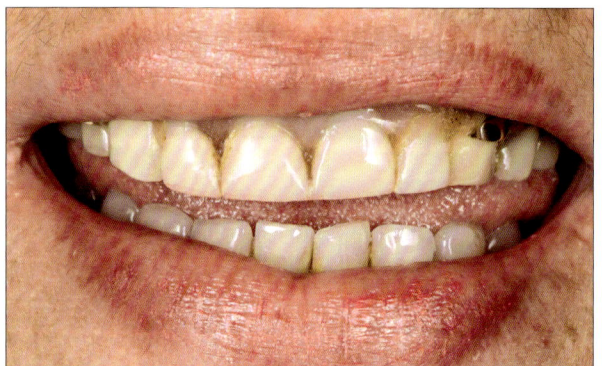

Fig 3   Frontal view of the patient's smile using her removable maxillary prosthesis.

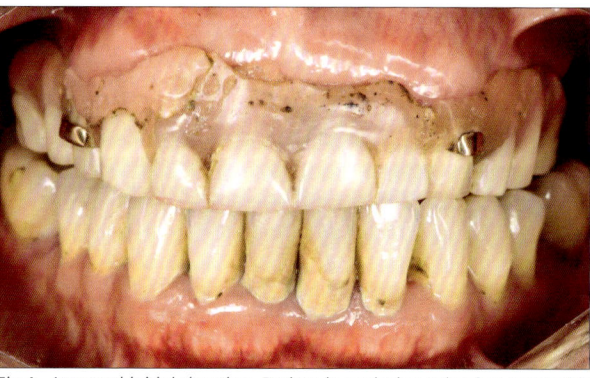

Fig 4   Intraoral initial situation. Patient in occlusion using her removable maxillary prosthesis.

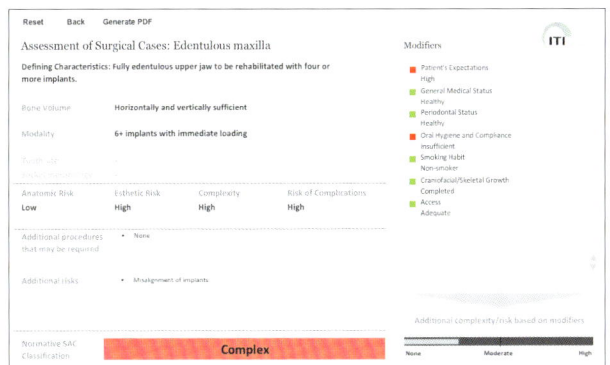

Fig 5   SAC assessment of the surgical case.

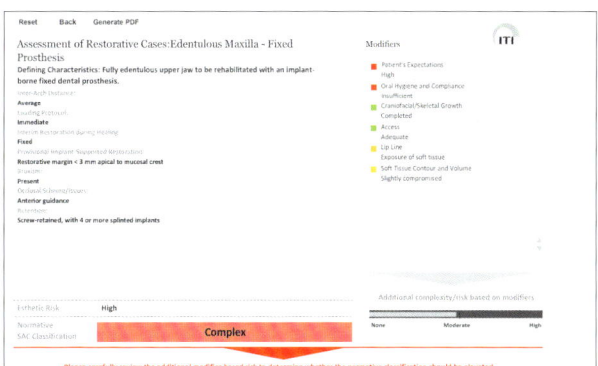

Fig 6   SAC assessment of the restorative case.

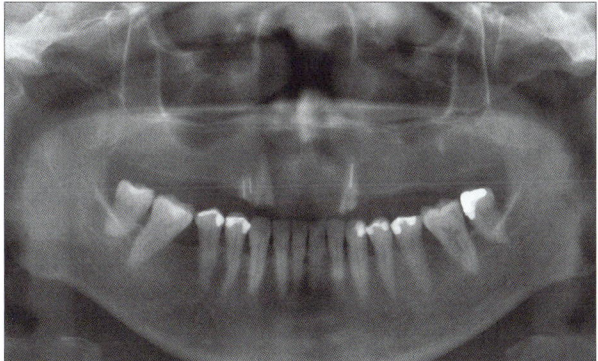

Fig 7   Patient's initial OPG.

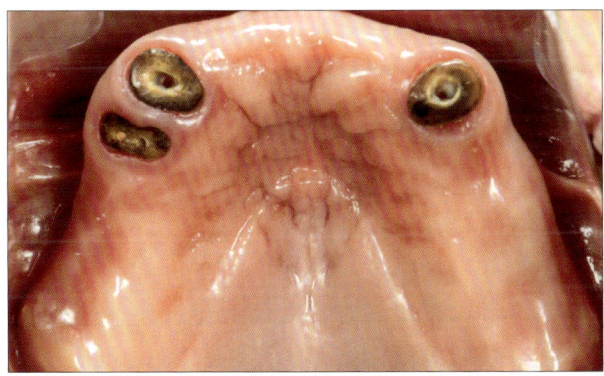

Fig 8   Occlusal view of the edentulous maxilla.

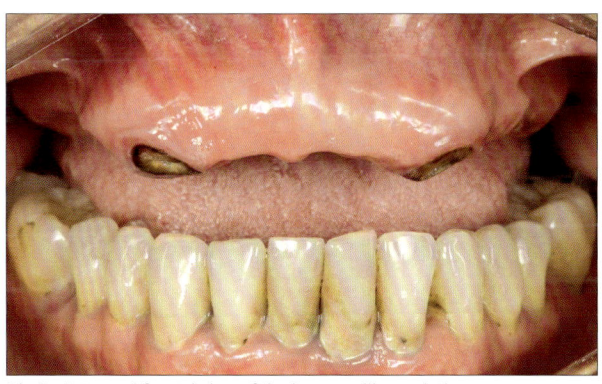

Fig 9   Intraoral frontal view of the intermaxillary relation.

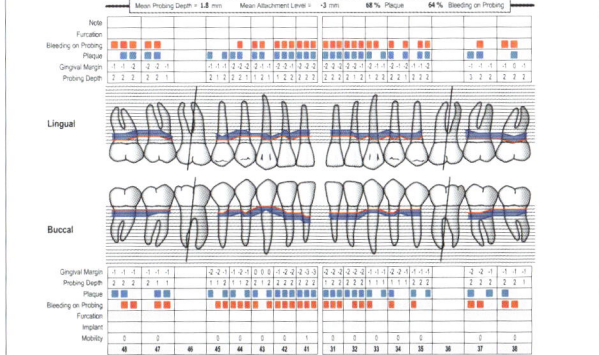

Fig 10   Maxillary periodontal assessment before periodontal treatment.

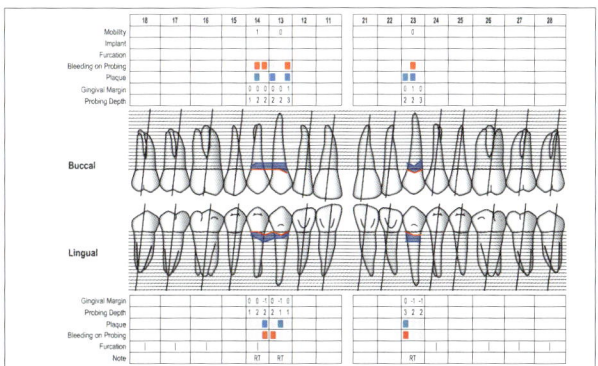

Fig 11   Mandibular periodontal assessment before periodontal treatment.

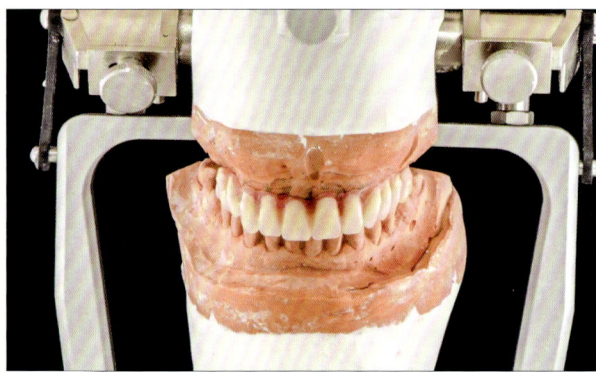

Fig 12   Maxillary set-up.

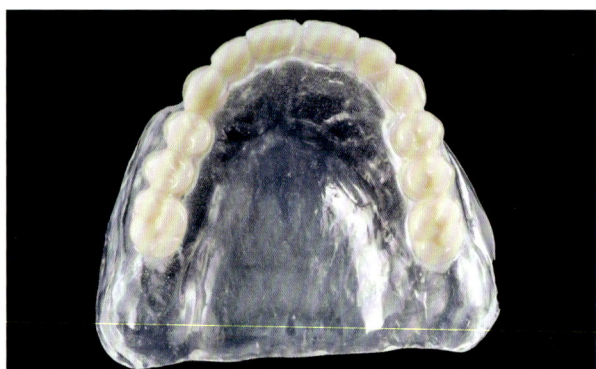

Fig 13   Maxillary radiographic template.

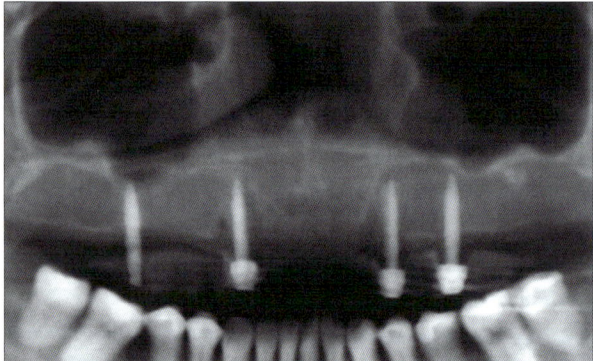

Fig 14   Panoramic CBCT view showing the four transitional implants in position, the O-rings, and the radiographic template. At site 15, limited vertical space prevented the installation of an O-ring.

The retained maxillary roots were removed and periodontal treatment performed. After four weeks of healing, a maxillary diagnostic prosthetic set-up was fabricated (Fig 12), clinically verified, and duplicated in translucent acrylic resin for a radiographic template (Fig 13). Steel ball bearings were added as radiopaque markers for the digitization process.

In the following appointment, four one-piece transitional implants (diameter 2 mm; Serson Implant, São Paulo, Brazil) were placed at sites 13, 15, 23, and 25 following the protocol proposed by Gallucci and coworkers (2015). This process aids in the stabilization of the radiographic template during CBCT scanning, improves the stability of the surgical guide during surgery, and provides retention and stability for the provisional restoration during the osseointegration period (Fig 14). O-ring attachments were included in the radiographic template.

CBCT scans were obtained following a dual-scan protocol. A first CBCT scan was taken of the patient wearing the template and a second scan of the radiographic template alone. The DICOM (Digital Communication in Medicine) files obtained by CBCT were imported into surgical planning software (coDiagnostiX; Dental Wings, Montreal, Quebec, Canada) for a complete virtual analysis and digital implant planning (Figs 15 and 16). The digitally designed surgical guide was then exported as an STL file and 3D-printed (Objet Eden 260VS; Stratasys, Eden Prairie, MN, USA). After cleaning, Guided Surgery T-Sleeves (Institut Straumann AG, Basel, Switzerland) were inserted into the surgical guide (Fig 17).

Rehabilitation of the edentulous maxilla was planned as the flapless computer-guided placement of seven Straumann Bone Level (BL) SLActive Guided Surgery implants (Institut Straumann AG). Following the mucosal-height information obtained from the digital analysis, screw-retained abutments (SRA; Institut Straumann AG) of appropriate heights were selected for full-arch splinted immediate loading. A full-arch CAD/CAM screw-retained metal-ceramic prosthesis was planned as the definitive restoration.

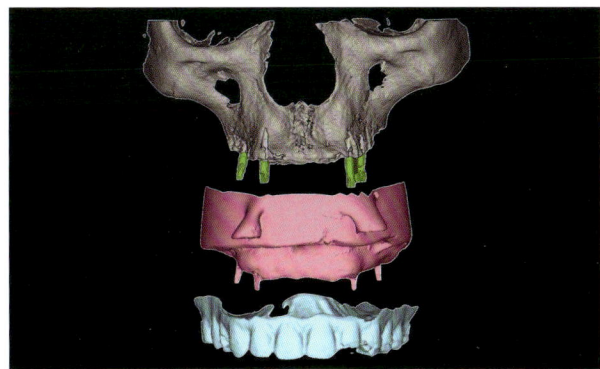

Fig 15 Digital 3D segmentation. Maxillary segmentation in gray. Transitional implants in green. Mucosal segmentation and transitional implants heads in pink. Radiographic template in light blue.

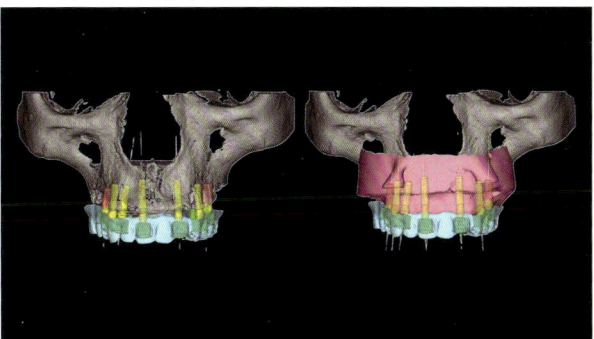

Fig 16 3D views showing superimposition of the different digital segmentations. Selected implants and abutments are included.

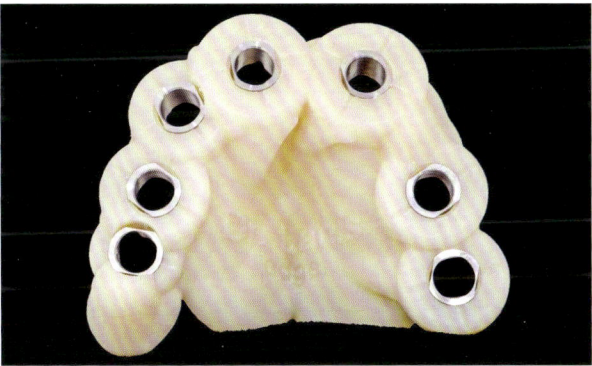

Fig 17 3D-printed surgical guide with Straumann Guided Surgery T-Sleeves.

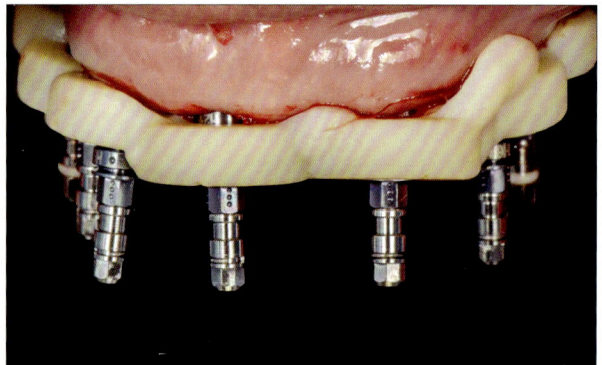

Fig 18   Flapless implant placement. Seven Straumann Bone Level Guided Surgery Implants in position.

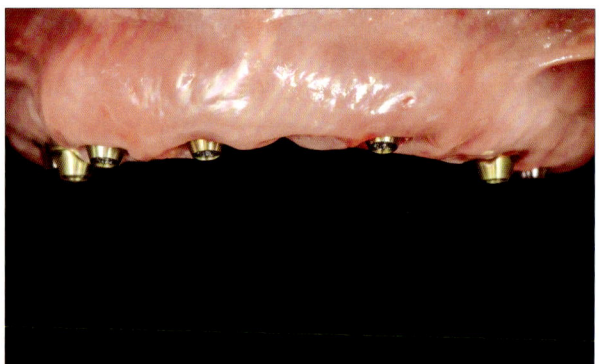

Fig 19   Intraoral frontal view of the preselected SRA abutments in position after implant placement.

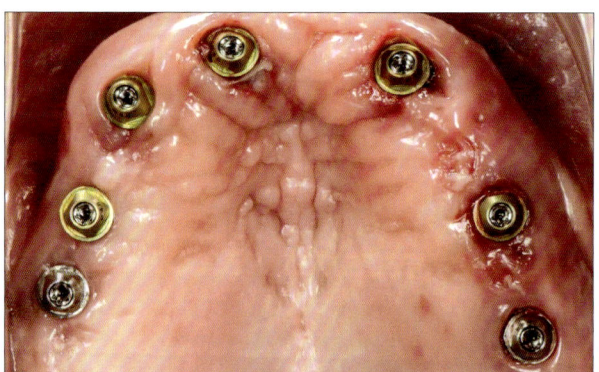

Fig 20   Occlusal view of the preselected SRA abutments in position after implant placement.

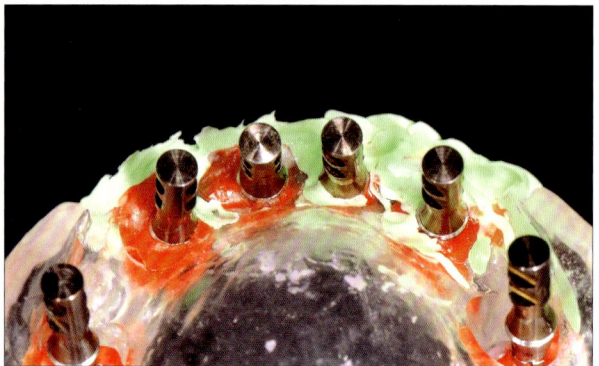

Fig 21   Inner view of the multifunctional tray with SRA analogs in position.

Surgical procedure

Local anesthesia was obtained with buccal and palatal infiltrations (Scandicaine 2%; Septodont, Lancaster, PA, USA). The surgical guide was attached to the maxillary transitional implants. Following the Straumann Guided Surgery Kit instructions, a circular scalpel was used to incise the keratinized tissue at each implant site. The surgical guide was then removed, and the precut soft tissue was removed with a Buser elevator (Hu-Friedy, Chicago, IL, USA). The surgical guide was then positioned once again over the transitional implants. Following the planned surgical protocol, osteotomies and implant placement were performed through the surgical guide, under a fully guided approach (Fig 18). The following implants were placed:

- BL NC, diameter 3.3.mm, length 12 mm, at sites 11 and 22
- BL NC, diameter 3.3 mm, length 10 mm, at sites 13, 14, and 24
- BL RC, diameter 4.1 mm, length 8 mm, at sites 16 and 26

(all Institut Straumann AG). All implants were inserted at a torque exceeding 50 Ncm. The implant transfer pieces, surgical guide, and transitional implants were then removed. The preselected SRA Abutments were positioned following the restorative protocol and torqued at 35 Ncm (Figs 19 and 20).

Based on the multifunctional tray protocol described by Leighton Fuentealba and Carvajal Herrera in 2013, the vertical dimension of occlusion, prosthetic teeth positions and implant/abutment positions were communicated to the lab technician (Fig 21). SRA cover screws (Institut Straumann AG) were placed over the abutments and the patient was dismissed until next day. 100 mg of ketoprofen (Profenid; Sanofi-Aventis, Bridgewater, NJ, USA) was prescribed to be taken twice per day for three days.

Using the multifunctional tray impression, the technician made a master cast and mounted it in an articulator (Whip Mix 2000; Whip Mix, Louisville KY, USA). A metallic framework was fabricated with titanium bar sections welded to temporary titanium cylinders (Institut Straumann AG). Using a silicon index as reference, the laboratory technician applied acrylic over the structure to create the same tooth shapes and positions as designed in the initial prosthetic set-up.

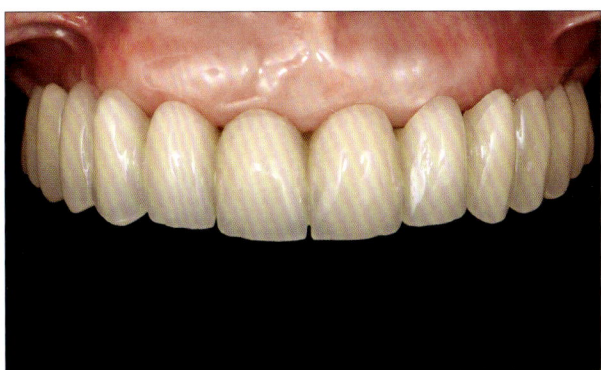

Fig 22 Intraoral frontal view of the provisional immediately loaded screw-retained restoration 24 hours after implant placement.

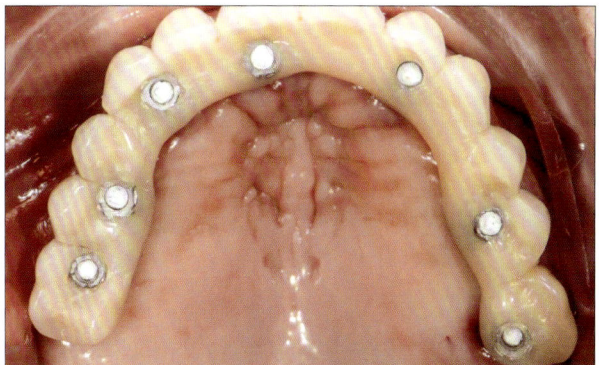

Fig 23 Intraoral occlusal view of the provisional immediately loaded screw-retained restoration 24 hours after implant placement.

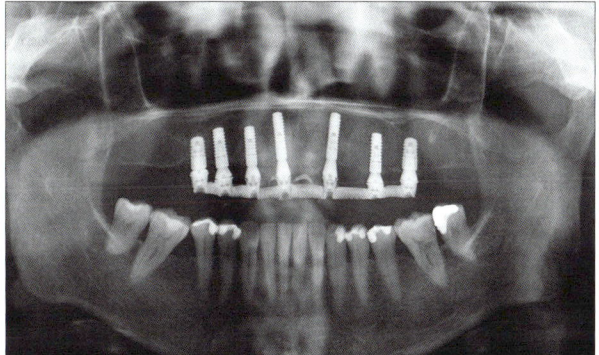

Fig 24 Panoramic radiograph after immediate prosthetic loading.

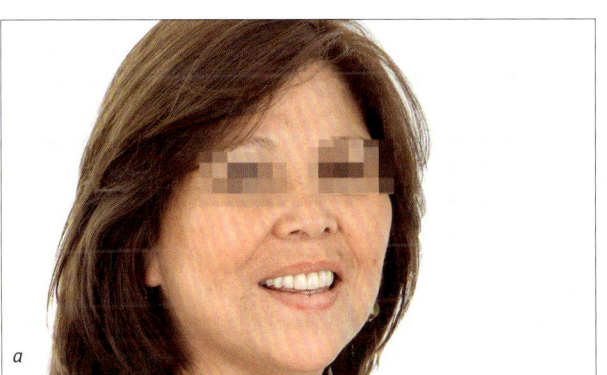

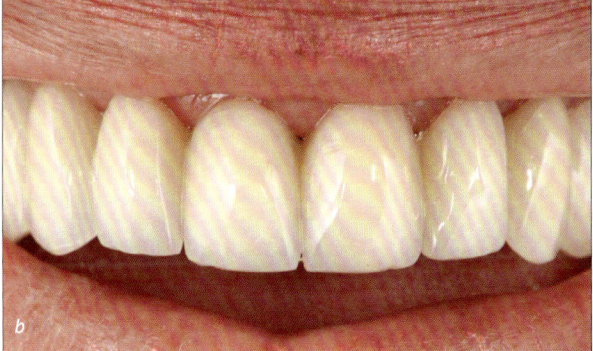

Figs 25a-b Extraoral view of the patient after immediate prosthetic loading (24 hours after implant placement) (a). Smile close-up view after immediate loading (b).

The patient was seen again 24 hours after implant placement for immediate loading with a titanium-reinforced screw-retained full-arch interim acrylic prosthesis (Figs 22 to 25).

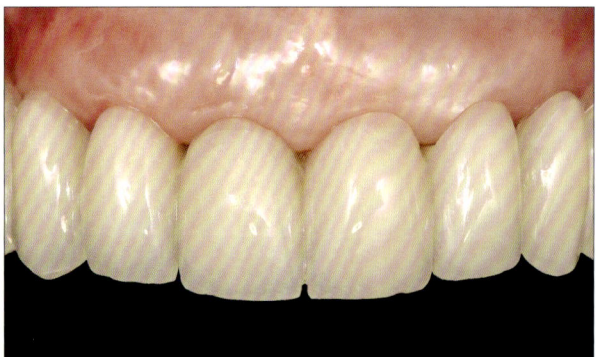

Fig 26   Frontal view of the provisional restoration at the 50-day follow-up.

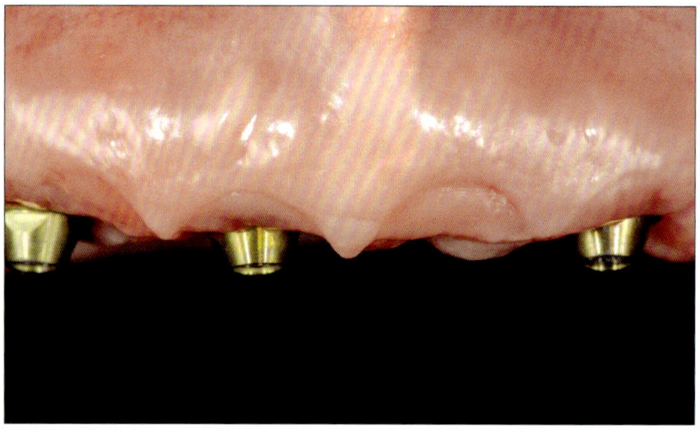

Fig 27   Soft-tissue condition after removing the provisional restoration at the 90-day follow up.

The patient was recalled at 3, 10, 14, 30, 50, 70, and 90 days; there were no complications. At the 30-days follow-up, soft-tissue contouring commenced by modifying the provisional emergence profiles with either the addition of composite resin (Tetric N-Ceram; Ivoclar Vivadent, Schaan, Liechtenstein) or by removing acrylic. This process was repeated at the following appointments until the desired soft-tissue profile was obtained (Figs 26 and 27).

At the 90-day follow-up, an abutment-level impression was taken using an open-tray technique and a master cast was made. Using the interim prosthesis as reference, the master cast was mounted in an articulator and a prosthetic wax-up performed (Fig 28). The wax-up was duplicated in acrylic resin for an intraoral verification. Minor modifications were performed by adding resin (Tetric N-Ceram; Ivoclar Vivadent) or by removing acrylic (Figs 29 and 30).

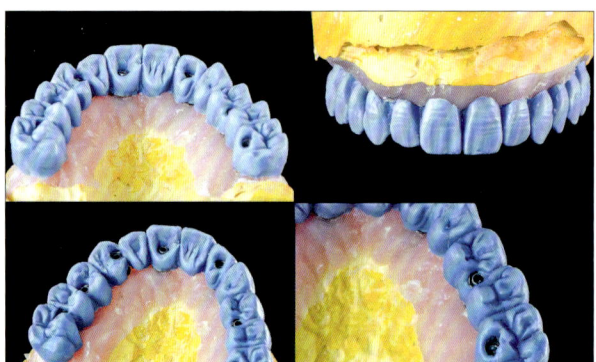

Fig 28   Full prosthetic wax-up over the master cast.

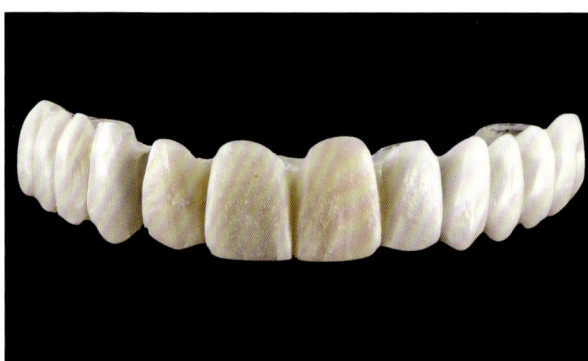

Fig 29   The wax-up was turned into acrylic for intraoral approval.

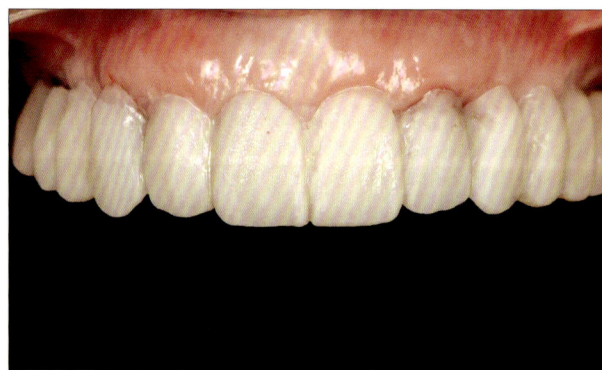

Fig 30   The acrylic structure was checked intraorally. Minor modifications were performed by adding resin or removing acrylic until the desired shape was obtained.

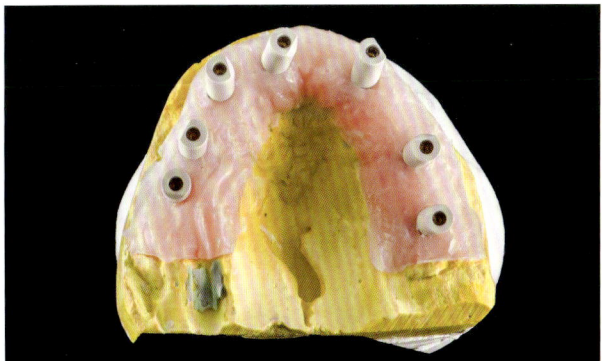

Fig 31   Master cast with SRA scanbodies in position for the scanning process.

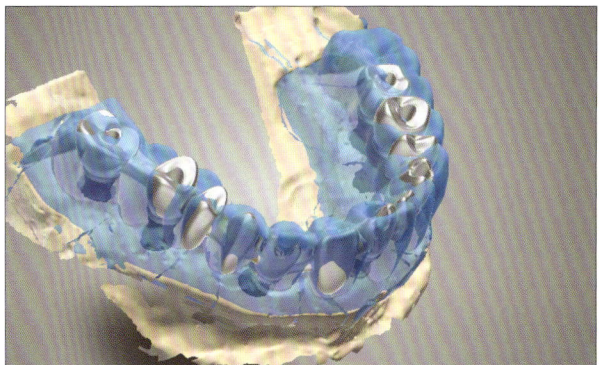

Fig 32   Straumann CARES digital design process. The prosthetic framework is designed based on the prosthetic wax-up with consideration for ceramic wall thicknesses.

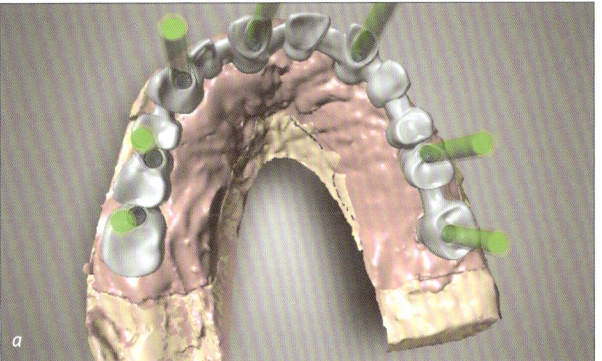

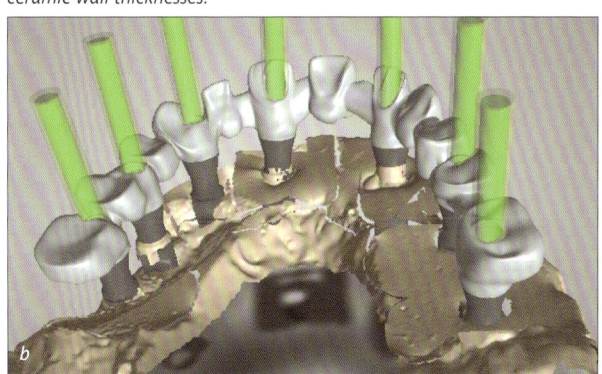

Figs 33a-b   Straumann CARES digital design process.

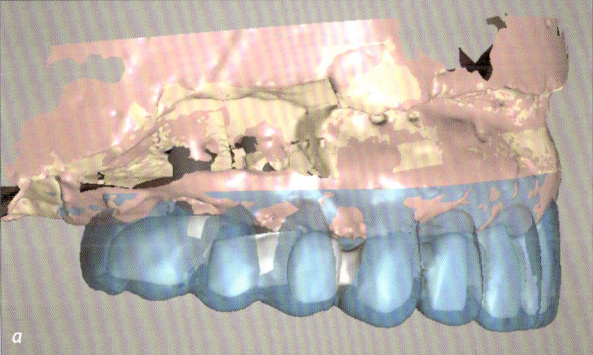

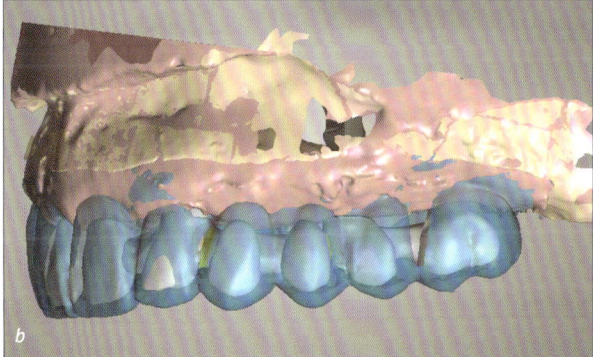

Figs 34a-b   Right (a) and left (b) lateral view of the digital prosthetic framework. The blue zone represents the wax-up. The gray zone represents the metallic framework.

The master cast with SRA scanbodies (Institut Straumann AG), antagonist model, and acrylic set-up were scanned with a lab scanner (3Series; Dental Wings). The resulting STL files were exported and sent to the Straumann CARES Milling Center in Curitiba, Brazil, for CAD/CAM fabrication of the definitive metallic framework (Figs 31 to 35).

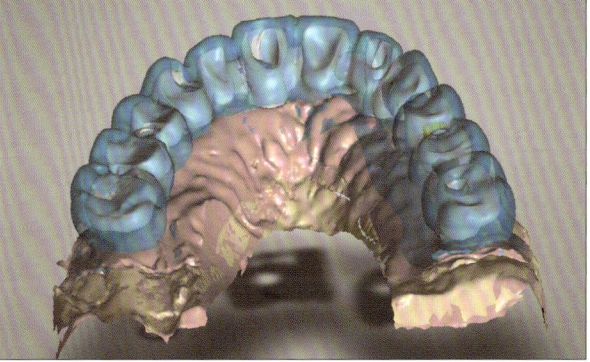

Fig 35   Posterior view of the digital prosthetic framework. The blue zone represents the wax-up. The gray zone represents the metallic framework.

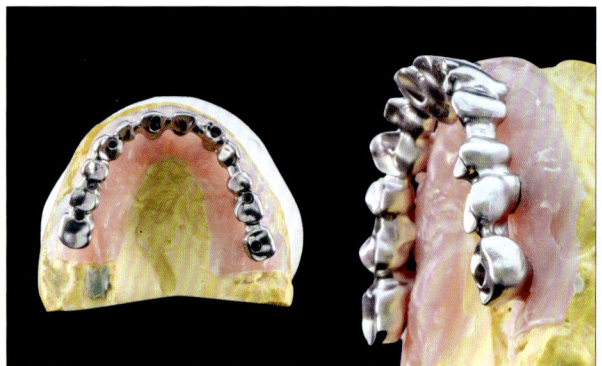

Fig 36   Cobalt-chromium milled full-arch structure.

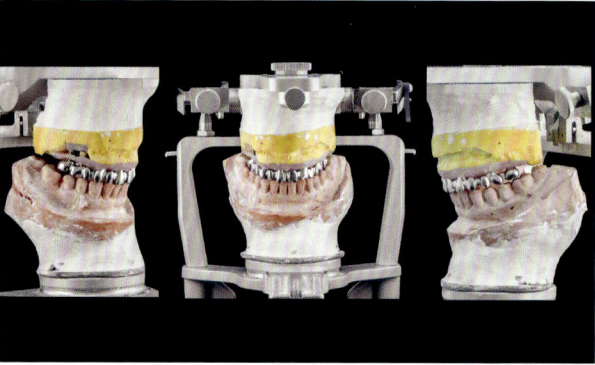

Fig 37   Cobalt-chromium milled full-arch structure checked in an articulator.

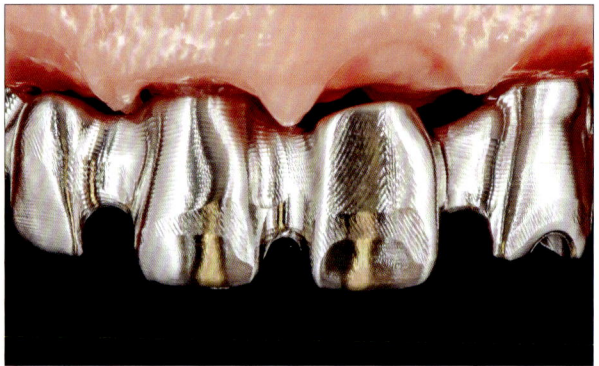

Fig 38   Frontal intraoral view of the milled structure in place.

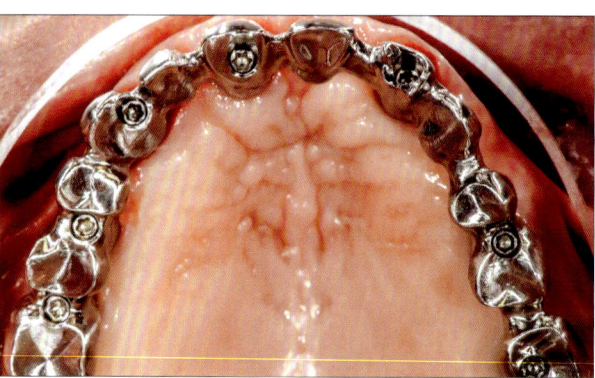

Fig 39   Occlusal intraoral view of the milled structure in place.

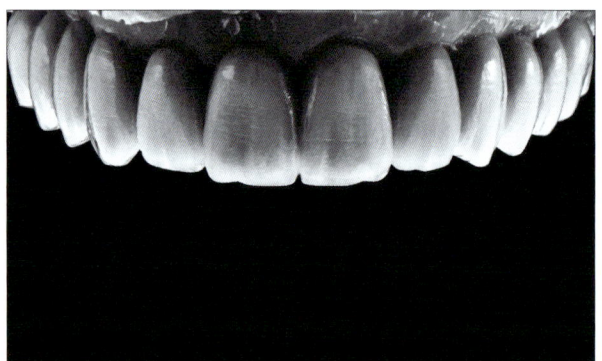

Fig 40   Based on the prosthetic set-up, Ceramco 3 Ceramic was built up on the metallic framework.

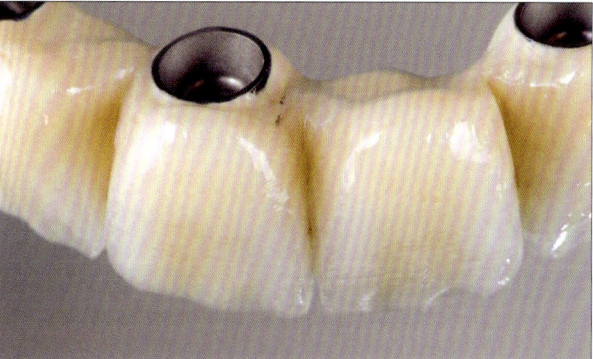

Fig 41   Close-up of the definitive restoration.

A milled cobalt-chromium full-arch structure was received ten days later. It was checked in the articulator and intraorally for adequate passive fit between components (Figs 36 to 39). Based on the wax-up, a silicone index was created as a reference for the build-up. Ceramco 3 (DentsplySirona, York, PA, USA) ceramic was selected as the veneering material (Figs 40 and 41).

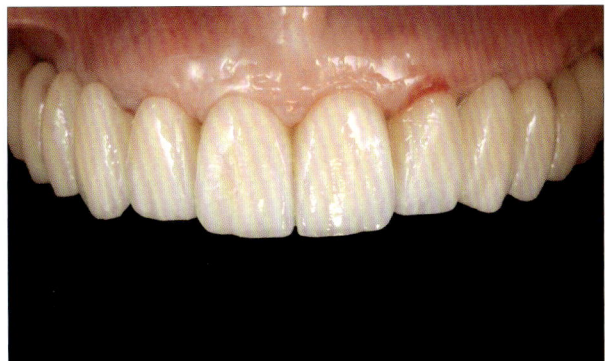

Fig 42   Delivery of the definitive restoration.

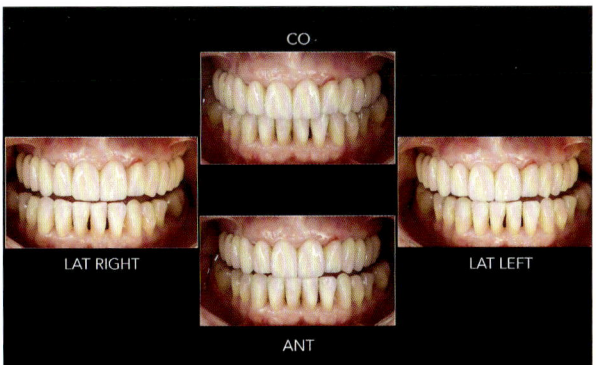

Fig 43   Function check of the definitive restoration. A mutually protected occlusion with anterior and canine guidance was selected as occlusal scheme.

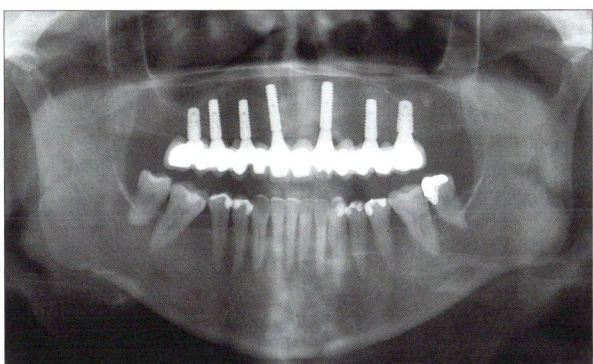

Fig 44   Panoramic control radiograph of the definitive restoration on the day of delivery.

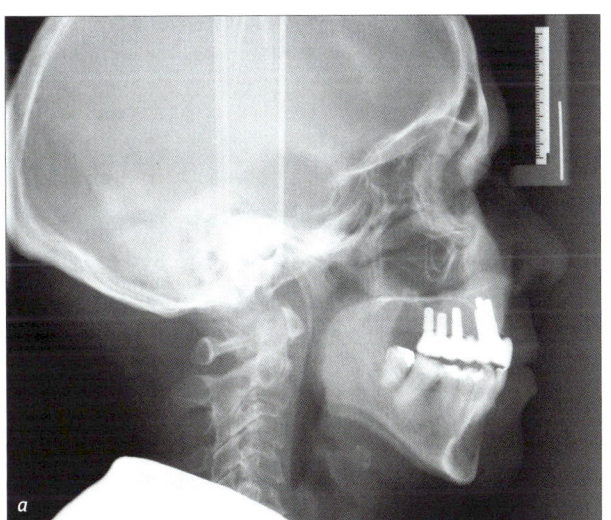

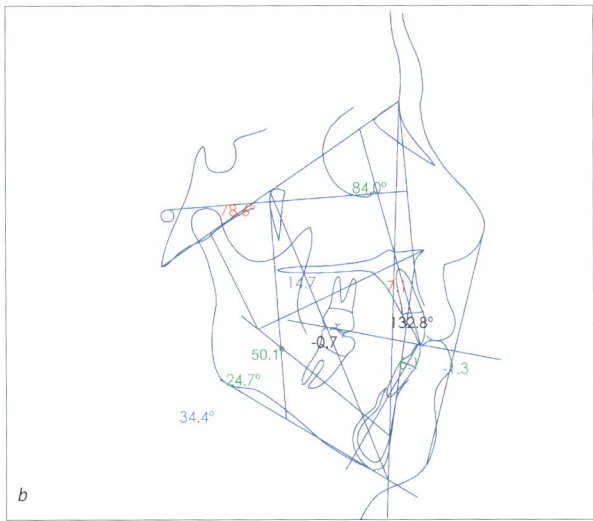

Figs 45a-b   Lateral control radiograph and cephalometric analysis on the day of delivery.

Following clinical try-in visits, the final restoration was delivered to the patient and tightened to 35 Ncm. The screw access holes were covered with PTFE plugs and composite resin (Tetric N-Ceram; Ivoclar Vivadent) (Fig 42). A mutually protected occlusion with anterior and canine guidance was selected as occlusal scheme, taking into consideration the periodontal proprioception provided by the natural antagonist dentition (Fig 43). An OPG and a lateral teleradiograph with a cephalometric analysis was performed (Fig 44 and 45a-b) to check if the prosthetic proposal was in concordance with normal cephalometric parameters. The patient was dismissed and followed for two years, with no complications reported (Figs 46 to 50).

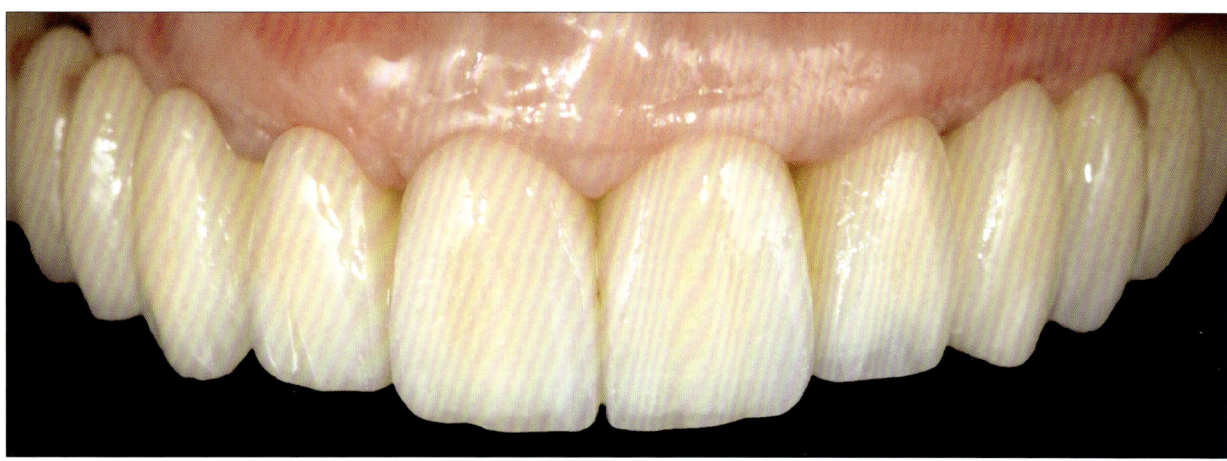

Fig 46   Intraoral frontal view of the definitive restoration at the 2-year follow-up.

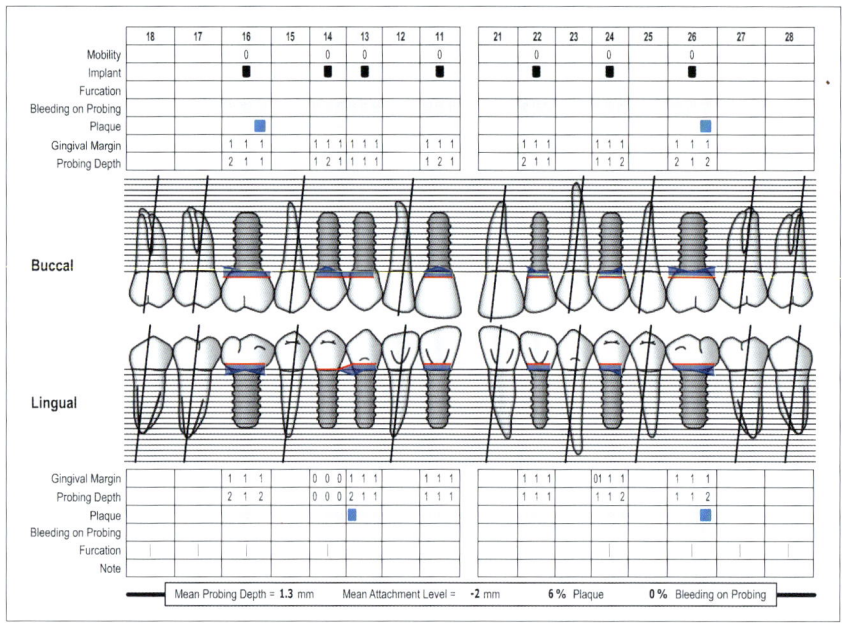

Fig 47   Maxillary periodontal assessment chart after implant treatment (at the 8-month follow-up).

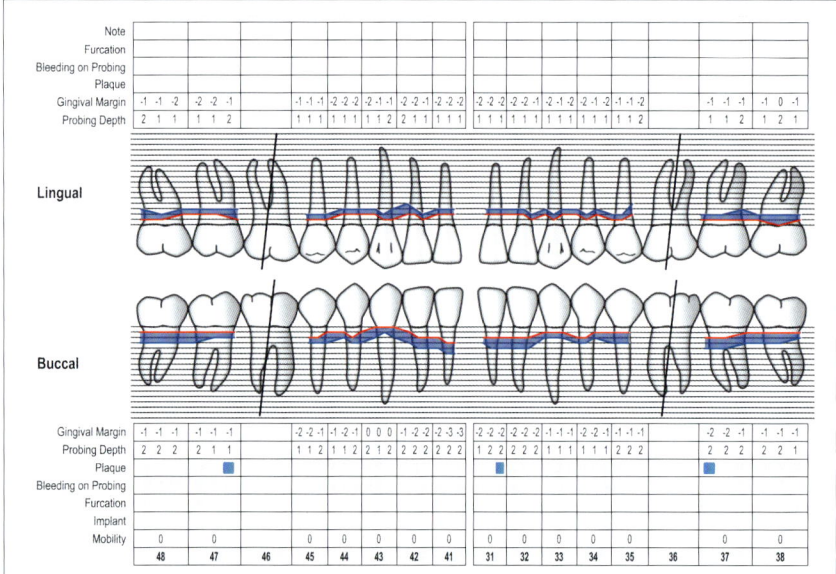

Fig 48   Mandibular periodontal assessment chart after treatment (at the 8-month follow-up).

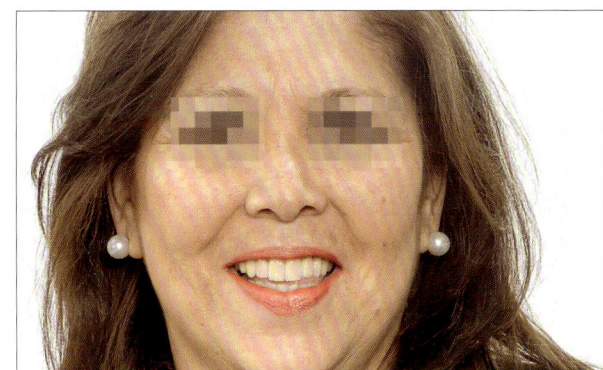

Fig 49   Extraoral photograph of the final result on the day of the prosthetic delivery.

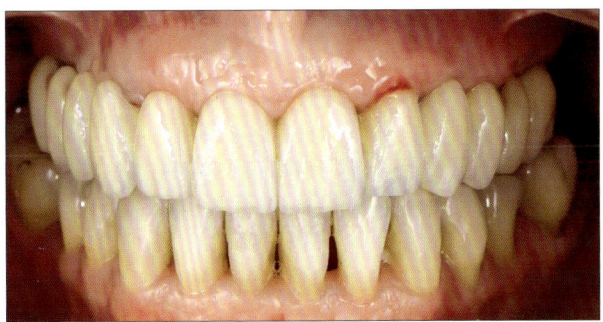 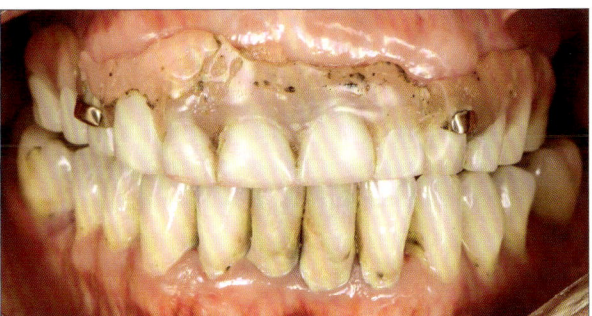

Fig 50   Intraoral photograph of the definitive restoration at the delivery day and the initial clinical situation.

Discussion

Computer-guided implant surgery allows for detailed surgical planning and accurate implant placement. This technique may also permit a less invasive surgical procedure by using a flapless approach. Since flapless surgery is a "blind" technique, it is highly recommended that the procedure be performed using a strict surgical guide, avoiding intraoperative complications such as fenestrations, dehiscences, or important anatomical structures. The computer-guided planning process facilitates the assessment of considerable surgical and prosthetic information prior to the actual surgery and should therefore enable accurate surgery while minimizing surgical risks.

Opinions are divided regarding the number of implants required to rehabilitate edentulous patients with fixed restorations. The number of implants used is usually determined based on multiple factors such as the prosthetic design and its extent, the distribution of implants, restorative materials used, shape of the maxillary arch, nature of the antagonist dentition, as well as patient-related and economic factors.

It is recognized that occlusal proprioception is considerably diminished with implant-supported restorations, affecting the mechanosensory balance. The absence of a periodontal ligament around dental implants and the consequent lack of proprioception could lead to occlusal overload, with biological and technical complications. In the clinical situation described, the maxillary rehabilitation was designed to be completely supported by osseointegrated implants. Accordingly, seven implants were planned and distributed to reduce interimplant distances, decreasing the width of connectors and providing maximal support for the prosthetic framework. The rehabilitation was designed to counteract the effects of any occlusal overload and to reduce stresses during function or parafunction.

The stiffness and durability of a multi-unit prosthetic framework is based on the material composition and on the height and width of the connectors. Consequently, an adequate prosthetic design and splinting are important for the performance of the structures in immediate loading. Different prosthetic materials have been proposed for full-arch immediate functional loading.

Amongst other authors, Tarnow and coworkers (1997), Gallucci and coworkers (2004), and Thomé and coworkers (2015) described different splinting techniques using metal or acrylic resin, respectively, reporting similar implant survival rates.

Even though the composition of the material seems to have no direct correlation with implant survival, care should be taken when using reduced connector dimensions, for example with fixed PF1 acrylic interim restorations. The rigid-splinting philosophy was originally described to equally distribute occlusal loads on recently placed implants, avoiding overloads on individual implants. Fracture of the prosthetic component as a result of reduced connector strength could overload individual implants during the early stages of osseointegration, leading to early implant failure.

Evidently, many factors should be considered before deciding on the material to be used for full-arch immediate functional loading with a provisional prosthesis to ensure adequate splinting during implant osseointegration.

In the clinical situation described, a rigid one-piece metallic framework was utilized as an interim restoration to reduce the risk of fracture associated with the selected prosthetic design. The availability of suitable sites for implant placement influenced the number of implants and their distribution, enabling the use of a one-piece milled metallic framework as the definitive option, which avoided the undesirable cantilevers that might have been required by a segmented bridge design.

Acknowledgments

Clinical procedures and photography
Dr. Orlando Álvarez del Canto – Santiago, Chile
Dr. Rodrigo Danesi – Santiago, Chile

Laboratory procedures
Dental Technician Victor Romero – Santiago, Chile
Dental Technician Geraldo Thomé Junior – Curitiba, Brazil

13.10 Oral Rehabilitation Aided by Digital Dentistry: Immediate Functional Loading with a Prefabricated Provisional Restoration

A. Lanis

Evaluation, data acquisition, and stabilization

A 45-year-old female patient was referred to the Advanced Prosthodontics and Digital Dentistry Clinic in Santiago, Chile for evaluation. Her main complaints were the long-term esthetic and functional problems related to advanced oral deterioration. In addition, the patient described low-intensity permanent bilateral pain in the TMJ region (Figs 1 to 6).

After a clinical analysis and preliminary imaging, articular, periodontal, muscular, and prosthetic diagnoses were performed (Figs 7 and 8). As part of the clinical examination, an SAC assessment was performed, which classified the case as Complex with regard to the surgical and restorative risk.

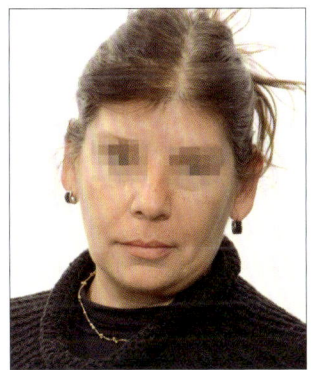

Fig 1   Patient's face at baseline.

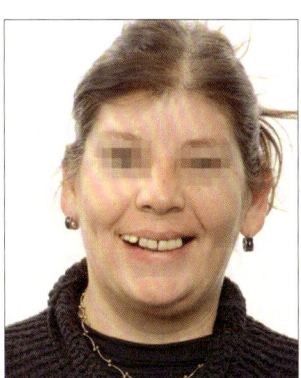

Fig 2   Patient's smile at baseline.

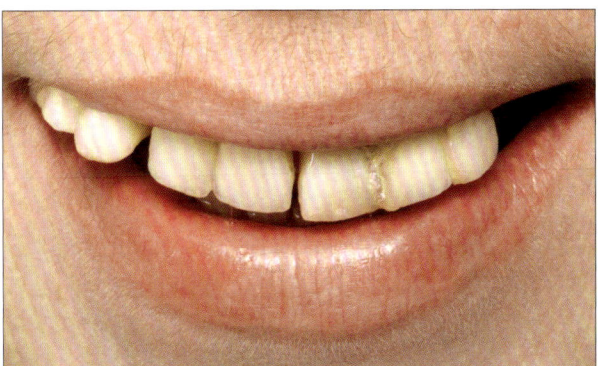

Fig 3   Baseline smile close-up.

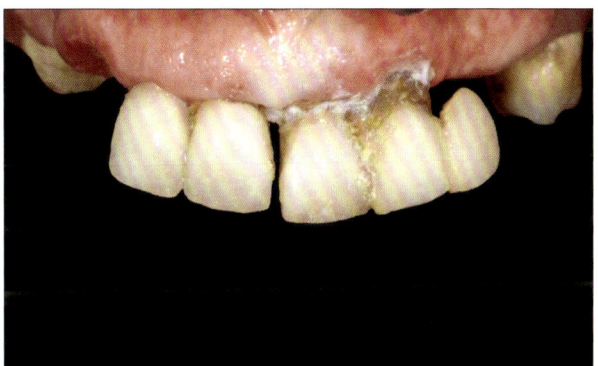

Fig 4   Maxillary baseline situation.

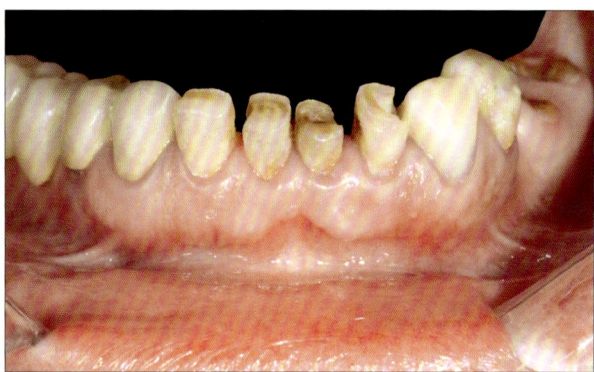

Fig 5   Mandibular baseline situation.

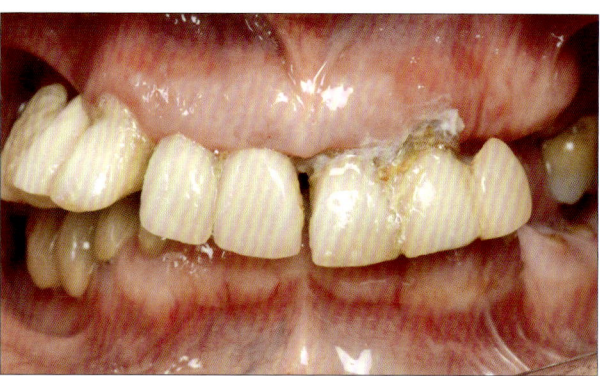

Fig 6   Maximum intercuspation.

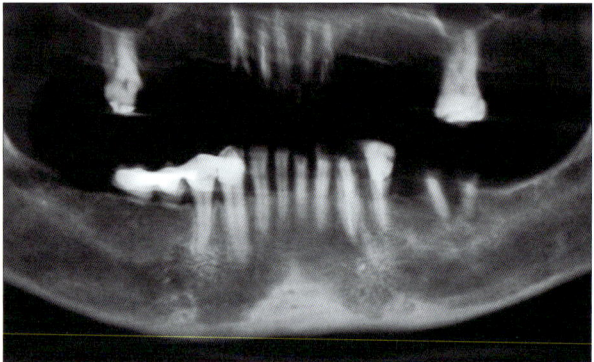

Fig 7   Baseline OPG.

Based on the initial situation, it was decided for the first phase of treatment to consist of comprehensive periodontal treatment, endodontic retreatment of teeth 31 – 33 and 41, and extraction of the non-restorable 13 – 24, 34 – 36, and 44. The patient wore several tooth-supported ceramic bridges with a poor prosthetic and periodontal prognosis. Since her occlusion had been unstable for a prolonged period, the initial plan was to focus on providing a stable occlusion.

Prior to the extractions, conventional alginate impressions were taken (Tropicalgin; Zhermack, Badia Polesine, Italy) and cast in stone (EliteRock; Zhermack). Using wax rims and a facebow, the models and casts were mounted in an articulator (Whip Mix 2000; Whip Mix, KY, USA) to obtain a tentative vertical dimension and sagittal maxillomandibular relation. The non-restorable teeth were then trimmed from the casts and modified zones were contoured, simulating the soft-tissue profile after the extractions.

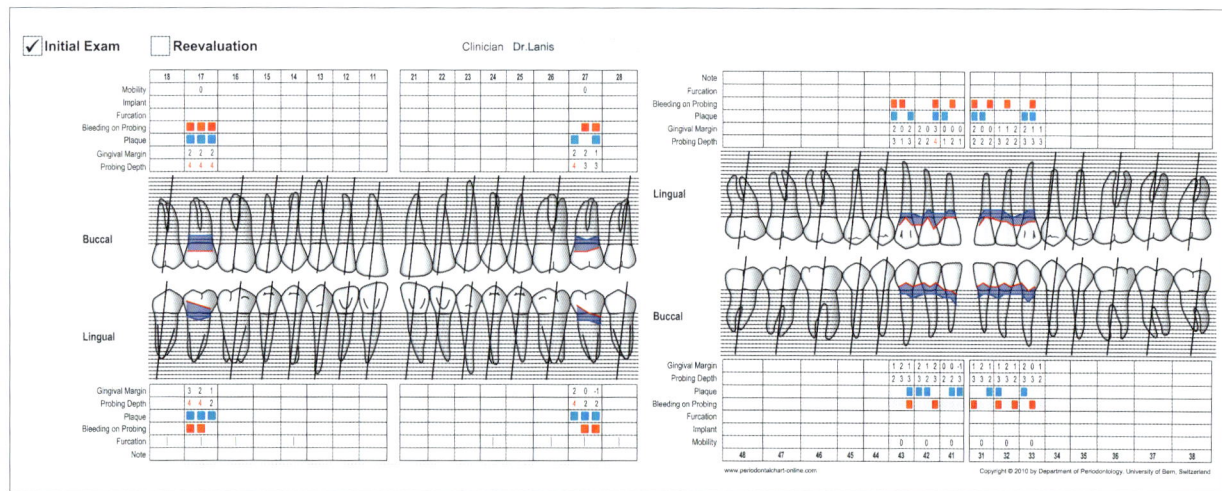

Fig 8   Periodontal chart of the restorable teeth.

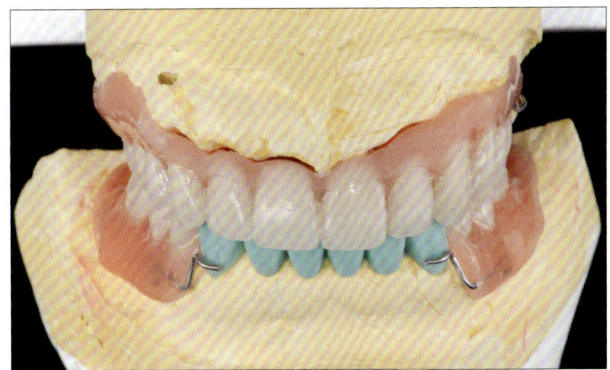

Fig 9 Mounted casts and models without the trimmed cast teeth. Diagnostic wax-up of the restorable lower anterior teeth. Maxillary and mandibular provisionals.

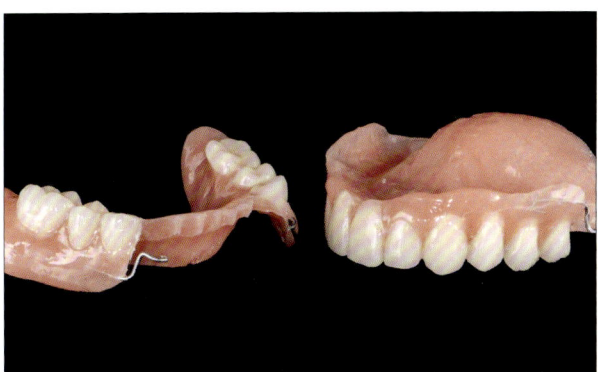

Fig 10 Immediate prostheses as provisionals.

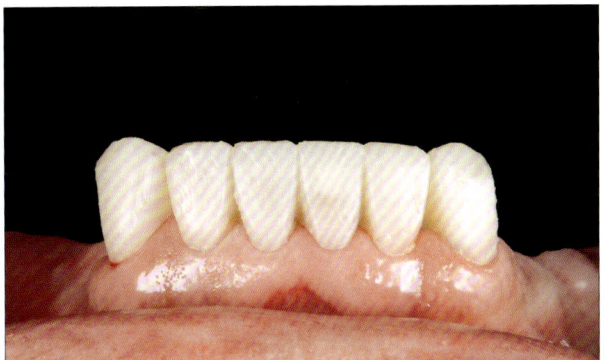

Fig 11 Mandibular anterior mock-up based on the wax-up. After endodontic retreatment, these teeth were adhesively reconstructed on fiber posts.

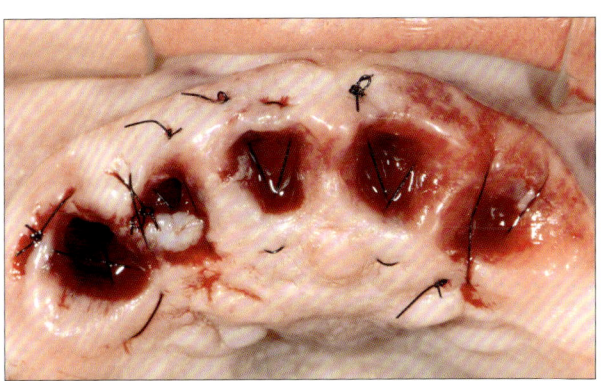

Fig 12 Maxillary non-restorable teeth extracted and sockets sutured.

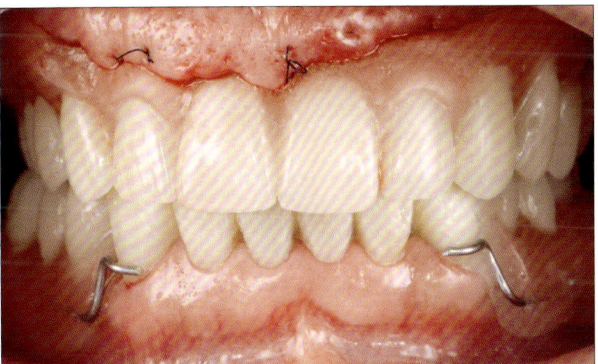

Fig 13 Installed provisionals after the extractions, following the proposed restorative plan.

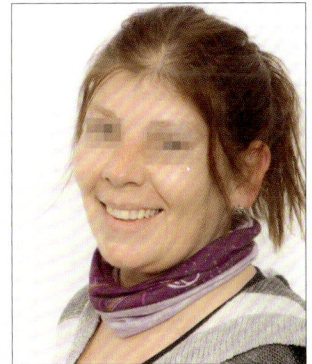

Fig 14 At the 21-day follow-up. The patient is wearing the provisionals.

Maxillary and mandibular immediate acrylic provisional restorations were fabricated (Figs 9 and 10). In addition, a functional wax-up of the restorable mandibular anterior teeth was performed.

Following the endodontic retreatment of teeth 31–33 and 41, the mandibular anteriors were restored with fiber posts and reconstructed with bisacryl (Luxatemp Star A1; DMG, Hamburg, Germany) based on the wax-up (Fig 11). Under local anesthesia (Scandicaine 2%: Septodont, PA,

USA), teeth 13–24, 34–36, and 44 were extracted as planned. Sutures were placed across the maxillary sockets for clot maintenance (Perma-Hand Silk 4-0; Ethicon, Johnson & Johnson, NY, USA) (Fig 12). The maxillary and mandibular prostheses were fitted (Fig 13). 100 mg of ketoprofen (Profenid; Sanofi-Aventis, NJ, USA) twice a day for three days was prescribed. The sutures were removed at the seven-day follow-up. The patient was reviewed at 14, 21, 30, and 45 days; no biological or prosthetic complications were observed (Fig 14).

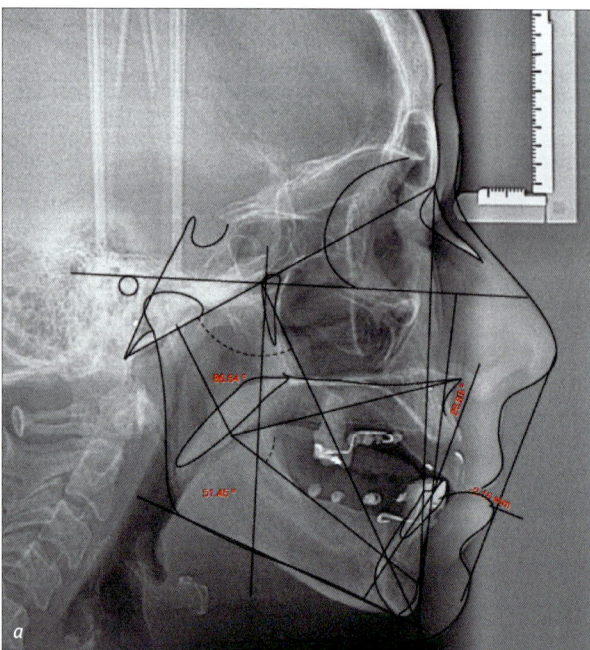

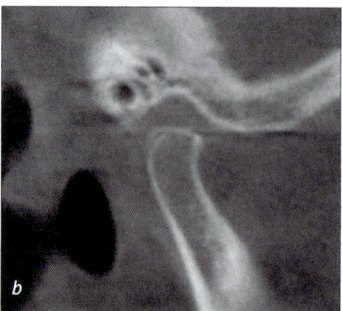

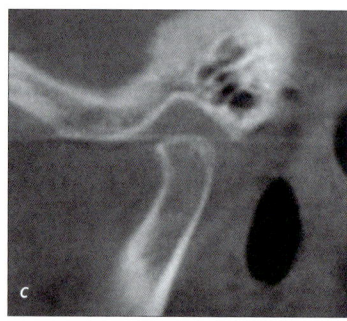

Figs 15a-c Cephalometric analysis and TMJ CBCT, with the patient wearing the provisionals.

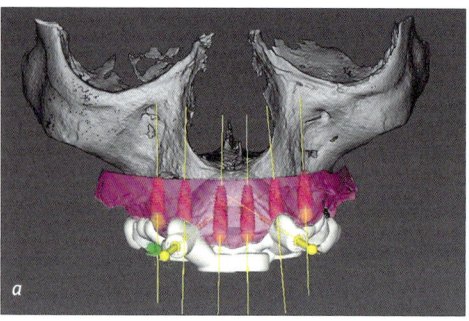

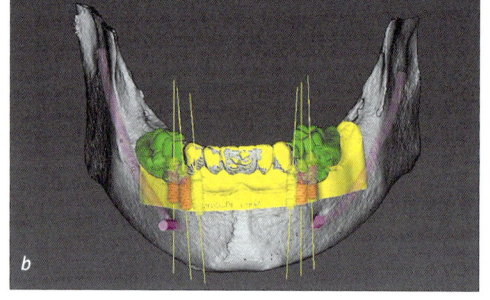

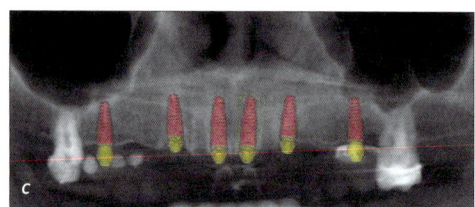

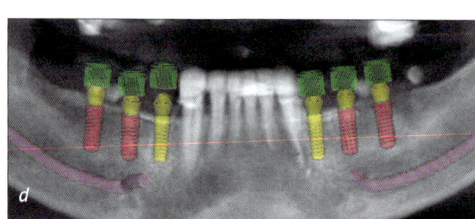

Figs 16a-d Maxillary and mandibular virtual implant planning.

Articular, muscular, functional, and phonetic evaluations were performed at each review to determine whether the vertical dimension and sagittal and transversal maxillomandibular relations were appropriate. Minor modifications were made by occlusal adjustment.

After 45 days of occlusal stabilization, cephalometric analysis (Fig 15) and cone-beam computer tomography (CBCT) images of both temporomandibular joints (TMJ)

were obtained to evaluate the new condylar positions in the glenoid fossae. Both condyles appeared in an adequate centric relation, in accordance with an adequate initial treatment position. The patient did not show any signs or symptoms of articular or muscular pathology during this phase. The previous diffuse TMJ pain also disappeared approximately two weeks after occlusal stabilization.

After the provisionals had been approved functionally and esthetically by the patient, both restorations were converted into radiographic templates by adding rounded steel balls, 2 mm in diameter, as radiopaque markers. A dual-scan protocol was indicated. A CBCT scan was taken with the patient wearing the templates and two additional CBCT scans were taken of each radiographic template, respectively. Then a second set of alginate impressions were taken of the maxilla and mandible, poured, and scanned with an optical laboratory scanner (3Series; Dental Wings, Montreal, Canada). The Digital Communication in Medicine (DICOM) files from the CBCT scans and the Standard Triangle Language (STL) files obtained with the optical scanner were imported to surgical planning software (coDiagnostiX; Dental Wings) for a complete virtual analysis and for digital implant planning (Fig 16).

Planning phase

To treat the partially edentulous mandible, a flapless, computer guided implant placement of six implants (Straumann BL SLActive; Institut Straumann AG, Basel, Switzerland) implants at sites 34 – 36 and 44 – 46 was planned. An early loading protocol was prescribed for the mandibular implants. Three-unit splinted screw-retained monolithic zirconia CAD/CAM restorations were planned bilaterally, to be retained at implant level. The lower anterior teeth were to be restored with monolithic lithium disilicate CAD/CAM crowns.

For the edentulous maxilla, flapless computer-guided placement of six implants (Straumann BLT SLActive; Institut Straumann AG) was planned. An immediate-loading protocol with a PMMA CAD/CAM screw-retained functional provisional restoration was proposed. Based on the digital analysis of the mucosal thickness, different heights of screw-retained abutments (SRA; Institut Straumann AG) were selected.

The provisional CAD/CAM restoration was designed and fabricated prior to implant placement based on the radiographic templates (Table 1). A full-arch screw-retained zirconia CAD/CAM structure was planned as the definitive prosthetic solution. For an optimum esthetic result, it was decided to manually build up ceramic on the buccal surfaces of the milled structure. Two posterior molars on each side (17 and 27) were to be maintained to preserve periodontal proprioception, with tooth 27 being restored with a monolithic zirconia CAD/CAM crown.

Table 1 Protocol summary for CAD/CAM provisionals prior to implant surgery.

Clinical examination
Prosthetic planning
CBCT and STL data acquisition
Digital planning
Surgical guide and master model design
Surgical guide and master model 3D printing
Implant replica insertion through surgical guide
Articulator mounting
Abutments installation over implant replicas
Model scanning
Provisional restoration design
Provisional restoration milling
Cementation of interfaces
Articulator checking

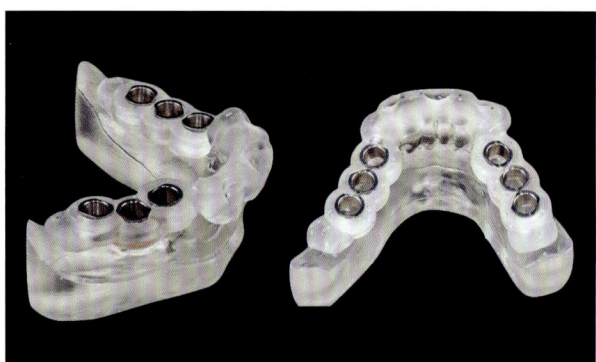

Fig 17   Mandibular surgical guide over a 3D-printed model.

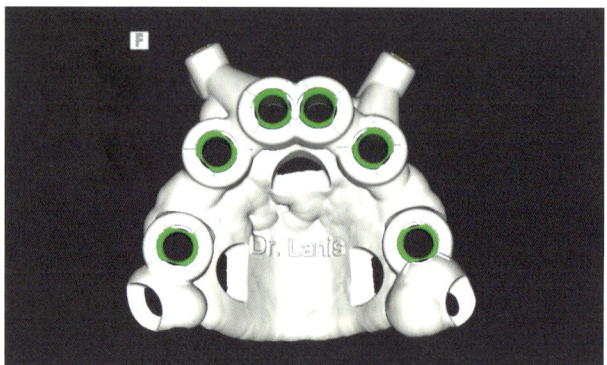

Fig 18   Digital design of the maxillary surgical guide.

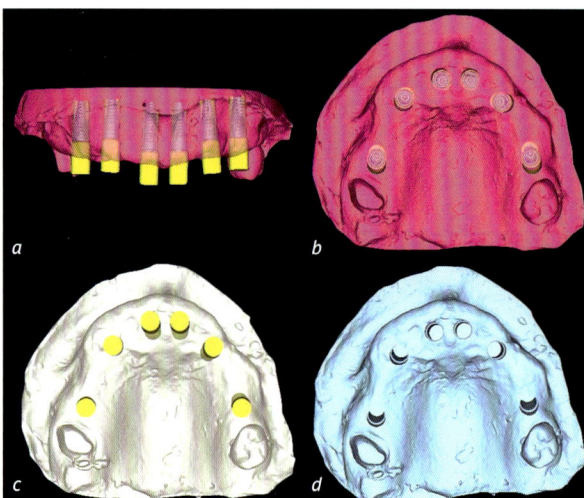

Figs 19a-d   Advanced virtual segmentation to incorporate implant replicas into the 3D soft-tissue model.

Surgical guides, master model, and fabrication of the provisional restorations

Following digital implant planning, the mandibular surgical guide was designed and 3D-printed using a FDA-approved resin material (PreForm, Formlabs 2, Dental SG Resin; Formlabs, MA, USA). Guided-surgery T-sleeves (Institut Straumann AG) were press-fitted into the guide's sleeve holes (Fig 17).

The maxillary guide was designed based on an advanced segmentation of the internal region of the radiographic template combined with a STL file of the maxillary edentulous ridge. Two anchor pins with appropriate sleeves (Neodent, Curitiba, Brazil) were digitally placed buccal to sites 13 and 23 to optimize the retention of the surgical template (Fig 18). Using a feature included in coDiagnostiX 9, it was possible to incorporate implant replicas into the 3D soft-tissue segmentation, following the implant coordinates as determined during planning. After subtraction of the implant replicas, a virtual model with spaces or "holes" could be generated where "real" implant replicas would be inserted (Fig 19). Because the implant replicas were of a standardized size, all digital analogs were designed the same — 4.1 mm in diameter and 10 mm in length. Since the selected SRA abutments have a 4.6-mm profile and the planned implants have a 4.1-mm platform diameter, a circumferential profile 4.8 mm in diameter and 6 mm in height profile was designed at the implant platform level (Fig 20). The proposed profile design would help achieve a correct fit of the SRA abutments and the replicas in the 3D-printed model. The surgical guide and master model were then exported in STL format and imported into 3D printing software. Both were then 3D-printed (Fig 21).

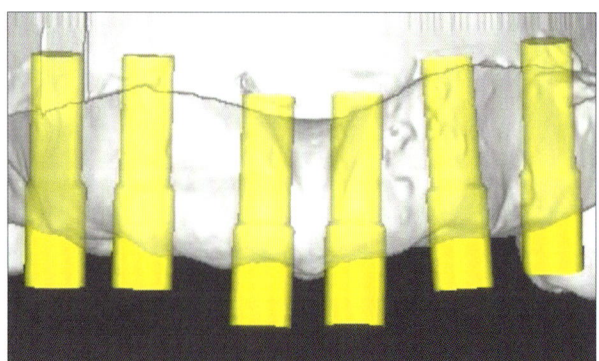

Fig 20   A circumferential profile 4.8 mm in diameter and 6 mm in height profile was designed at the implant platform level.

Once both 3D printed devices were cleaned, guided-surgery T-sleeves (Institut Straumann AG) and Neodent fixation pin sleeves (Neodent, Curitiba, Brazil) were pressed into the surgical guide, which was then mounted on the printed master model and secured with the anchor pins (Neodent, Curitiba, Brazil). Following the insertion protocol and using guided-surgery implant mounts (Institut Straumann AG), implant replicas were inserted through the designed holes, respecting the planned implant depth (Fig 22). The implant mounts and the surgical guide were then removed.

The surgical templates were tested intraorally for correct fit. After checking, a new facebow record was made with the patient's maxillary prosthesis as an occlusal reference. An occlusal index was also performed by registering the previously defined intermaxillary relation (Occlufast; Zhermack). The maxillary and mandibular interim prostheses were then removed and placed on the 3D-printed master model and the mandibular cast, respectively. Both were then mounted in an articulator (Fig 23).

The individual models, both prostheses, and their occlusal relationships were scanned (3Series; Dental Wings). To transfer the implant and abutment positions, SRA scanbodies (Institut Straumann AG) were positioned over the SRA abutments. All digital information was imported into a CAD software package (Dental System; 3Shape, Copenhagen, Denmark).

Based on the denture tooth positions and their occlusal relations, an implant-supported bridge was designed and functionally checked in a virtual articulator (Fig 24). The digital structure was then exported as an STL file and milled (K5; VHF, Ammerbuch, Germany) in PMMA (AnaxCAD; Anaxdent, Stuttgart, Germany). Once finished, it was cleaned and stained. Metallic interfaces (Institut Straumann AG) were cemented into the inner zone of the prosthetic connections of the PMMA framework (Multilink; Ivoclar Vivadent, Schaan, Liechtenstein) (Fig 25). The provisional CAD/CAM restoration was mounted on the 3D master model and functionally checked in the analog articulator (Fig 26).

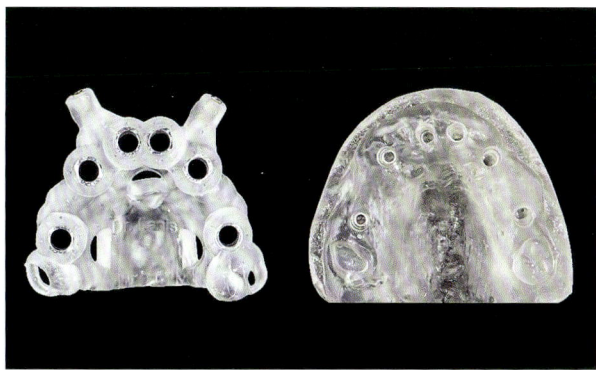

Fig 21   3D-printed surgical guide and 3D-printed master model with hollow cylinders for placing the implant replicas.

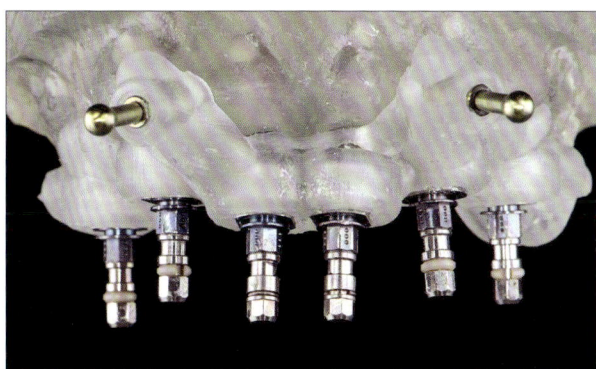

Fig 22   Implant replicas were placed through the surgical guide into the designed spaces of the master model and replicas secured with liquid adhesive through external holes.

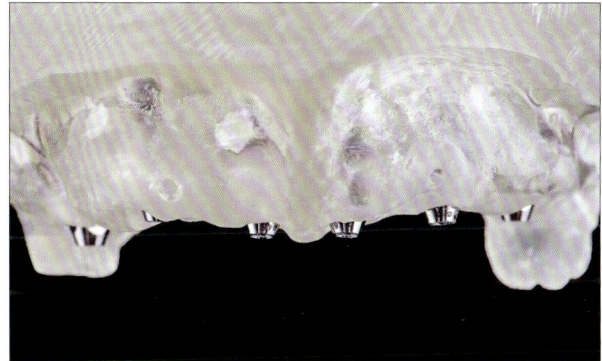

Fig 23   With the 3D-printed master model mounted in the analog articulator, SRA abutments were positioned following the restorative protocol.

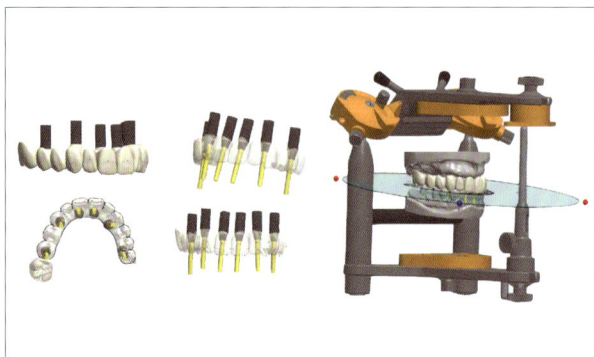

Fig 24   CAD design of the provisional restoration, which was checked for function in a virtual articulator.

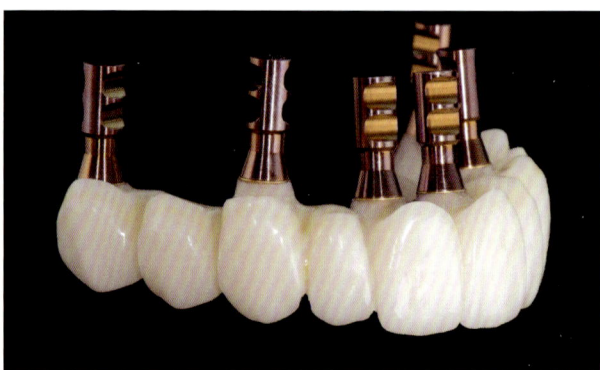

Fig 25   PMMA CAD/CAM provisional after milling and staining. SRA analogs were positioned on the structure to visually check the future implant positions in relation to the prosthetic profiles.

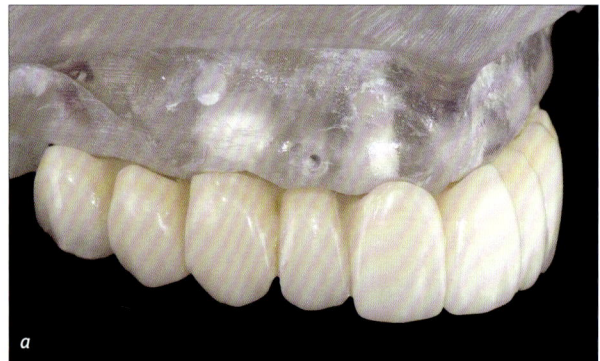

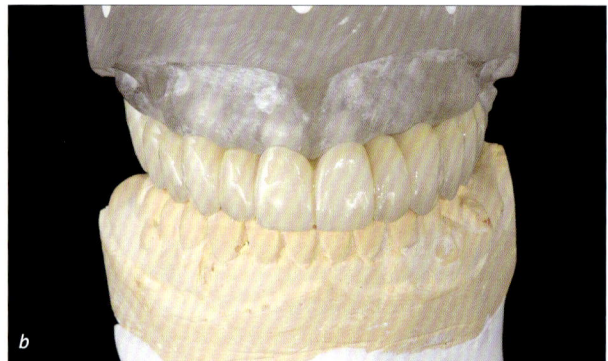

Figs 26a-b   CAD/CAM provisional on the 3D printed model (a), then checked in the analog articulator (b) to compare it with the virtual articulator analysis. The result was similar.

Mandibular surgical procedure

For the mandibular surgical procedure, a local anesthetic was administered buccally and lingually to the edentulous ridges (Scandicaine 2%; Septodont). After fifteen minutes, the surgical guide was positioned on the mandible. Following the Straumann guided surgery kit instructions, keratinized tissue was excised with a circular scalpel. The surgical guide was removed and the precut soft tissue extracted with a Buser elevator. The surgical guide was positioned on the mandibular ridge. Following the surgical protocol, osteotomies and implant placement were performed through the surgical guide. All six implants were inserted at more than 50 Ncm of torque. Implant mounts and guides were removed. Healing abutments 4 mm in height were installed on the implants (Institut Straumann AG) (Fig 27). 100 mg of ketoprofen (Profenid; Sanofi-Aventis) was prescribed to be taken twice a day for three days. The patient was dismissed and recalled at three and seven days; no complications were observed.

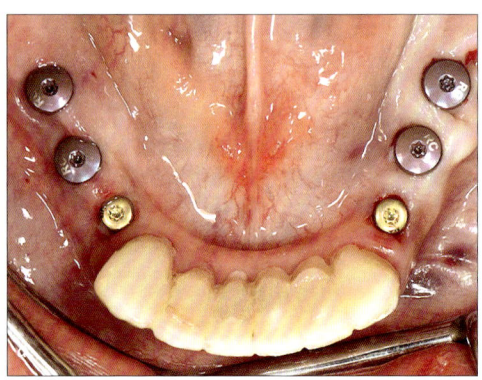

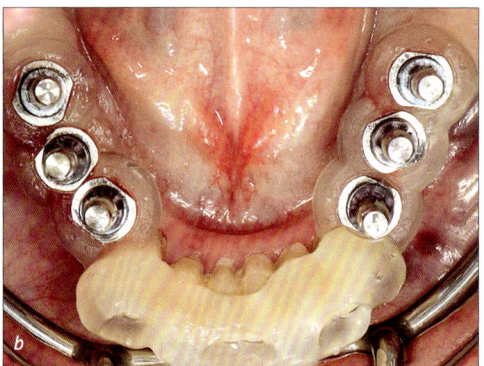

Figs 27a-b   Mandibular surgical procedure. Implants were placed through the surgical guide in a flapless approach.

Maxillary surgical procedure and immediate loading

Ten days after the previous surgery, the patient was scheduled for maxillary implant placement. Local anesthesia was infiltrated buccally and palatally to the edentulous ridges (Scandicaine 2%; Septodont). Mucosal surgery similar to that in the mandible was performed. The surgical guide was positioned over the maxilla and fixed with two anchor pins (Neodent, Curitiba, Brazil). Following the surgical protocol, osteotomies and implant placements were performed through the surgical guide. All implants were inserted with more than 50 Ncm of torque (Fig 28). The implant mounts and guide were removed. Selected SRA abutments were positioned following the restorative plan and torqued to 35 Ncm. (Fig 29). The PMMA CAD/CAM provisional bridge was then positioned on the SRA abutments and the prosthetic screws hand-tightened (Fig 30). The occlusion was checked and minor occlusal adjustments were performed. A mutually protective occlusion with bilateral group function was selected. PTFE plugs were placed on the prosthetic screws and sealed with a photopolymerizing resin material (Fermit; Ivoclar Vivadent). A small connective-tissue graft was performed to widen the ridge contour around sites 22 and 23 (Figs 31 and 32). A panoramic radiograph was requested (Fig 33). 100 mg ketoprofen (Profenid; Sanofi-Aventis) was prescribed to be taken twice per day for three days. The patient was dismissed and recalled at 3, 7, 14, 21, 30, and 45 days. No biological or prosthetic complications were observed.

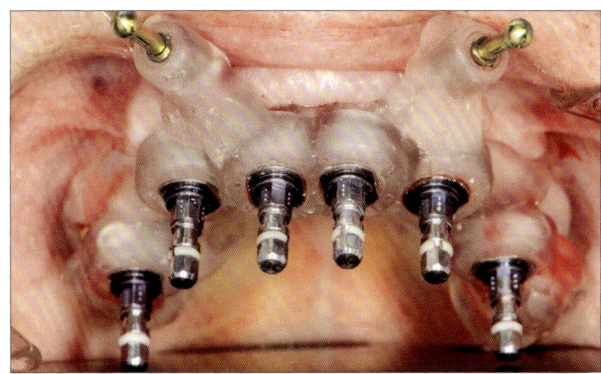

Fig 28 Maxillary surgical procedure. Implants were placed through the surgical guide in a flapless approach.

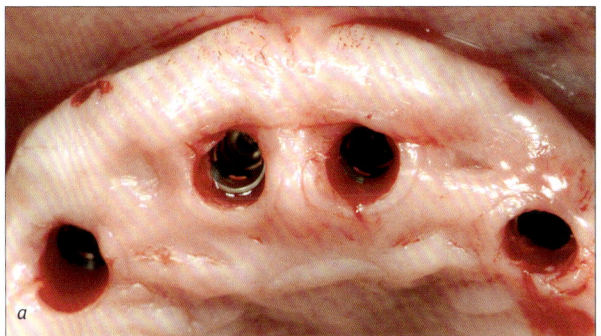

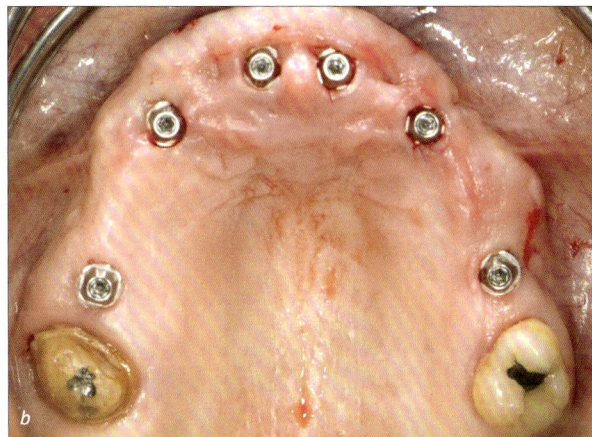

Figs 29a-b The surgical guide was removed and SRA abutments positioned and torqued following the restorative protocol.

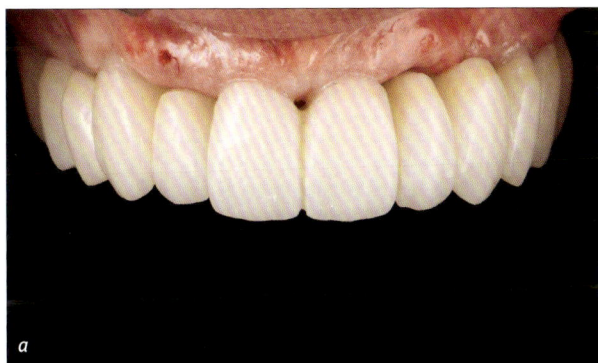

Fig 30 PMMA CAD/CAM provisional installed over the SRA abutments and hand-torqued.

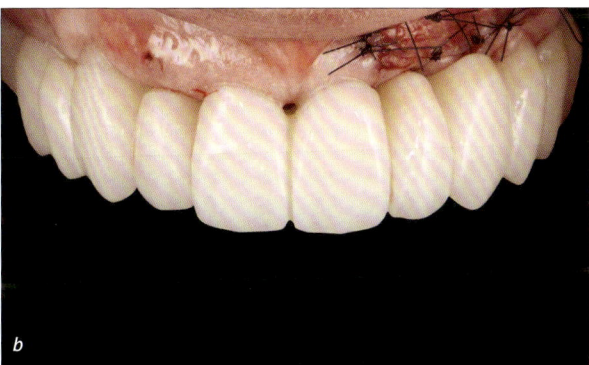

Fig 31 A connective-tissue graft was performed to obtain an ideal ridge contour around sites 22 and 23.

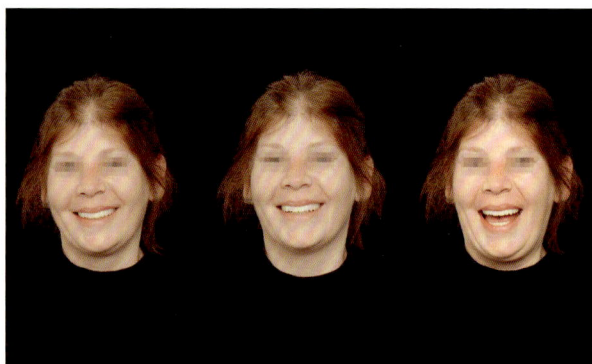

Fig 32   The patient 30 minutes after surgical procedure and immediate loading.

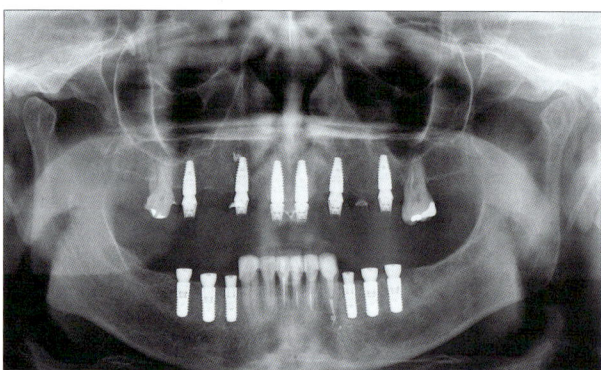

Fig 33   Panoramic radiograph after implant placement and immediate loading.

At the 30-day follow-up, soft-tissue contouring commenced, modifying the provisional emergence profile by adding composite resin (Tetric N-Ceram; Ivoclar Vivadent) or removing PMMA. The objective was to change the shape of the ridge-lap pontics to ovate. This was repeated at the following appointments until the desired soft-tissue profile was obtained (Fig 34). Articular, muscular, functional, and phonetic evaluations were also performed at each follow-up. No complications occurred during this process.

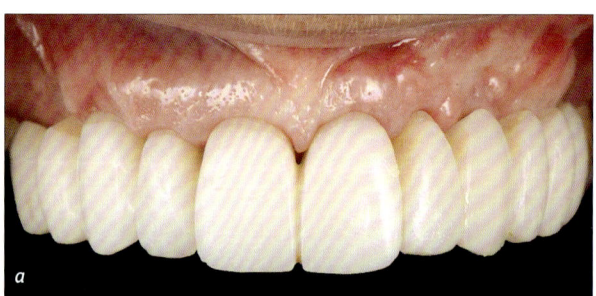

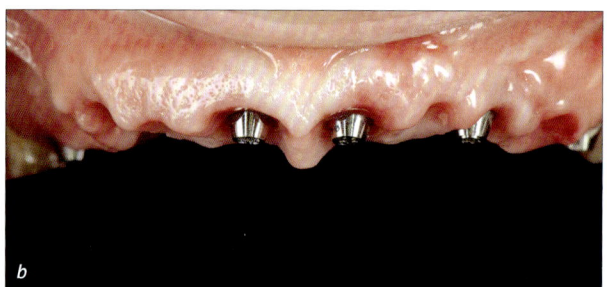

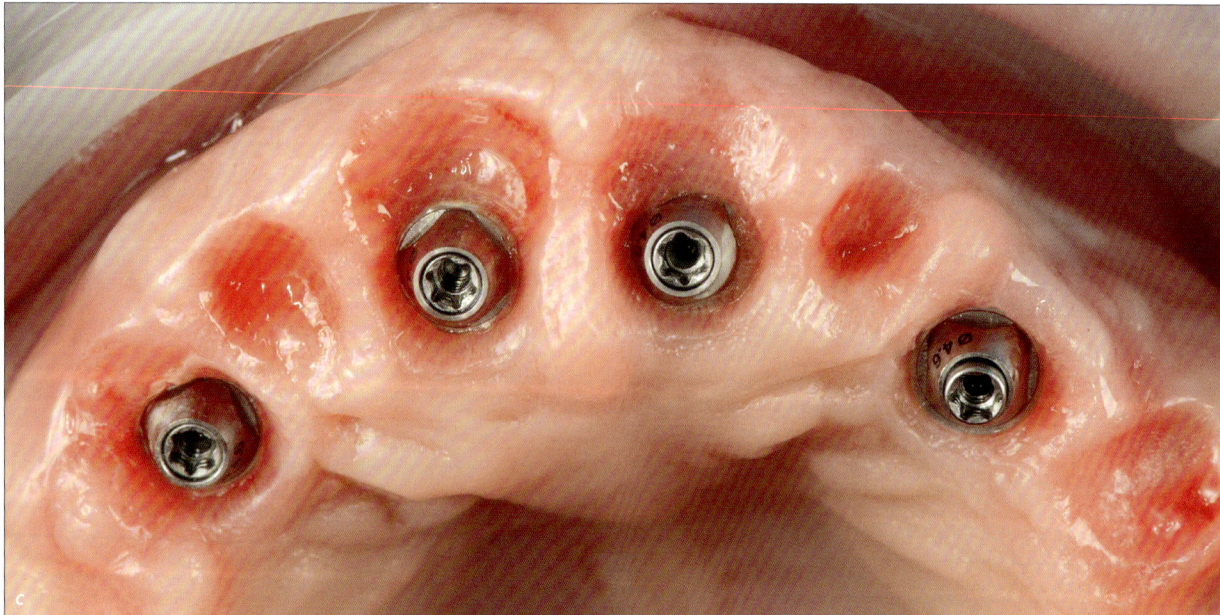

Figs 34a-c   Three months after implant placement. The desired gingival profile was achieved by soft-tissue conditioning with the provisional restoration.

Mandibular definitive restorations

Six weeks after the surgery, the posterior implants, maxillary PMMA structure, and occlusal relations were digitally recorded. Following the CAD design and milling process, the implants were restored with three splinted screw-retained CAD/CAM crowns on each side (Variobase, Institut Straumann AG; and Katana; KurarayNoritake, Tokyo, Japan) (Fig 35). Prosthetic screws were torqued to 35 Ncm and covered with PTFE plugs and composite resin (Tetric-N; Ivoclar Vivadent).

Once the posterior crowns had been installed and the occlusal relation functionally checked, digital impressions were taken of the anterior mock-up and tooth preparations (Trios; 3Shape) (Fig 36). The maxillary PMMA structure and its occlusal relations were also recorded digitally and the data imported into the CAD software (Dental System; 3Shape). The lower anterior restorations were designed according to the mock-up shape, imitating the initial wax-up. The designed restorations were milled (K5; VHF) from monolithic lithium disilicate (e. max CAD; Ivoclar Vivadent). After checking, they were cemented (Variolink Esthetic DC; Ivoclar Vivadent) under absolute isolation (Nic Tone Dental Dam; Nic Tone, Bucharest, Romania) (Fig 37).

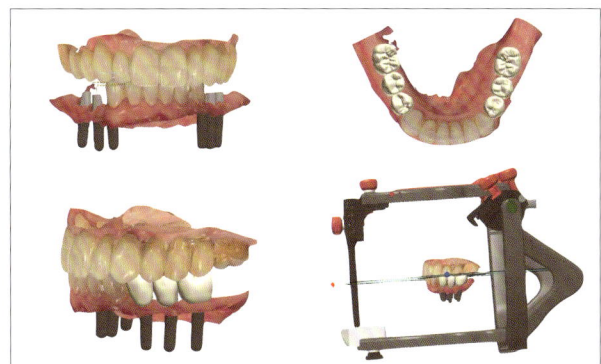

Fig 35   CAD design of the lower posterior implant-supported restorations.

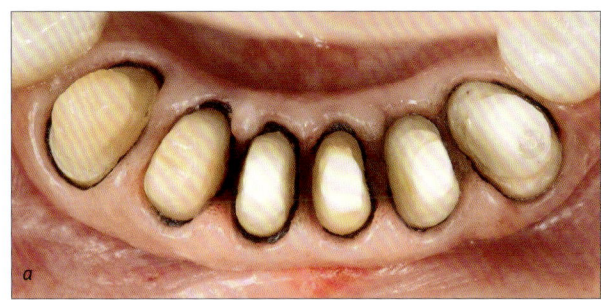

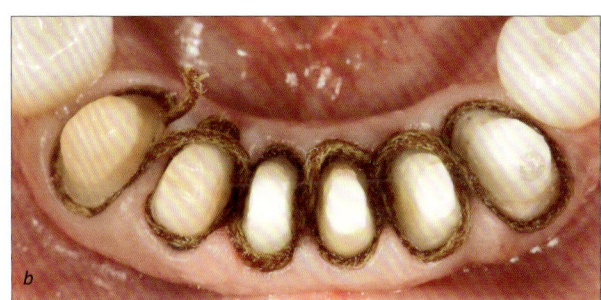

Figs 36a-b   Lower anterior preparations ready for digital impressions. 000 and 0 gingival cord was used.

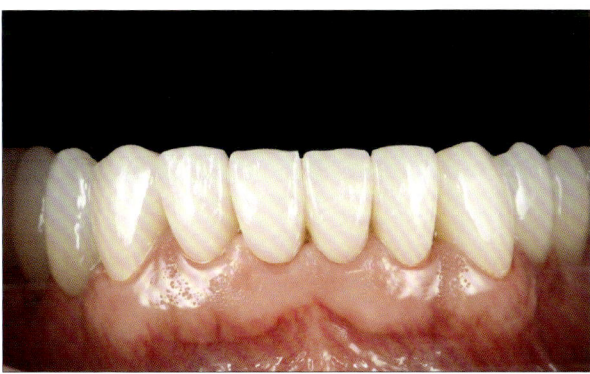

Fig 37   Cementation follow-up of the lower anterior CAD/CAM crowns.

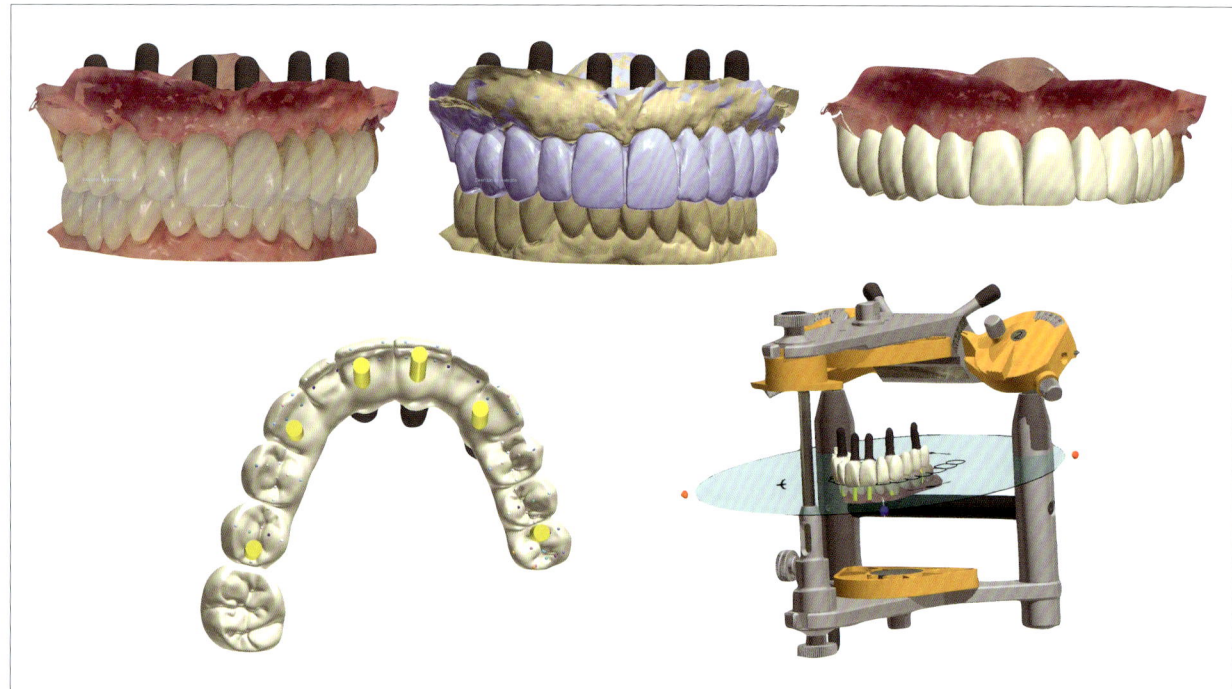

Fig 38   CAD design of the maxillary definitive implant-supported restoration.

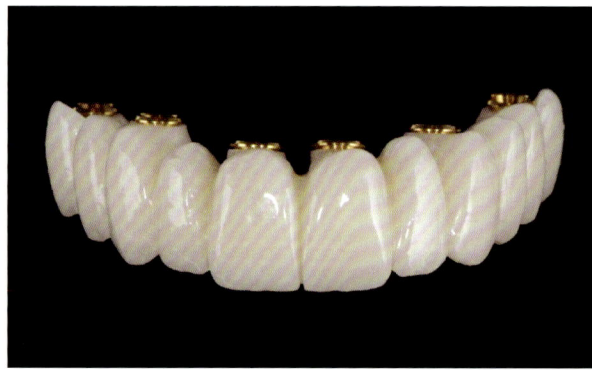

Fig 39   PMMA CAD/CAM definitive restoration prototype.

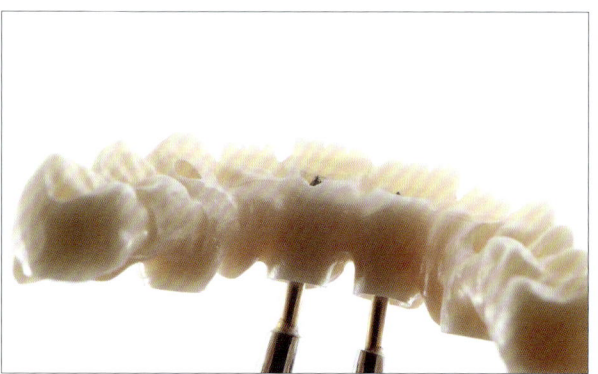

Fig 40   Definitive zirconia CAD/CAM restoration with reduced buccal and incisal space for porcelain layering based on the PMMA prototype shape.

Maxillary definitive restorations

Three months after implant insertion, the soft-tissue contours were complete, presenting the desired emergence profile for an optimal esthetic result. Digital impressions were taken of the implant-retained PMMA bridge, maxillary abutments (SRA scanbody; Institut Straumann AG), mandibular restorations, and the occlusal relation (Trios; 3Shape). Taking the PMMA interim prosthesis as reference, a full-arch implant-supported structure was designed, improving tooth shapes and positions. The digital structure was then functionally checked in a virtual articulator (Fig 38). The file was exported and a new PMMA restoration milled. After cleaning, metallic interfaces (Institut Straumann AG) were cemented into the prosthetic connections of the PMMA framework (Multilink; Ivoclar Vivadent). The new PMMA restoration was installed in the patient's mouth, and a complete functional, esthetic, and phonetic analysis was performed (Fig 39). The PMMA structure was used to check every clinical detail before converting it into a definitive restorative material; minor modifications were performed. Following approval, the virtual design was modified, subtracting approximately 1.5 to 2 mm from the buccal surface and incisal edges. No occlusal surfaces were changed from the initial design. Buccal and incisal spaces were created to leave enough room for the ceramic build-up. The modified virtual

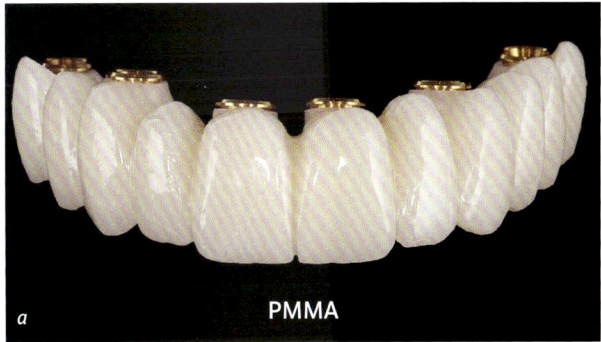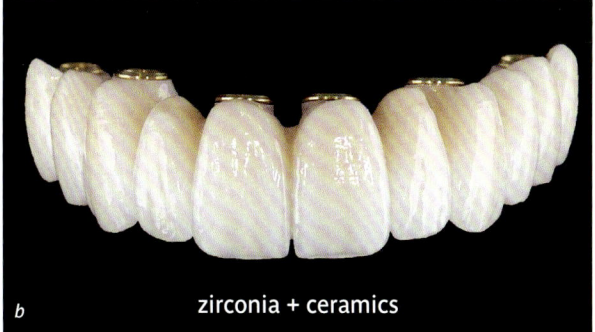

Figs 41a-b   PMMA prototype and definitive zirconia/ceramic CAD/CAM restoration.

structure was exported and milled in zirconia (Katana; KurarayNoritake) (Fig 40). The PMMA and zirconia restorations were sent to the laboratory for ceramic veneering, using a silicon index to transfer the PMMA shape to the zirconia bridge (e.max Ceram; Ivoclar Vivadent) (Fig 41). Metallic interfaces (Institut Straumann AG) were cemented into the prosthetic connections. The definitive restoration was checked in the patient's mouth and screwed onto the SRA abutments. No occlusal modifications were performed. The prosthetic screws were torqued to 35 Ncm. Screw holes were sealed with PTFE plugs and composite resin (Tetric-N; Ivoclar Vivadent). A monolithic zirconia CAD/CAM crown was cemented on tooth 17 (Multilink; Ivoclar Vivadent) (Figs 43 to 49). The patient was followed at 3, 7, 15, and 30 days, when no complications were noted, and then recalled at 6, 12, and 18 months for maintenance. No complications were reported.

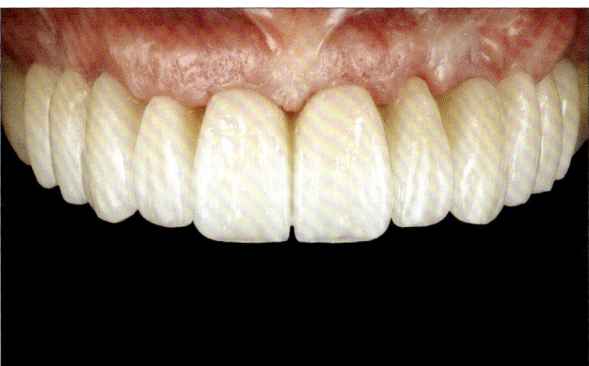

Fig 42   Follow-up 7 days after the delivery of the maxillary restoration.

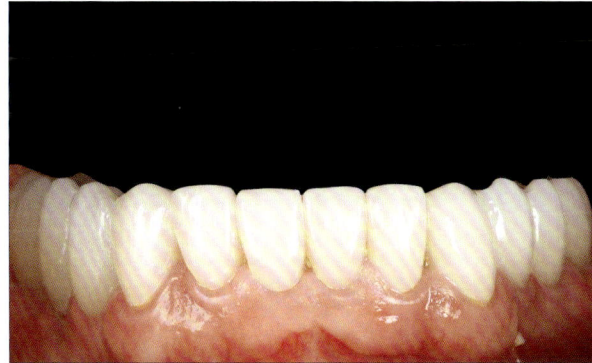

Fig 43   Follow-up 7 days after the delivery of the mandibular restoration.

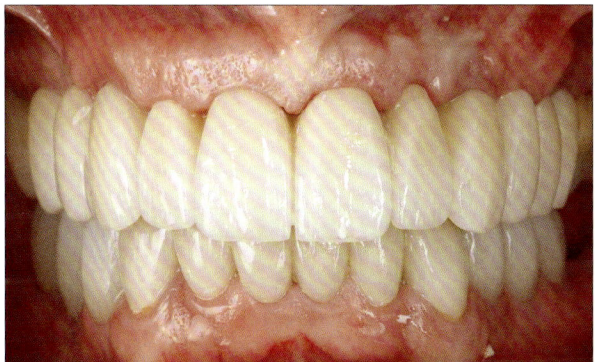

Fig 44   7-day follow-up. Occlusal relation.

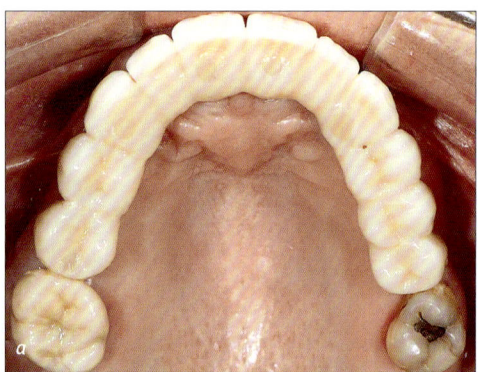

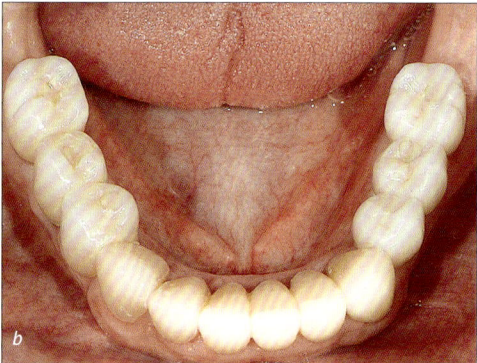

Figs 45a-b   14-day follow-up. Occlusal view of the maxillary and mandibular restorations.

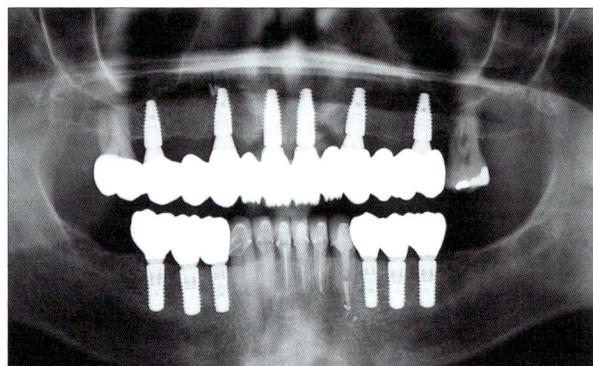

Fig 46   Final OPG showing different components of the prosthodontic treatment.

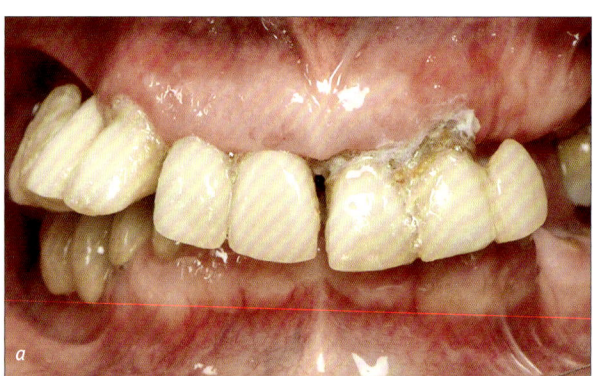

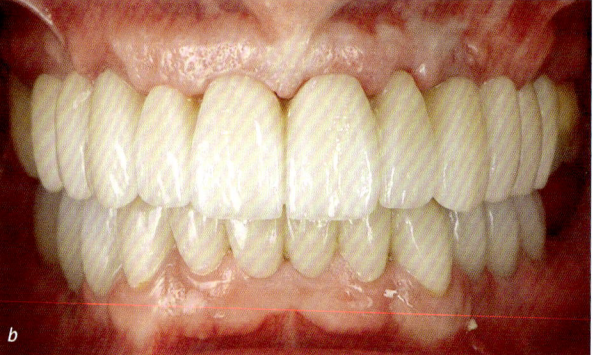

Figs 47a-b   Intraoral comparison between the initial situation and the situation after treatment.

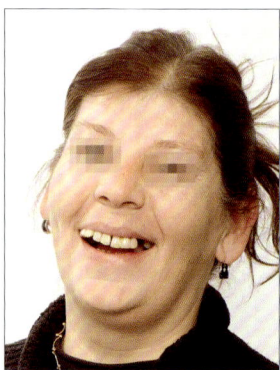

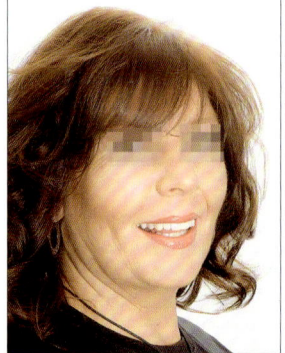

Figs 48a-b   Extraoral comparison between the initial situation and the situation after treatment.

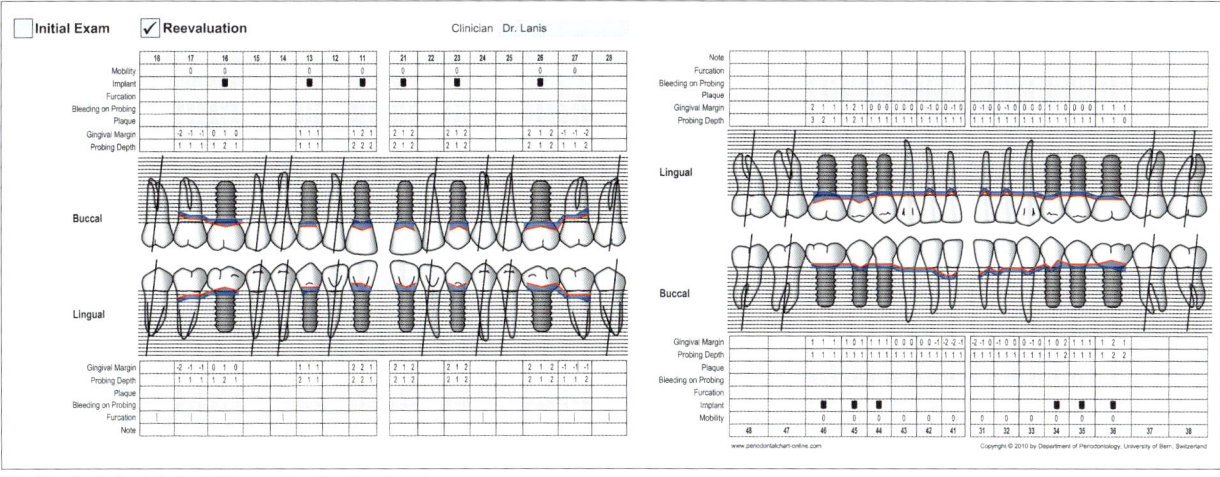

Fig 49   Periodontal chart 18 months after treatment.

Discussion

Computer-guided implant placement facilitates detailed surgical planning and accurate implant insertion through a custom surgical template (Bornstein 2014, Lanis 2015b, Jokstad 2017). This technique may also permit a less invasive, flapless surgical procedure (Arısan 2013, Lin 2014). Computer-assisted planning allows the visualization of considerable surgical and prosthetic data prior to the actual surgery, helping to perform an accurate procedure based on the prosthetic plan (Brodala 2009; Becker 2009; Lanis and coworkers 2017).

In the present case, the use of this technology not only contributed to a non-invasive and precise implant placement but also yielded a functional design of the provisional restoration based on the projected implant positions. The correct fit of the provisional restoration on the implants is dependent on the correlation between the digital surgical plan and the actual surgical outcome. Therefore, the use of a computer-generated surgical template is mandatory (Neumeister 2018). Every detail in designing, printing, and securing the surgical template, both on the model and intraorally, should be carefully considered. Moreover, the pre-designed prosthetic structure should also consider the patient's capability for appropriate cleaning and the viability for clinical probing and maintenance.

It is well documented that a fracture of an immediately loaded full-arch restoration during the early phases of osseointegration could overload some implants, leading to early failure (Tarnow et and coworkers 1997; Jaffin and coworkers 2004; Misch and coworkers, 2004; Maló and coworkers 2005; Widmann and Bale 2006; Leighton and Carvajal 2013; Gallucci 2014). Several factors should therefore be considered before deciding on a splinting technique and restorative material to ensure prosthetic integrity during the osseointegration process. It is recommended that the patient periodontal biotype, the type of antagonist, the number distribution of implants, the prosthetic design, and connector height and width should all be considered in selecting the appropriate material and prosthetic design (De Bruyn 2014).

In the present case, PMMA was selected for an immediately loaded functional provisional, based on the esthetic and biomechanical properties of the material, but also because it is possible to design digitally before milling (Chung 2011). The versatility of CAD permits custom designs and the fabrication of a milled monolithic PMMA structure to optimize the structural characteristics of the restoration. Connector height and width were carefully considered during the digital designing phase (Sanz-Sánchez 2015).

3D printers are revolutionizing the manufacturing industry. The option of personalized fabrication processes for different components and products is changing the way we consume services and products. In implant dentistry, 3D printers facilitate the creation of diverse prototypes, components, and devices, helping to plan and implement clinical procedures faster and more safely (Alharbi 2017; Matta 2017). In the present case, the digitally designed 3D-printed master model saves considerable time compared to conventional master models, as previously reported for computer-guided surgery techniques. Moreover, the fact that the model is CAD/CAM designed and made reduces any distortion produced by the interaction of different materials and the manual processes needed for conventional fabrication (Gillot 2010). The fabrication of the provisional restoration prior to surgery was considerably easier, faster, and cheaper overall.

One disadvantage of this technique is that shape of the provisional restoration is determined by the consistency of the 3D-printed model. The model used here was made of resin and therefore rigid, so it was impossible to fabricate a prosthetic structure with an ideal prosthetic emergence profile and soft-tissue adaptation. That is why the ridge-lap pontic shape designed initially was later modified to an ovate pontic during soft-tissue contouring. This shortcoming could be resolved by modifying the 3D-printed model digitally before printing or manually before scanning. This would give the temporary restorations ideal prosthetic and soft-tissue profiles. Novel printing materials or technologies could help overcome this inconvenience.

CAD/CAM and its application in dentistry are revolutionizing our profession. The amount of information that can be easily managed and stored is changing the way we practice. It also affects the way laboratories work and patients perceive our efforts. Digital photography, intraoral scanners, lab scanners, CAD software, milling machines, and 3D printers in combination with developments in dental materials optimize treatment time, cost, and predictability. In the present case, digital technologies were successfully used in every treatment step, from initial evaluation to the delivery of the definitive restorations. Their application also promoted patient understanding and involvement. However, these powerful tools should be used following stringent prosthetic and surgical principles.

In summary, digital technologies will be of great help to clinicians who are well-prepared. But they will not save those who are not.

Acknowledgments

Clinical procedures and photography
Dr. Orlando Álvarez del Canto – Santiago, Chile
Dr. Sofia Kupfer – Santiago, Chile

Laboratory procedures
Dental Technician Victor Romero – Santiago, Chile

13.11 Rehabilitating an Edentulous Maxilla with a Conventional Removable Denture and an Edentulous Mandible with a Fixed Dental Prosthesis Using s-CAIS

W.-S. Lin, W. Polido, J. R. Charette, D. Morton

A 72-year-old male patient was referred to the prosthodontic clinic for possible implant treatment. He presented with a partially edentulous maxilla and mandible. The clinical and radiographic examination showed generalized chronic severe periodontitis with tooth mobility, dental caries, and direct composite restorations in three teeth. Pre-treatment periapical and panoramic radiographs revealed horizontal bone loss associated with all remaining teeth and vertical bone loss associated with the anterior teeth and confirmed the presence of generalized carious lesions. Pneumatization of the right and left maxillary sinuses resulted in minimal posterior ridge height (Figs 1 and 2).

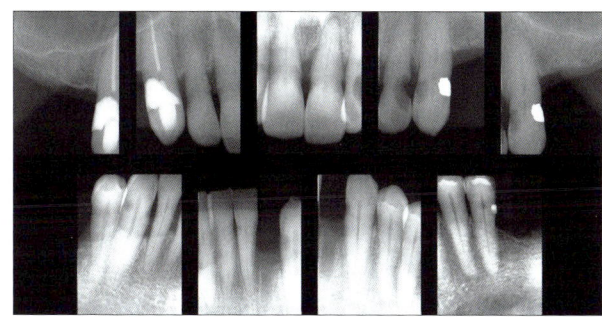

Fig 1   Baseline periapical radiographs.

The periodontal evaluation showed maxillary probing depths from 4 to 6 mm, with an isolated 9-mm pocket on the mesiolingual aspect of tooth 21. All teeth exhibited gingival recession, bleeding on probing, and class I to II mobility. Mandibular probing depths ranged from 3 to 4 mm, with all teeth exhibiting gingival recession, bleeding on probing, and class I to II mobility (Figs 3 and 4).

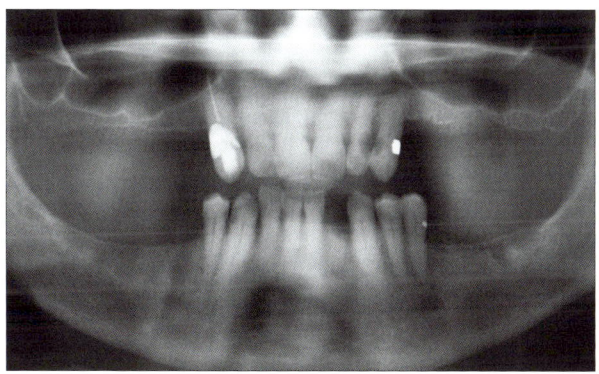

Fig 2   Baseline panoramic radiograph.

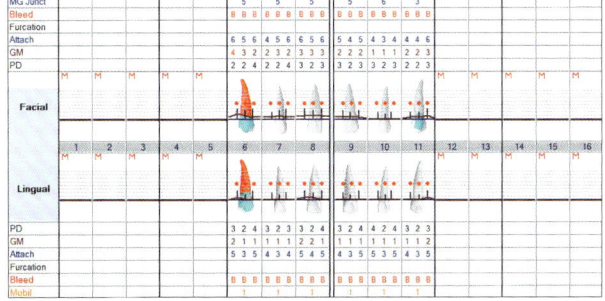

Fig 3   Periodontal chart, maxillary arch.

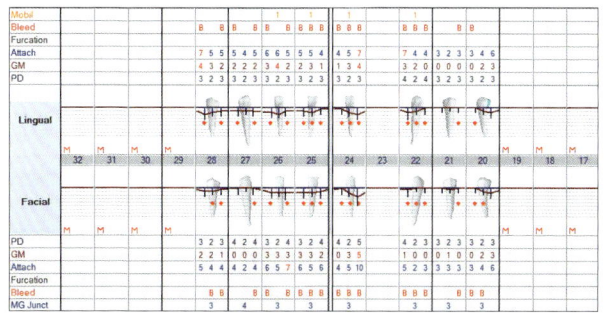

Fig 4   Periodontal chart, mandibular arch.

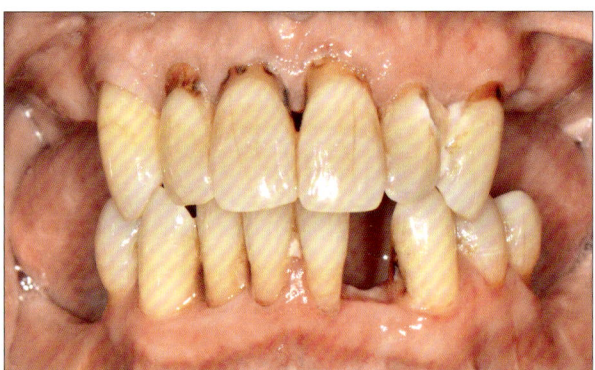

Fig 5   Frontal view of the baseline situation with the patient in centric occlusion (CO). Three composite resin restorations in teeth 22, 23, and 35.

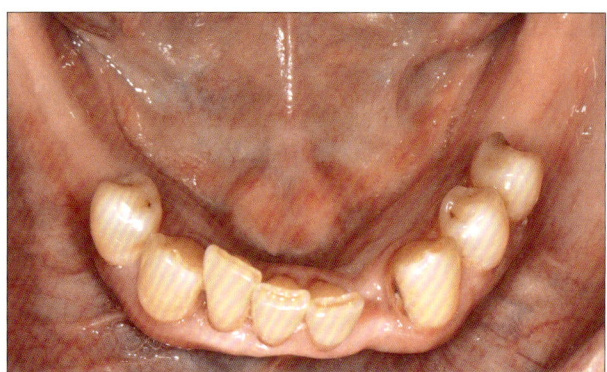

Fig 6   Mandibular occlusal view of the baseline situation.

The detailed dental history obtained from the patient and referring dentist showed that the patient had experienced a lapse in routine dental care that had contributed to the progression of the periodontal disease and dental caries, resulting in the eventual loss of most posterior teeth and compromising the remaining dentition, which had a poor long-term prognosis (Figs 5 and 6).

The patient's medical history presented no contraindication to implant treatment. Different treatment options were discussed with the patient, along with their associated costs, risks, and benefits, including conventional complete removable dental prostheses (CRDPs), implant-supported overdentures (IODs), and implant-supported complete fixed dental prostheses (ICFDPs). The patient indicated a preference for a fixed solution and accepted a treatment plan that called for a maxillary conventional CRDP and a mandibular ICFDP supported by five implants.

Intraoral and extraoral examinations confirmed that the desired vertical dimension of occlusion and a stable maxillomandibular relationship could be achieved with the existing dentition. There were no posterior occlusal interferences, and the maximal intercuspal position (MIP) and centric occlusion (CO) coincided.

The patient was referred for cone-beam computed tomography (CBCT) at the existing maxillomandibular relationship. The resulting DICOM (Digital Imaging and Communications in Medicine) files and clinical digital photographs were forwarded to a dental laboratory (NDX nSequence; Reno, NV, USA) to complete the segmentation of the CBCT volume and for a virtual diagnosis and implant planning using the selected software package (Maven Pro; NDX nSequence). The first assessment based on the DICOM files showed no additional pathologic findings. The patient had enough remaining bone for potential immediate implant placement.

The existing dentition was segmented to ensure that the maxillomandibular relationship during CBCT imaging coincided with the desired final occlusal position (Fig 7).

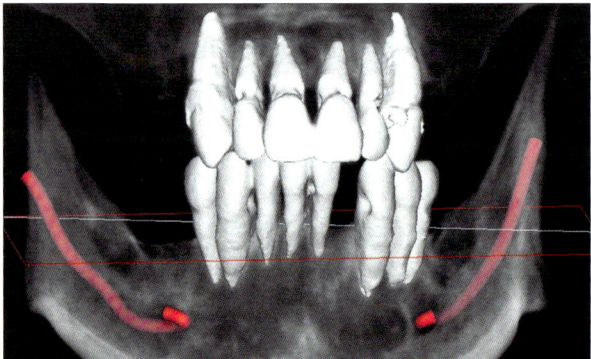

Fig 7   The existing dentition (white) was segmented from the DICOM files and used to confirm the maxillomandibular relationship.

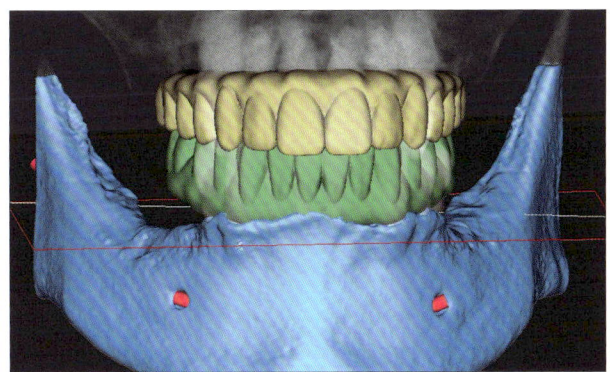

Fig 8   Maxillary (yellow) and mandibular (green) virtual diagnostic tooth set-up.

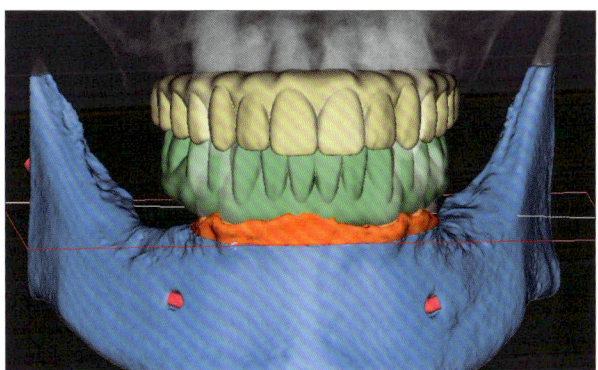

Fig 9   Simulated virtual bone reduction (orange) to create the desired prosthetic space.

Maxillary and mandibular virtual diagnostic tooth set-ups were created for the prosthetically driven implant planning (Fig 8). Simulated bone reduction was performed to obtain the necessary restorative space (Fig 9) as part of the prosthetically driven surgical plan (Fig 10).

Online collaboration platforms such as TeamViewer (TeamViewer US, FL, USA) allow clinicians to communicate with dental technicians and to receive immediate feedback and validation of the implant surgical plan.

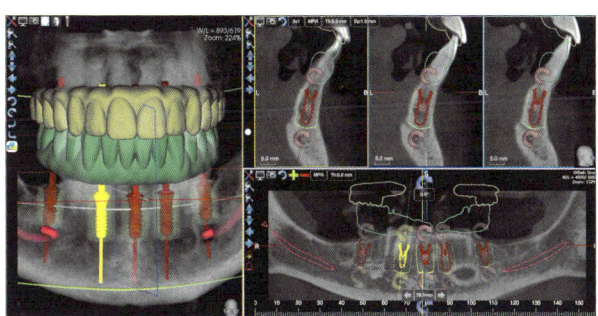

Fig 10   Virtual prosthetically driven surgical plan.

Using the DICOM datasets, the dental technician identified and traced the soft-tissue outline on the axial, coronal, and sagittal views (Figs 11 and 12). Soft-tissue tracing in the DICOM files eliminated the need for intraoral impressions or digital scans. For the interim removable dental prostheses, soft relining material can be used after tooth extraction for more accurate soft-tissue adaptation.

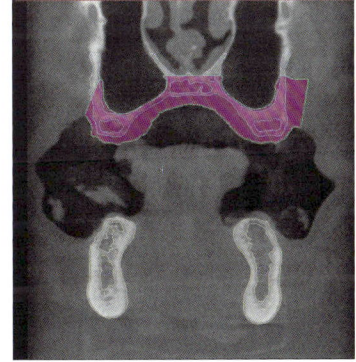

Fig 11   Identification of the soft-tissue outline from cone-beam computed tomography data, coronal view.

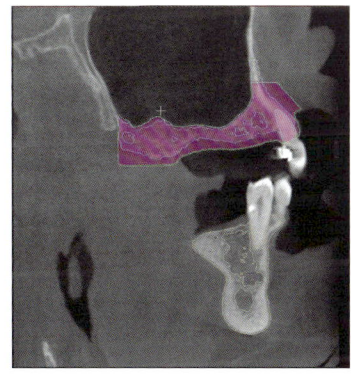

Fig 12   Identification of the soft-tissue outline from cone-beam computed tomography data, sagittal view.

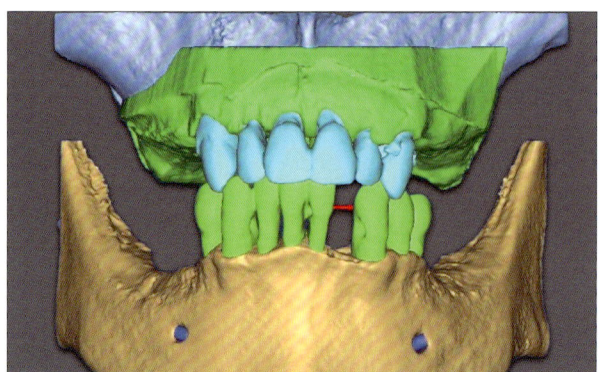

Fig 13   Maxillary virtual diagnostic cast with remaining dentition and reconstructed soft-tissue profile (green), facial view.

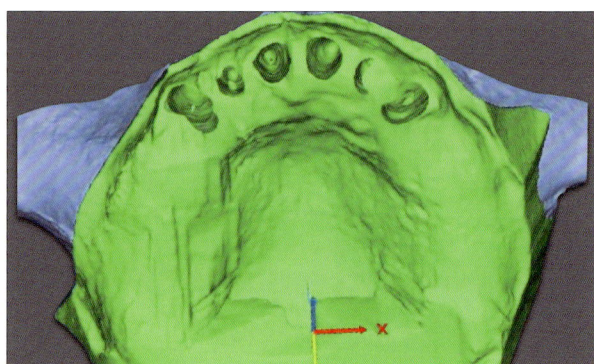

Fig 14   Maxillary virtual diagnostic cast with only reconstructed soft-tissue profile (green), occlusal view.

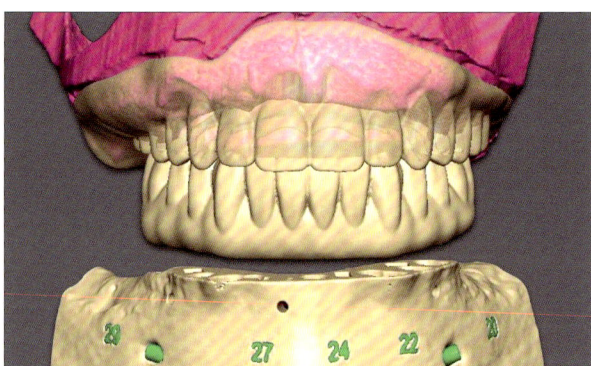

Fig 15   Designs of the CAD/CAM maxillary interim CRDP and mandibular interim ICFDP.

With the soft-tissue tracing, a virtual maxillary diagnostic cast was created in the CAD/CAM software (Maven Pro; nSequence) (Figs 13 and 14). A denture base was created on the virtual maxillary diagnostic cast with the reconstructed soft-tissue profile and merged with the virtual diagnostic tooth set-up (Fig 15).

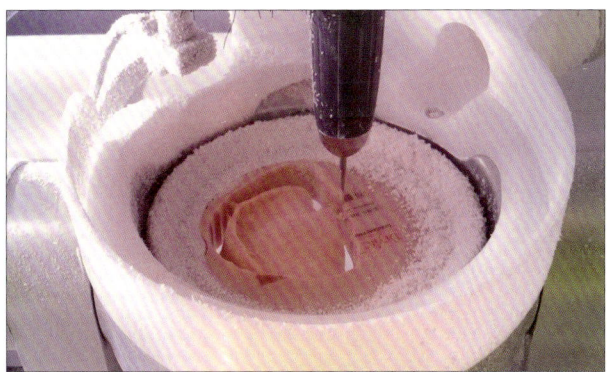

Fig 16   Computer-aided manufacturing.

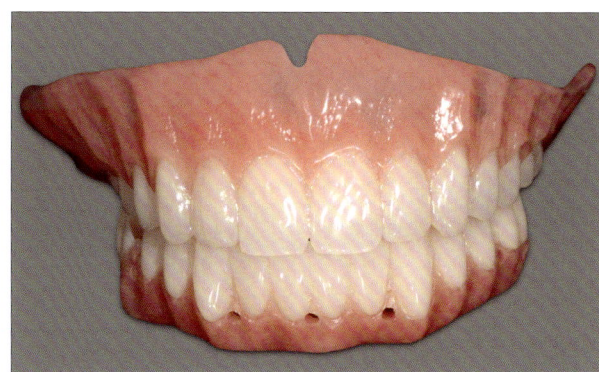

Fig 17   CAD/CAM interim prostheses.

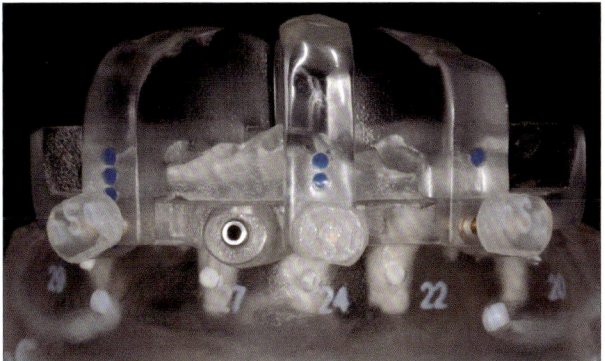

Fig 18   Bone-reduction template with three reposition devices repositioned on the mandibular cast (simulation cast with post-extraction alveolar ridge).

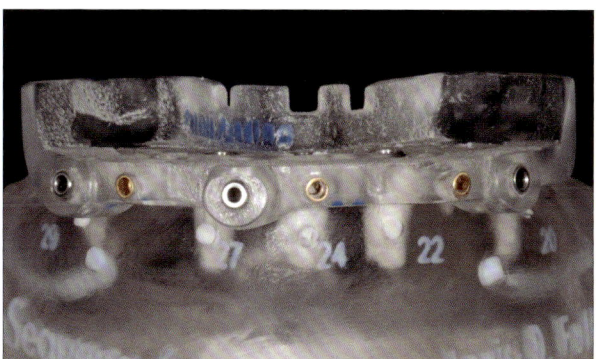

Fig 19   Bone-reduction template on CAD/CAM mandibular cast (simulation cast with post-osseous-recontouring alveolar ridge).

The completed virtual designs of the maxillary interim CRDP and mandibular interim ICFDP were exported to a milling unit (M5; Zirkonzahn, Gais, Italy) to fabricate the CAD/CAM prostheses using prefabricated PMMA-based resin blocks (Temp Basic; Zirkonzahn) (Fig 16). The milled interim prostheses were built up using light-polymerizing tooth-colored and pink resin (Gradia system; GC America, Alsip, IL, USA) to produce the desired esthetic outcome (Fig 17).

Based on the prosthetically driven implant plan, a two-piece CAD/CAM surgical template was fabricated (nSequence Guided Surgery; NDX nSequence), encompassing a bone-reduction template and an implant-placement template.

The bone-reduction template was to be fitted over the alveolar ridges after extractions and stabilized with anchor pins (Guided Anchor Pin; Nobel Biocare, Yorba Linda, CA, USA). Three repositioning jigs were designed based on the simulated post-extraction alveolar ridges contours of the CAD/CAM software (Maven Pro; NDX nSequence) to facilitate the correct seating of this bone-reduction template (Fig 18), and the flat platform on the occlusal aspect of the bone-reduction template served as a reference plane for bone reduction (Fig 19).

The implant-placement template was to be assembled on the bone-reduction template after bone reduction and osseous recontouring to provide guidance for implant placement.

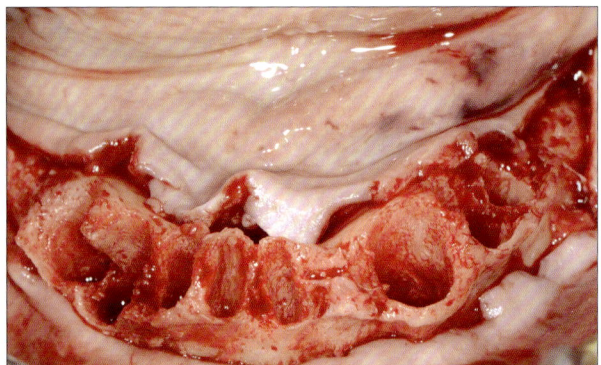

Fig 20   The remaining mandibular teeth were removed using a minimally traumatic approach to avoid excessive deformation of the alveolar ridge.

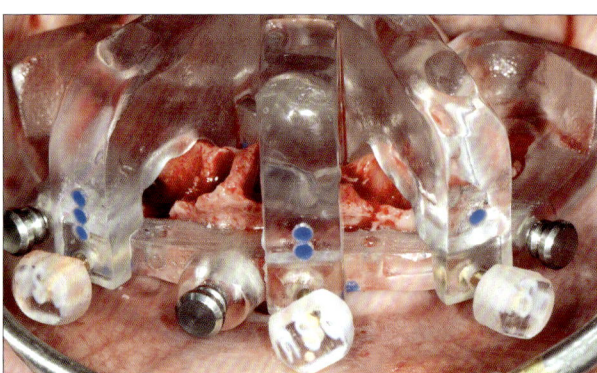

Fig 21   Repositioning jigs confirmed the seating of the bone-reduction template on the post-extraction alveolar ridge.

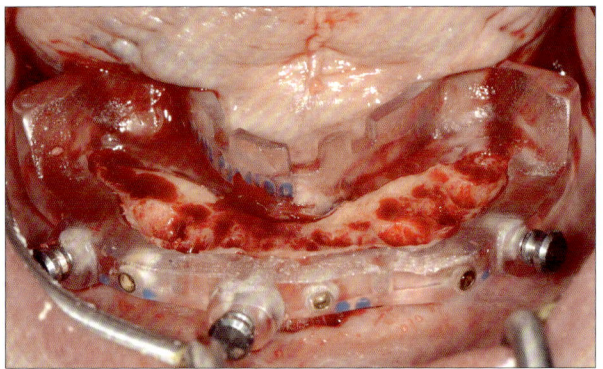

Fig 22   The bone-reduction template guided the planned osseous recontouring.

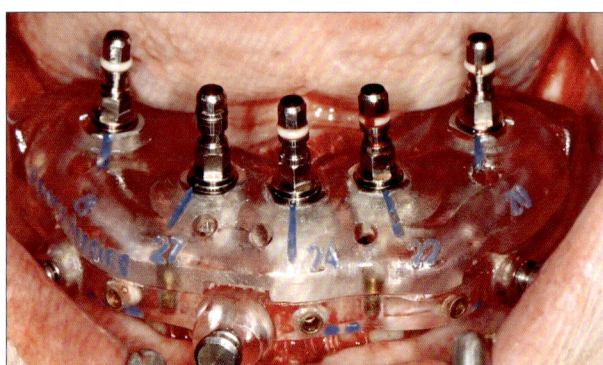

Fig 23   Mandibular implants placed as guided by the CAD/CAM two-piece surgical templates.

At the surgical appointment under local anesthesia and intravenous sedation, the remaining teeth were removed (Fig 20), the bone-reduction template with the three repositioning jigs was fitted onto the alveolar ridge and stabilized with anchor pins, and the planned osseous recontouring was completed (Figs 21 and 22). The implant-placement template was then fitted onto the bone-reduction template.

Five implants (Soft Tissue Level SLActive, guided RN, diameter 4.1 mm, length 10 mm or 8 mmm; and RN, diameter 3.3 mm, length 10 mm; Institut Straumann AG, Basel, Switzerland) were placed at insertion torques of 35 to 45 Ncm (Fig 23).

Following implant placement, 5 provisional abutments (RN synOcta post for temporary bridge restorations; Institut Straumann AG) were attached to the implants at a torque of 15 Ncm. A prefabricated polyvinylsiloxane shield was fitted over the provisional abutments to direct excess resin away from the implants and to facilitate re-positioning the mandibular interim ICFDP (Figs 24 and 25). The provisional abutments and mandibular interim ICFDP were connected with the autopolymerizing resin (Jet Tooth Shade Acrylic; Lang Dental Manufacturing, Wheeling IL, USA). The mandibular interim ICFDP was removed from the mouth for finishing and polishing in the dental laboratory. The bone-reduction template was removed and the flaps were sutured. The mandibular interim ICFDP was secured to the implants at a torque of 15 Ncm, and the screw access holes were sealed with cotton pellets and a single-component resin sealing material (Fermit; Ivoclar Vivadent, Schaan, Liechtenstein) (Fig 26).

Following removal of the remaining maxillary teeth, the CAD/CAM maxillary interim CRDP was relined with a soft reliner (Coe-Soft; GC America) (Figs 27 and 28).

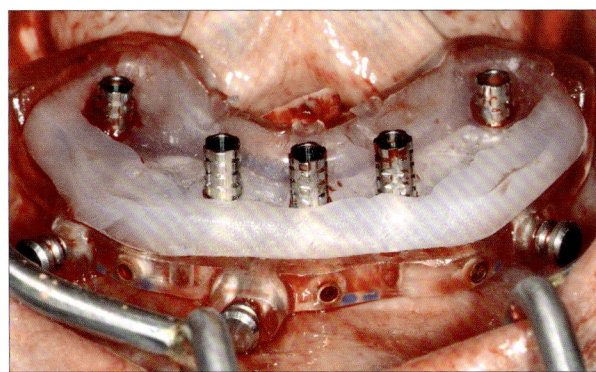

Fig 24 A laboratory-made polyvinylsiloxane shield fitted over the provisional abutments and onto the bone-reduction template.

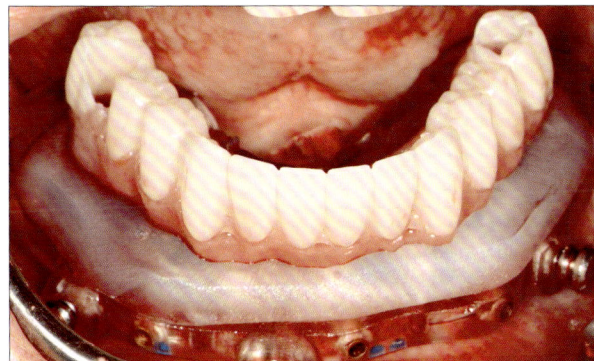

Fig 25 The CAD/CAM mandibular interim ICFDP was connected to the provisional abutments with autopolymerizing resin.

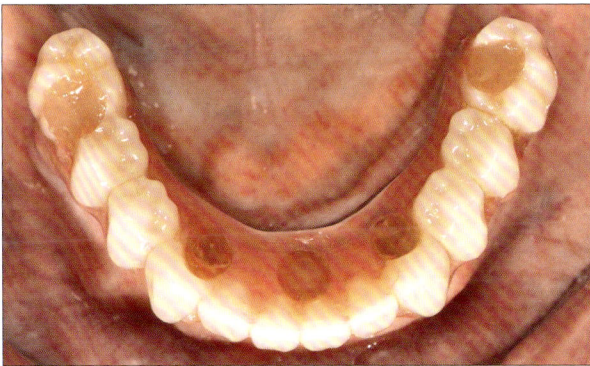

Fig 26 Occlusal view of the fitted mandibular interim ICFDP.

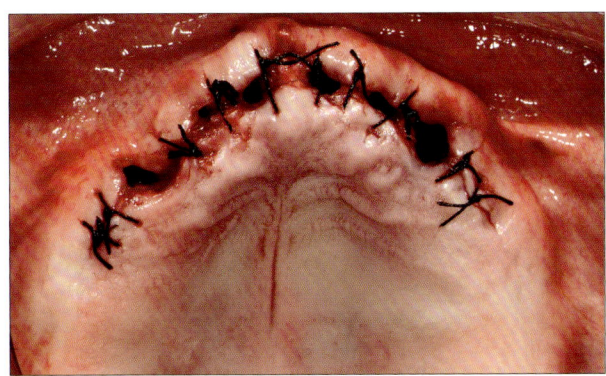

Fig 27 The remaining maxillary teeth were removed.

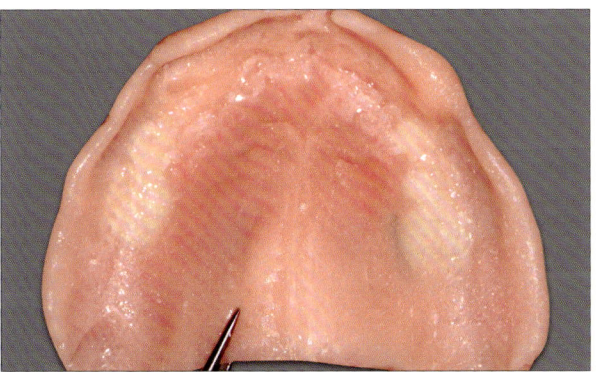

Fig 28 The CAD/CAM maxillary interim CRDP was relined with a soft liner.

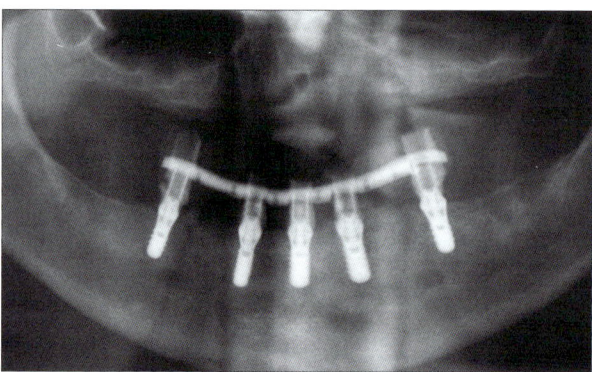

Fig 29   Postoperative panoramic radiograph showing complete seating of the mandibular interim ICFDP on the implants.

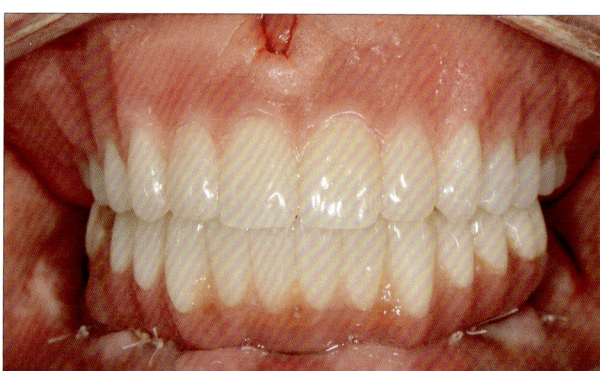

Fig 30   Facial view of the maxillary and mandibular interim prostheses.

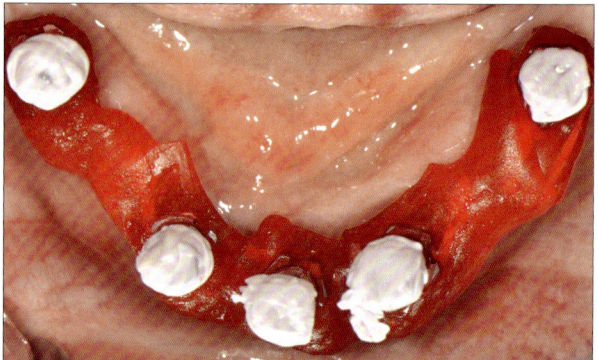

Fig 31   Impression copings were connected intraorally prior to the definitive impression.

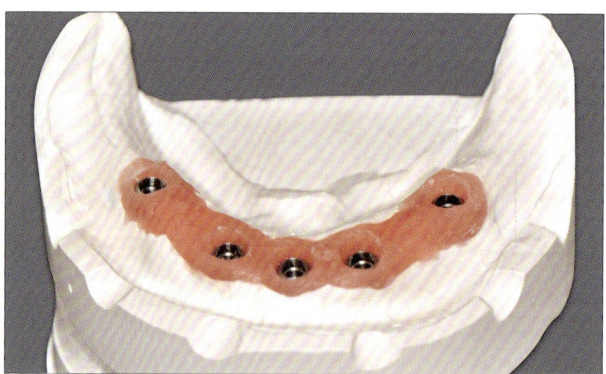

Fig 32   Definitive cast with implant analogs and removable soft tissue.

The placement of the implants was evaluated radiographically. The patient was satisfied with the esthetic and functional outcomes of the interim prostheses. Home-care instructions were given that provided for a soft diet and a 0.12% chlorhexidine digluconate mouthwash (CHG Oral Rinse; Xttrium Laboratories, Mount Prospect, IL, USA). The patient was scheduled for follow-up appointments at one day, at one week, and then every four weeks for twelve weeks before taking the definitive impression (Figs 29 and 30).

The patient returned for the maxillary and mandibular definitive impressions after three months. Custom trays were fabricated with light-polymerizing resin (Triad VLC; Dentsply Sirona, York PA, USA). A maxillary definitive impression was made in polyvinylsiloxane impression material (Virtual XD Heavy Body; Ivoclar Vivadent). Prior to the mandibular definitive impression, the impression copings were linked with autopolymerizing resin (Pattern Resin; GC America Inc) (Fig 31). A mandibular implant-level definitive impression was made using an open-tray impression technique and polyvinylsiloxane (Virtual XD Heavy Body and Extra Light Body; Ivoclar Vivadent). The corresponding implant analogs (RN analog; Institut Straumann AG) were connected to the impression copings and the impression was poured with

Type IV dental stone (ResinRock; Whip Mix, Louisville KY, USA) (Fig 32).

Light-polymerizing resin (Triad VLC; Dentsply Sirona) and dental wax were used to fabricate a baseplate and occlusal rim. Occlusal records and facebow recording were made and the maxillary and mandibular definitive casts mounted in an articulator (Stratos 300; Ivoclar Vivadent).

The mandibular interim ICFDP was repositioned on the definitive cast and a facial matrix made with laboratory polyvinylsiloxane putty (Sil-Tech; Ivoclar Vivadent), adapted around the facial surface of the interim ICFDP and mandibular definitive cast. The facial matrix was used to record the spatial orientation of the satisfactory tooth set-up of the interim prosthesis during laboratory procedures (Fig 33).

The maxillary and mandibular diagnostic tooth set-up was completed and the esthetic, phonetic, and functional clinical outcomes were confirmed by a trial insertion (Fig 34).

Following the trial insertion, the definitive casts and diagnostic set-ups were sent to a dental laboratory (Roy Dental Laboratory; New Albany, IN, USA). The

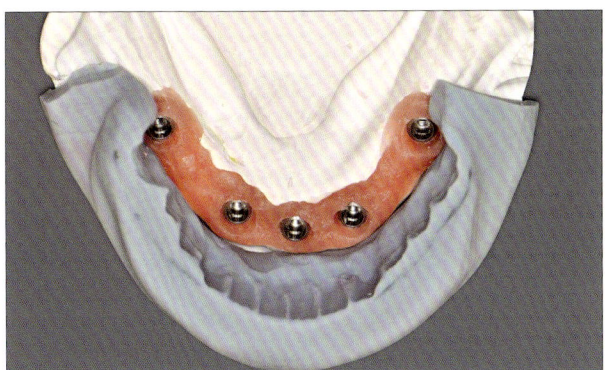

Fig 33 A facial matrix can serve as a reference during the tooth set-up process for the definitive prostheses.

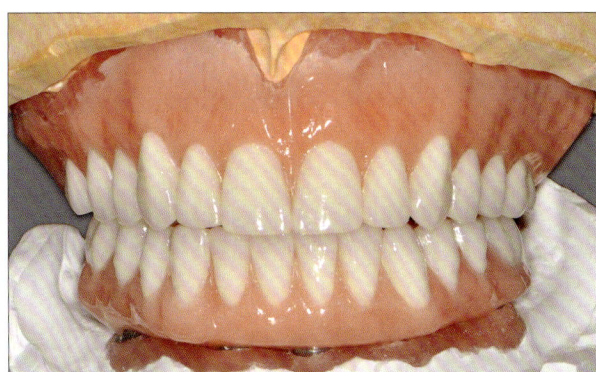

Fig 34 Maxillary and mandibular diagnostic tooth set-up for the definitive prostheses.

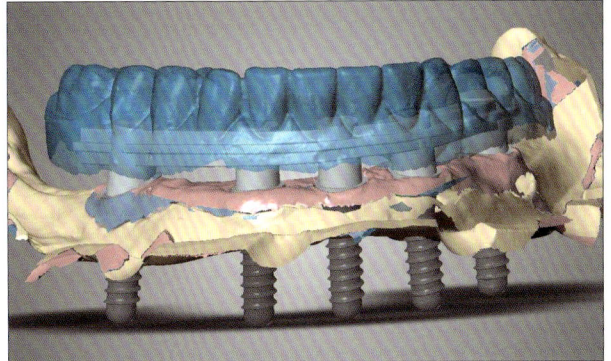

Fig 35 Design of the definitive CAD/CAM titanium framework with the scanned diagnostic tooth set-up in blue.

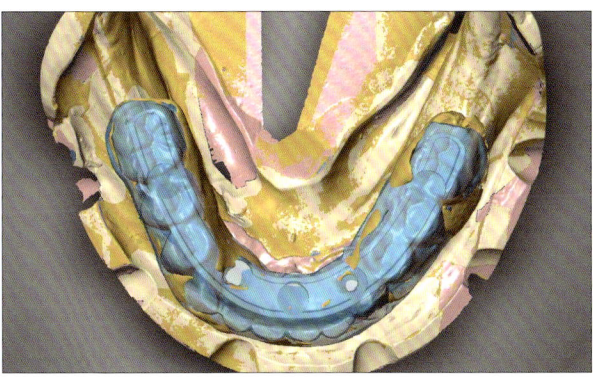

Fig 36 Design of definitive CAD/CAM titanium framework.

mandibular definitive cast and diagnostic set-ups were scanned with a laboratory scanner (7Series; Dental Wings, Montreal, Quebec, Canada). A mandibular CAD/CAM titanium framework was virtually designed using a scan of the diagnostic tooth set-up as reference (DWOS; Dental Wings) (Figs 35 and 36).

The completed mandibular CAD/CAM titanium framework was placed on the definitive cast to verify its accurate and passive fit. Since the maxillary and mandibular

diagnostic set-ups were finalized during and after the trial insertion, a new matrix was produced with laboratory polyvinylsiloxane putty (Sil-Tech; Ivoclar Vivadent) to more accurately transfer the set-up to the titanium framework. Using this matrix, the diagnostic set-up was transferred to the mandibular CAD/CAM titanium framework. Following the manufacturer's instructions, autopolymerizing injection-molded resin (IvoBase High Impact; Ivoclar Vivadent) was used to fabricate the definitive prostheses (Figs 37 and 38).

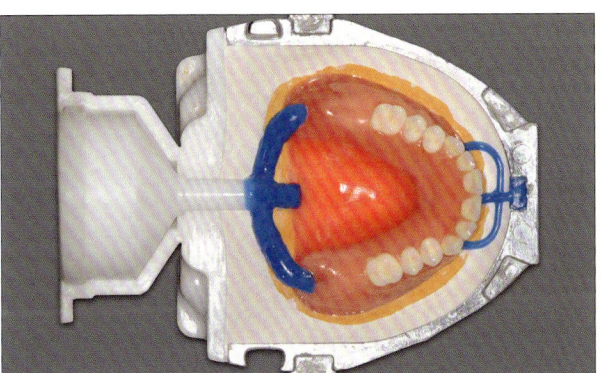

Fig 37 Invested maxillary tooth set-up and definitive cast in the processing flask.

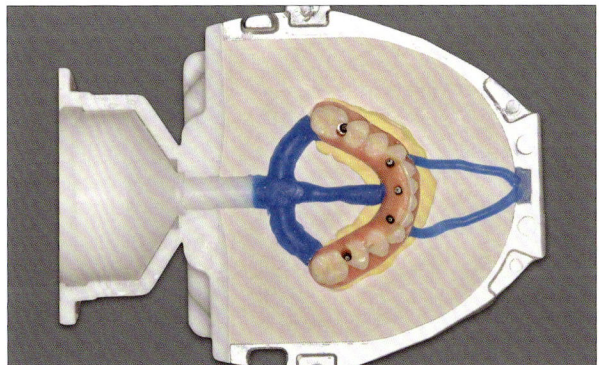

Fig 38 Invested mandibular set-up and CAD/CAM titanium framework assembly and definitive cast in the processing flask.

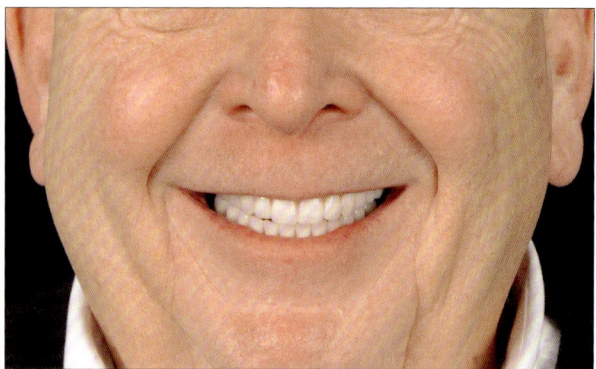

Fig 39   Patient's smile following delivery of definitive prostheses.

The definitive prostheses were adjusted on the articulator, finished, and polished in the dental laboratory before being returned to the clinician for insertion. The esthetic, phonetic, and functional clinical outcomes of the definitive prostheses were confirmed with the patient. The definitive mandibular ICFDP was secured to the implants at a torque of 35 Ncm and the screw access holes again sealed with cotton pellets and single-component resin (Fermit; Ivoclar Vivadent). The patient received home-care instructions and was scheduled for periodic maintenance appointments at six-monthly intervals (Figs 39 to 43).

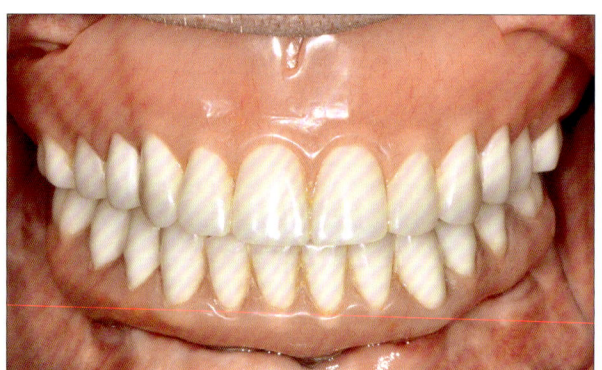

Fig 40   One year after the treatment. Frontal view of the maxillary CRDP and the mandibular ICFDP in centric occlusion (CO).

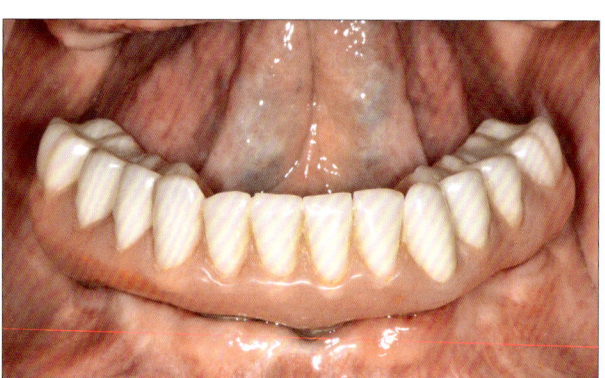

Fig 41   One year after the treatment. Mandibular ICFDP (frontal view).

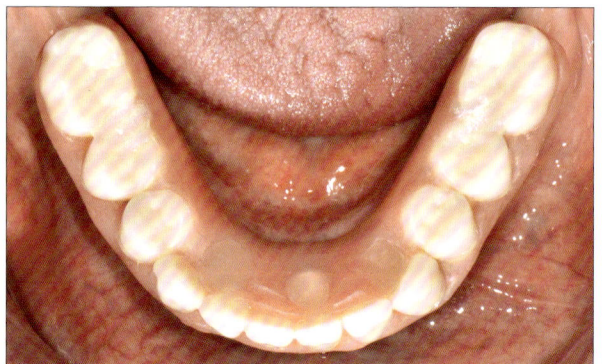

Fig 42   One year after the treatment. Mandibular ICFDP (occlusal view).

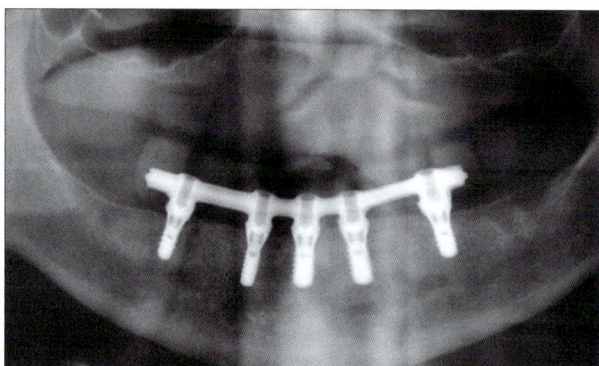

Fig 43   One year after the treatment. Panoramic radiograph.

Discussion

This case report described a partial digital workflow used in the treatment of a patient with a terminal dentition using a maxillary CRDP and a mandibular ICFDP on five implants. During the diagnostic and treatment-planning stages, CBCT volumetric data were utilized in the virtual planning of static computer-aided implant surgery (s-CAIS) and in the production of a CAD/CAM maxillary interim CRDP and mandibular interim ICFDP on the immediately placed and immediately loaded implants. A CAD/CAM titanium framework and autopolymerizing resin were used to complete the mandibular ICFDP.

CBCT imaging was used for the primary diagnostic record (dispensing with conventional diagnostic impressions and intraoral digital scanning). Thus, the DICOM volumetric dataset was the only digital diagnostic record used in the virtual implant planning and CAD of the interim prostheses.

Metallic restorations in the radiographic field of view (FoV) can cause scatter and affect the accurate interpretation of DICOM data in virtual implant planning. STL files derived from intraoral scanning or from laboratory scans of diagnostic stone casts can be imported and merged with the DICOM files to provide scatter-free surface profiles of the remaining dentition and surrounding soft tissue (Mora and coworkers 2014). The merged files will contain clearly defined soft-tissue and dental contours to assist both treatment planning and the subsequent fabrication of stereolithographic diagnostic casts and tooth-supported surgical templates (Stapleton and coworkers 2014).

The patient had only a few direct restorations, so minimal CBCT scatter was expected. The remaining dentition was compatible with the desired final and occlusal vertical dimension and maxillomandibular relationship. Bone-supported CAD/CAM surgical templates were intended for the s-CAIS, so a scatter-free surface profile of the baseline soft tissue and dentition was not required to design surgical guides. As no conventional diagnostic impressions or intraoral digital scans were required, the treatment time was shortened, and overall treatment efficiency was increased.

During CBCT imaging, clinicians were present to guide the patient into the desired vertical dimension of occlusion (preserving the existing dimension) and maxillomandibular relationship (maximal intercuspal position).

In virtual implant planning, the remaining teeth were segmented from the DICOM files to verify that the patient was in the desired occlusal position as intended. The segmented dentition was then used as reference for the planned final tooth set-up; simulated bone reduction and implant planning were performed according to that set-up.

ICFDPs have been proposed as a predictable treatment modality for edentulous patients. It has been reported, based on the evaluation of patient-reported outcomes, that immediate loading and immediate provisionalization improve patient satisfaction and self-perceived comfort, function, and cosmetic outcomes for patients (Dierens and coworkers 2009). Mandibular ICFDPs in particular have demonstrated high implant and prosthesis survival rates of more than 96% at 10 years (Papaspyridakos and coworkers 2014). Implant survival rates appear to be unaffected by the different fabrication techniques employed in CAD/CAM and conventionally fabricated prostheses (Kapos and Evans 2014).

With a mandibular ICFDP opposing a maxillary CRDP, most patients appear to be satisfied with the masticatory function and retention of the maxillary CRDP, with only a few patients reporting esthetic or phonetic problems (Davis and coworkers 2003; Wennerberg and coworkers 2001). In addition, screw-related complications with the mandibular ICFDP were found to be less likely, regardless of the patient's age or cantilever length (Purcell and coworkers 2015).

No esthetic, technical, or mechanical complications were observed at the twelve-month follow-up appointment. Clinical and radiographic examinations showed stable peri-implant soft-tissue and hard-tissue conditions.

Acknowledgments

Treatment planning and surgical procedures
Dr. Ryan Lewis – Longmont, CO, USA
Dr. Jack Goldberg – Mexico City, Mexico
Dr. Bryan Harris – Louisville, KY, USA

Part of this clinical case was previously published in Charette (2016). The reproduction of this article and photographs was approved by the Editorial Council for The Journal of Prosthetic Dentistry, Incorporated, on February 2, 2017.

13.12 Rehabilitating an Edentulous Maxilla with a Fixed Dental Prosthesis Using a DSD-Guided Approach

N. Sesma, W. Polido

A 60-year-old man was referred to the Center of Excellence for Prosthodontics and Implant Dentistry (CEPI) of the School of Dentistry of the University of São Paulo, Brazil for implant therapy. Anamnesis, clinical examination, and radiographs revealed esthetic and functional problems, the absence or structural compromise of various teeth (16 – 11, 21, 22, 24, 25, 37, 45, and 48), periodontal and endodontic problems (17 and 27), implant fracture (46), and occlusal disorders (Figs 1 and 2a). The patient reported that he was undergoing treatment for cardiovascular diseases. Periodontal probing depth, bleeding score, and plaque score were recorded on the periodontal chart available at *www.periodontalchart-online.com* (Department of Periodontology, University of Bern, Switzerland) during the initial examination (Fig 2b).

Conventional impressions, occlusal registration, panoramic radiographs, photographs, videos, intraoral and model scans, and cone-beam computed tomography (CBCT) scans were acquired to provide data for treatment planning. After consultation with specialists in other disciplines, different treatment options were presented to the patient and the following treatment plan was agreed:

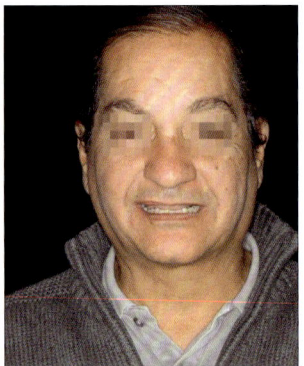

Fig 1   Pre-treatment, facial view.

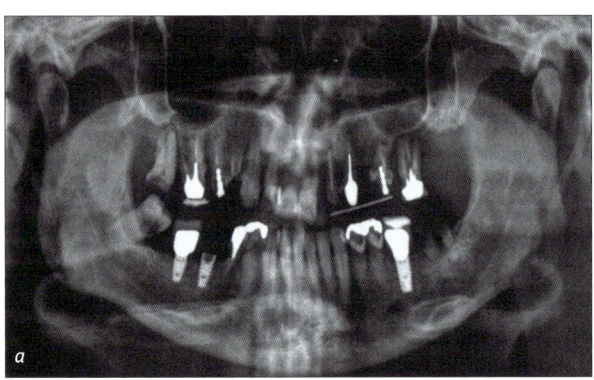

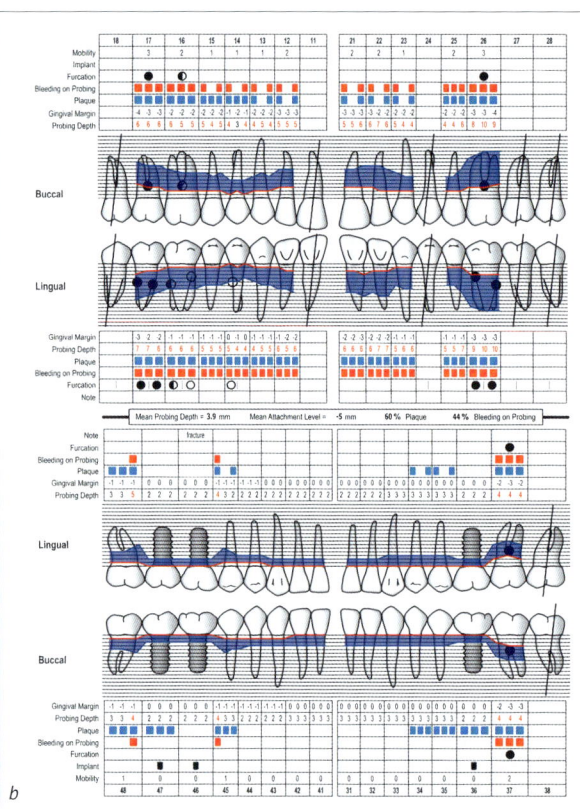

Figs 2a-b   Pre-treatment panoramic radiograph (a). Periodontal and peri-implant chart of the baseline clinical examination (b).

- *Phase 1 — Preparatory therapy.* Basic periodontal treatment, extraction of all maxillary teeth except 13, 23 and provision of an provisional removable upper partial denture. Extraction of teeth 37, 45, 48 and removal of the fractured implant 46.
- *Phase 2 — Planning and implant surgery.* Six months after the extractions: Implant planning, extraction of teeth 13 and 23, flapless implant placement supported by digital technologies, and delivery of an immediately loaded provisional full-arch screw-retained prosthesis.
- *Phase 3 — Final rehabilitation.* 10 months after loading with a provisional prosthesis: Definitive computer-aided designed and manufactured (CAD/CAM) maxillary hybrid full-arch fixed prosthesis.

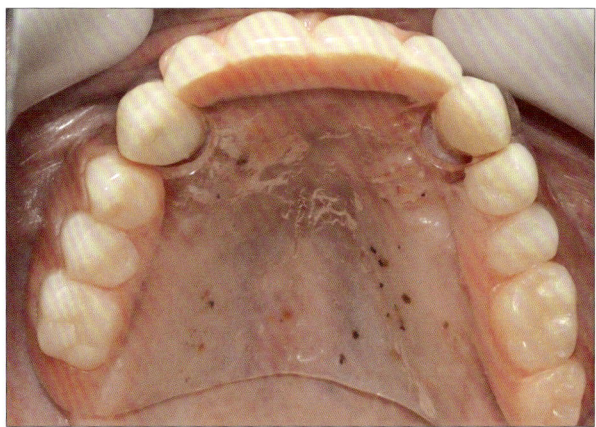

Fig 3   Provisional removable partial denture, occlusal view.

Phase 1 — Preparatory therapy

The vertical dimension of occlusion (VDO) and the centric relation (CR) were recorded clinically and the stone casts were accordingly in a semi-adjustable articulator. Teeth 13 and 23 were retained for strategic reasons to support the surgical template, their extraction being planned for the day of implant surgery. A maxillary provisional removable partial denture was fitted immediately after the extraction of teeth 16 – 12, 21, 22, 25, and 26 to reestablish the VDO, anterior guidance, and occlusal plane (Fig 3). Teeth 37, 45, and 48 were extracted; the fractured implant 46 was removed. We decided to keep the implants and crowns at sites 36 and 47 because they were osseointegrated and clinically acceptable despite the marginal bone loss.

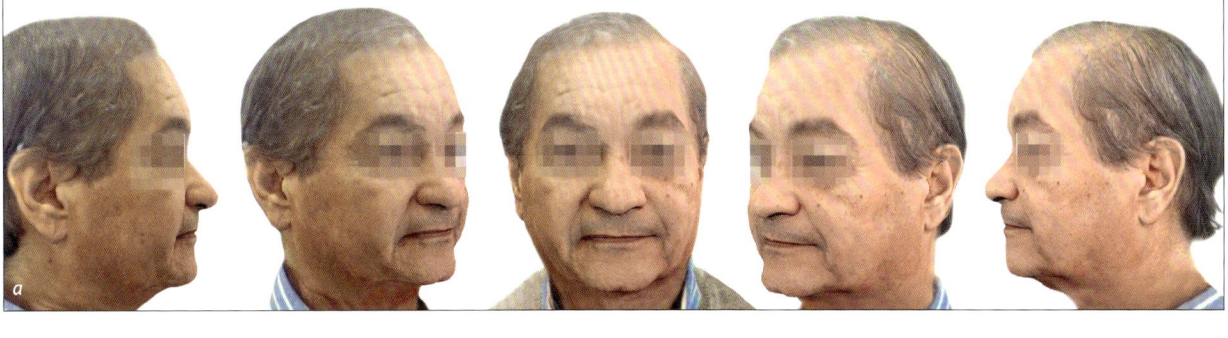

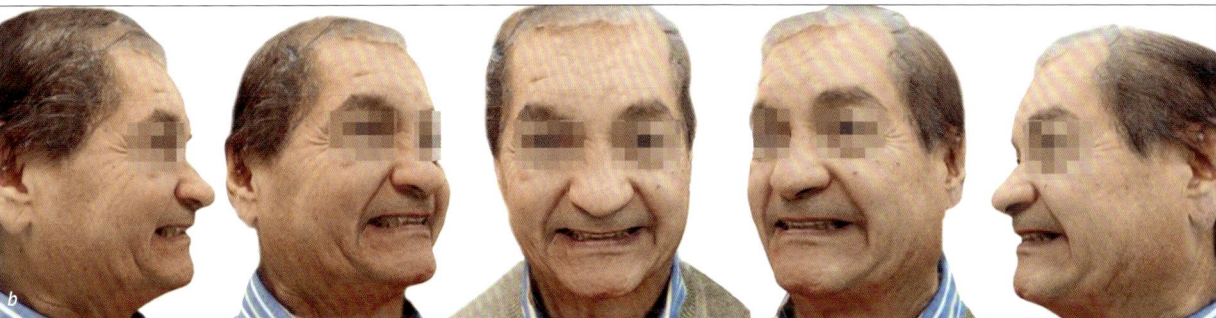

Figs 4a-b   3D digital files of the face at rest (a). Forced smile (b).

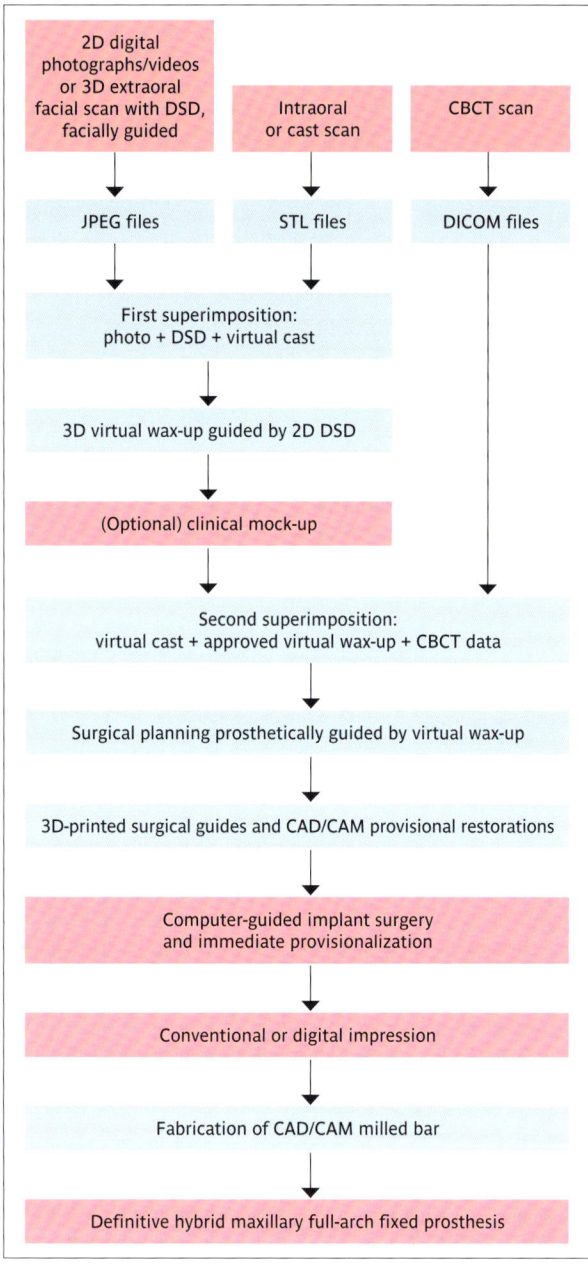

Fig 5   Digital workflow guided by facial references (adapted from Coachman and coworkers 2017). Clinical appointments are shown in pink.

Phase 2 — Implant planning and implant surgery

Six months after the preparatory phase, digital clinical information was transferred to a software program (Nemo Smile Design; Nemotec, Madrid, Spain). These included digital photographs and screenshots exported from smartphone videos, IOS (STL) files of scanned casts, and extraoral photographs of the face converted into three-dimensional (3D) STL files (Remake; Autodesk, San Rafael, USA) (Figs 4a-b), and CBCT scan (DICOM) files.

The starting point for the proposed digital workflow was the Digital Smile Design (DSD) guided by facial references such as the facial midline, bipupillary line, smile curve, and smile height (Fig 5). Frontal photographs of the face were taken with and without lip retractors, keeping the camera and the patient's head still to create photographs with similar distances, angles, and distortions. Using Nemo Smile Design software (Nemotec), the photographs were adjusted and merged. Facial reference lines were drawn over the smiling photograph and transferred to the photographs using lip retractors. These facial references guided the 2D smile design and the 3D virtual wax-up (Figs 6 and 7). Superimposition of the scanned casts on the DSD facilitated a virtual wax-up, correcting the occlusal plane and harmonizing the position of the teeth with the face and smile (Figs 8 to 10). Although the DSD is subject to limitations inherent in the photographic process and in the superimposition of 2D to 3D files, it is a useful planning tool that assists decision-making, improves diagnostic vision, and facilitates education and communication between professionals and patients

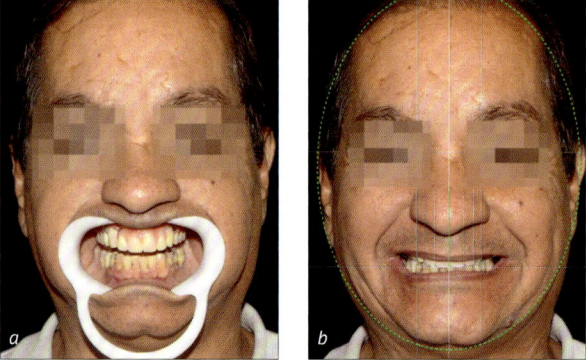

Figs 6a-b   View of the face with lips retracted (a). Facial reference lines drawn over the 2D photograph of the face to create a smile frame (b).

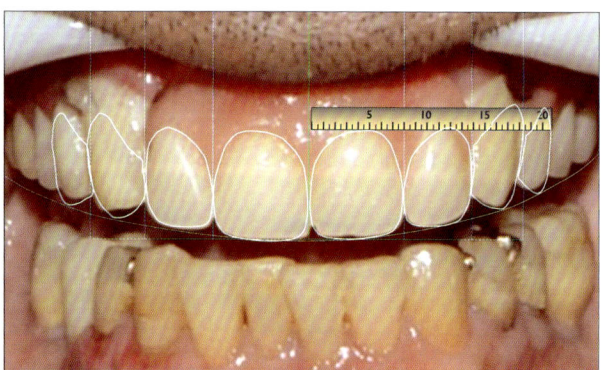

Fig 7   Generated 2D digital smile design according to the facial reference lines transferred from smile photograph to retracted photograph.

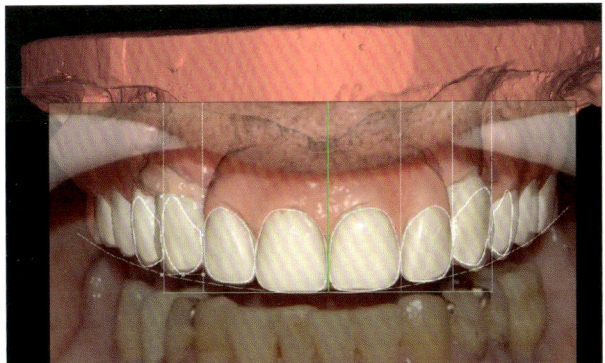

Fig 8   Scanned cast data superimposed on 2D digital smile design using the teeth of the provisional denture as reference points.

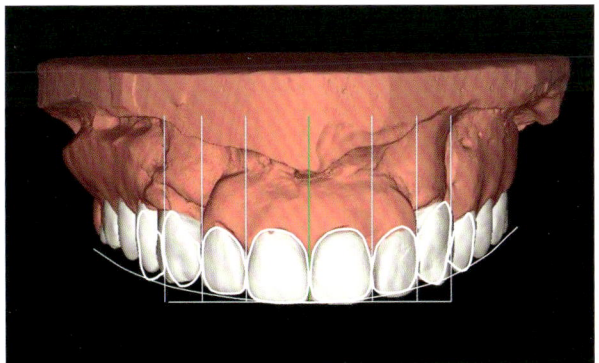

Fig 9   Scanned cast with 3D virtual waxing guided by 2D digital smile design.

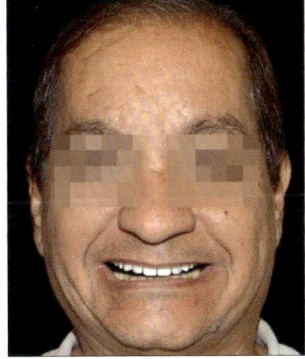

Fig 10   Overlapping digital wax-up and facial photographs for a digital esthetic evaluation before inserting the implants.

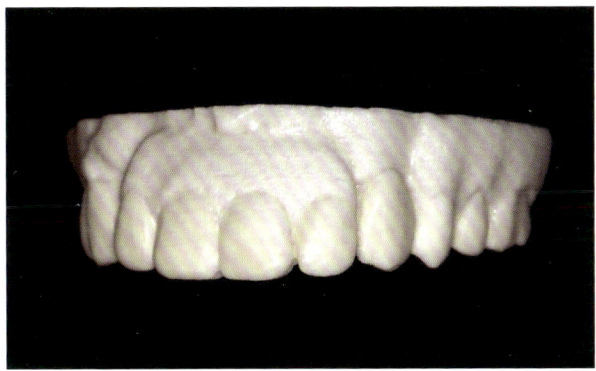

Fig 11   3D-printed cast.

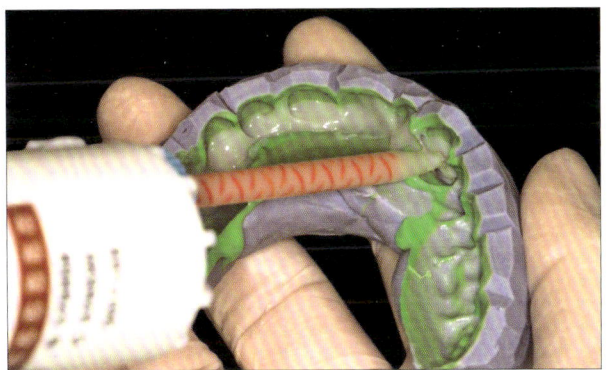

Fig 12   Silicone index and Protemp 4 bisacryl composite resin (3M Espe, Maplewood, MN, USA) for a diagnostic preview.

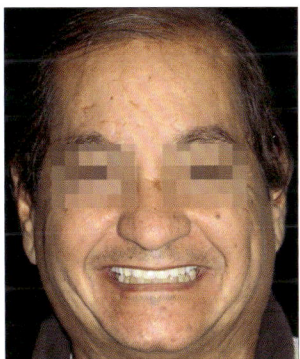

Fig 13   Trial restoration in harmony with the face.

The maxillary digital wax-up was exported as an STL file to be 3D-printed. A silicone index was prepared for the fabrication of trial restorations (Figs 11 to 13). This clinical step was very useful for the esthetic evaluation; however, this step will not always be possible (especially not in patients with excessive hypereruption or abnormal tooth angulations) as the silicone index will not fit properly over the remaining teeth in such situations.

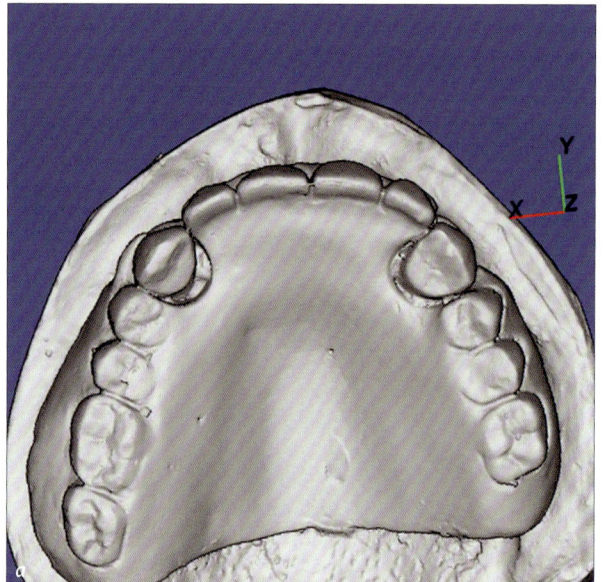

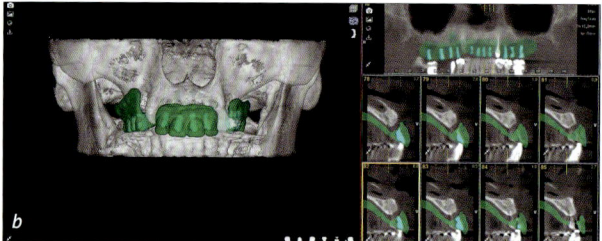

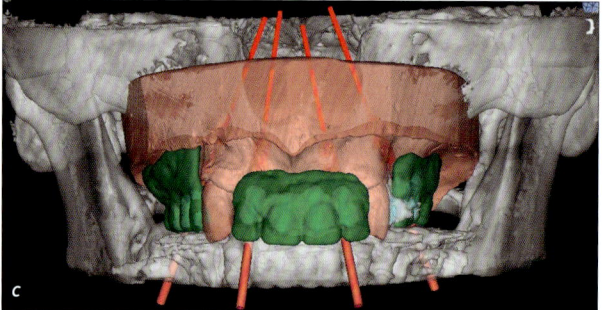

Figs 14a-c   STL of the scanned cast (a). Merged anatomical (CBCT) and prosthetic data (radiographic template) (b). Superimposition of CBCT and virtual-cast data (c).

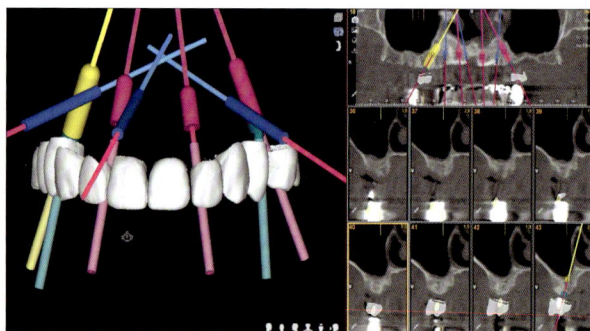

Fig 15   Prosthetically driven surgical planning.

Once the trial restorations were approved by the patient, the surgical steps were planned.

Impressions were taken with the provisional denture in place and the resulting cast was scanned in a lab scanner (7-series; Dental Wings, Montreal, Canada) (Fig 14a). The provisional denture was also used as a radiographic template, using denture teeth filled with radiopaque composite resin. A CBCT scan was obtained using the double-scan technique: The patient was scanned with the radiographic template in the first scan and the radiographic template was scanned separately, extraorally, in the second scan (Fig 14b). The radiopaque fiducial marks were the references for data matching. Using the Nemo Smile Design-DSD software (Nemo Smile Design; Nemotec), the data were superimposed, merging the cast with the virtual wax-up and CBCT data with the denture teeth as reference points, thus allowing prosthetically driven planning of the position of implants (Figs 14c and 15). Implant planning provided for the placement of four implants (Bone Level; Institut Straumann AG, Basel, Switzerland), two placed axially in the anterior region and two distally tilted implants in the posterior region (Straumann Pro-Arch protocol), using computer-guided flapless implant surgery.

From this planning, two surgical guides and a provisional denture were designed in a CAD software package (Nemo Smile Design; Nemotec) (Figs 16a-c). The surgical guides were 3D-printed (Digital Wax; DWS Systems, Vicenza, Italy), and the CAD/CAM provisional denture was milled from the 3D virtual wax-up (Ceramill Motion2; Amann Girrbach, Pforzheim, Germany), all with sleeves for anchor guide pins in the predetermined positions (Fig 17).

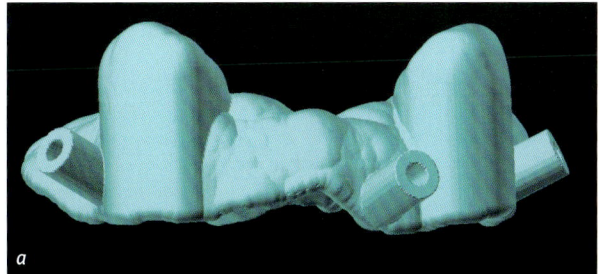

Following administration of a local anesthetic, the first tooth-supported guide (Fig 18) was positioned on the remaining maxillary teeth. This guide was used to secure the position of the anchoring guide pins, so that the second guide for implant placement (used after removing the teeth) and the dental prosthesis itself would use the same positional references as indicated by these pins.

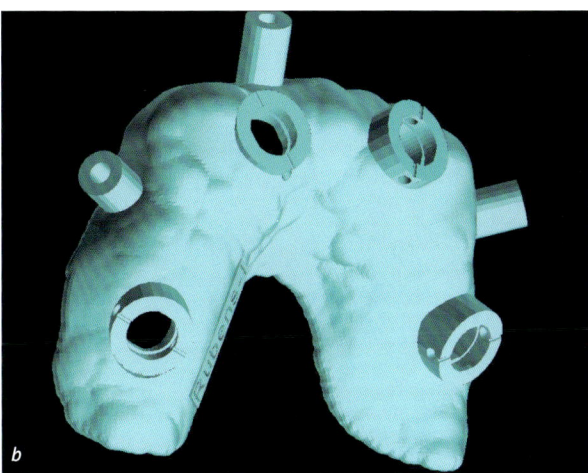

Teeth 13 and 23 were extracted (Fig 19) and the mucosa-supported surgical guide was positioned according to the anchor guide pins. Two bone-level implants (Bone Level RC, diameter 4.1 mm, length 8 mm; Institut Straumann AG, Basel, Switzerland) were placed in the anterior region and two additional bone-level implants (Bone Level RC, diameter 4.1 mm, length 12 mm; Institut Straumann AG) were placed in the posterior maxilla in a flapless approach (Fig 20). All implants displayed a high insertion torque and adequate primary stability, so immediate provisionalization was possible.

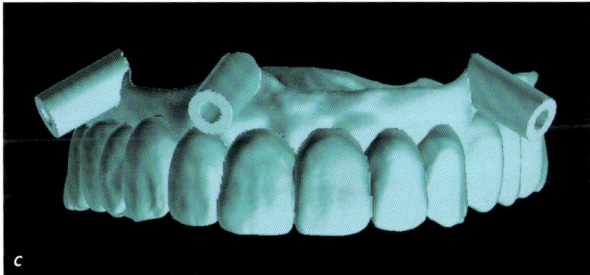

Definitive screw-retained abutments (SRA; Institut Straumann AG) were tightened on the implants at a torque of 35 Ncm. The provisional restoration was positioned in the mouth using the anchor guide pins, and provisional titanium cylinders were connected to the prosthesis with autopolymerizing acrylic resin.

Figs 16a-c STL image of the tooth-supported guide (a). STL image of the mucosa-supported guide for implant placement (b). STL image of the provisional prosthesis (c).

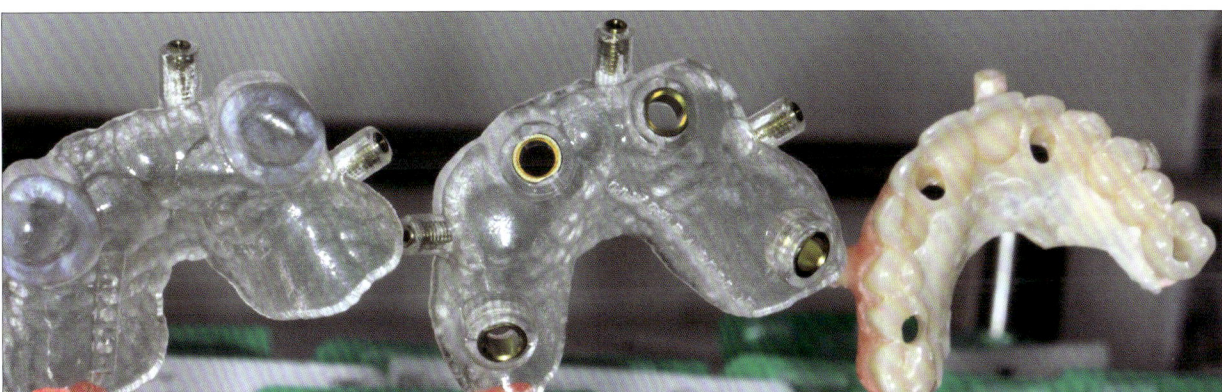

Fig 17 Printed guides and milled provisional denture.

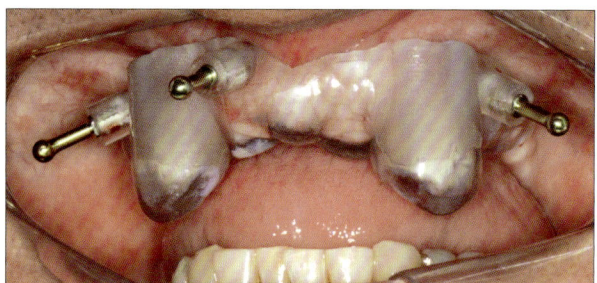

Fig 18   Tooth-supported guide used to determine position of anchor guide pins.

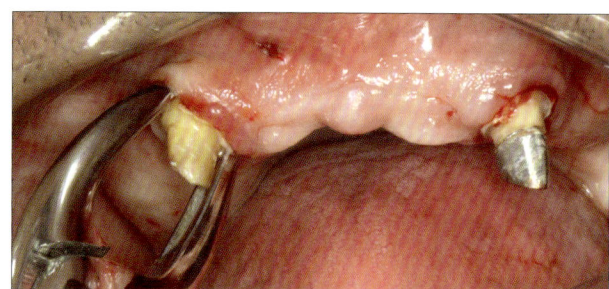

Fig 19   Extraction of teeth 13 and 23.

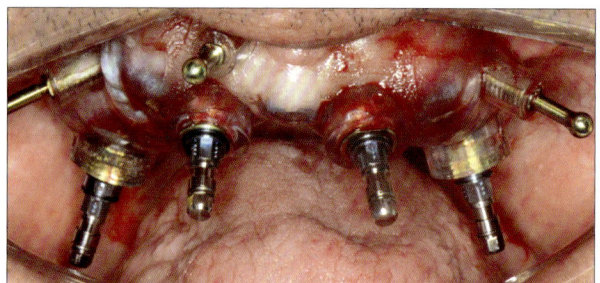

Fig 20   Guided flapless implant placement.

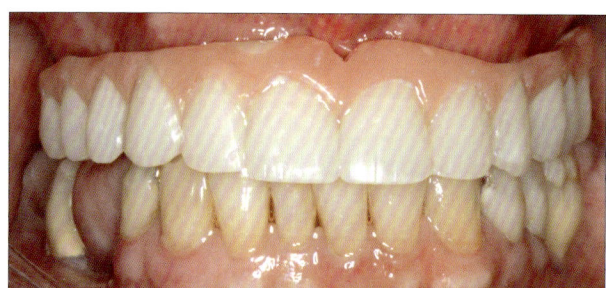

Fig 21   CAD/CAM provisional maxillary fixed dental prosthesis, frontal view.

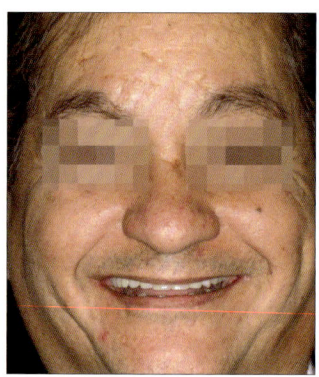

Fig 22   Postoperative view of the face.

The anchor guide pins were removed together with the corresponding guide sleeves in the denture. The occlusion was checked and adjusted and the prosthesis was polished before being screwed in place at a torque of 15 Ncm (Fig 21). The screw access holes were sealed with PTFE tape and composite resin, and the patient was given postoperative instructions. Clinical and radiographic postoperative evaluations (Figs 22 to 24) were performed during the 10 months until the definitive prosthesis was fabricated.

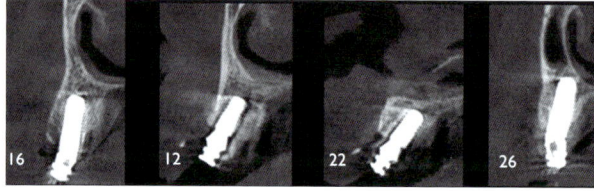

Fig 24   Postoperative CBCT scan.

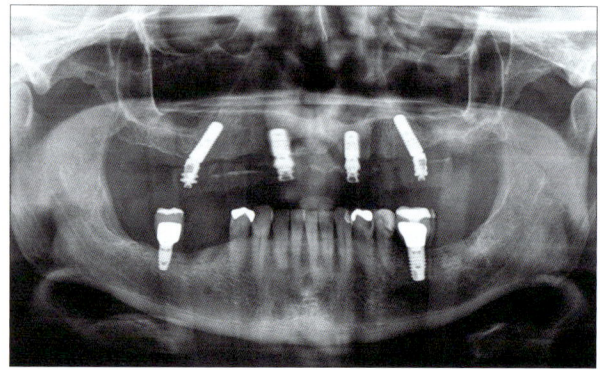

Fig 23   Postoperative radiograph.

Phase 3 — Final rehabilitation

In the mandible, two bone-level implants (Bone Level NC, diameter 3.3 mm, length 10 mm; Institut Straumann AG) were placed at sites 45 and 46 in a conventional manner after computer-assisted planning (Fig 25).

Two months after mandibular implant placement, an implant-level digital impression was taken with scanbodies inserted into the implants (Scan Body; Institut Straumann, AG) using an intraoral scanner (Straumann Cares/Dental Wings; Institut Straumann AG). Using the resulting STL file, the single crowns were designed digitally. Monolithic zirconia crowns (Prettau; Zirkonzahn, Gais, Italy) were fabricated by CAM, cemented to the Variobase abutments, and screwed onto the implants (Figs 26a-b).

For the maxillary rehabilitation, a conventional abutment-level impression was taken and a working model made 10 months after implant placement and loading with the provisional prosthesis. A trial wax set-up was tested and adjusted in the mouth. A silicone index was made to evaluate the space available for the bar (Figs 27a-e).

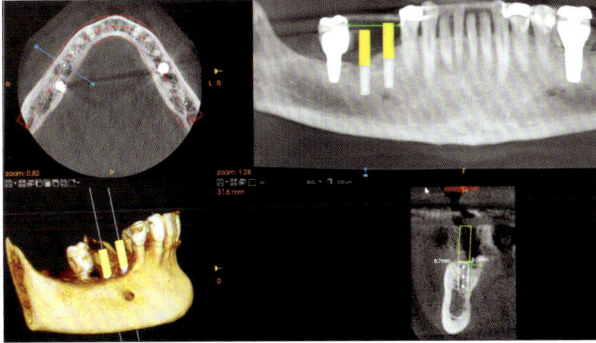

Fig 25   Surgical planning of the mandibular implants assisted by software.

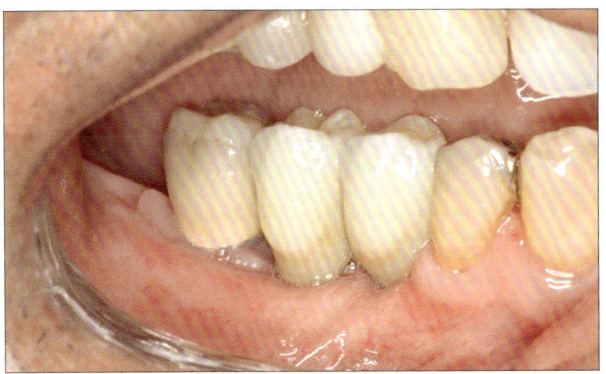

Fig 26a   Zirconia crowns cemented onto Variobase abutments and screw-retained on the implants.

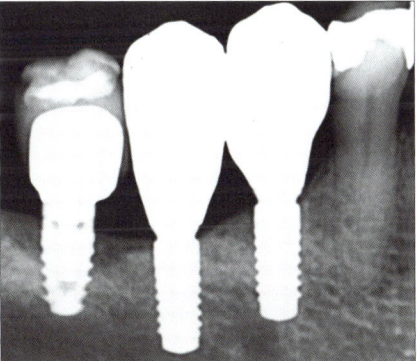

Fig 26b   Periapical radiograph.

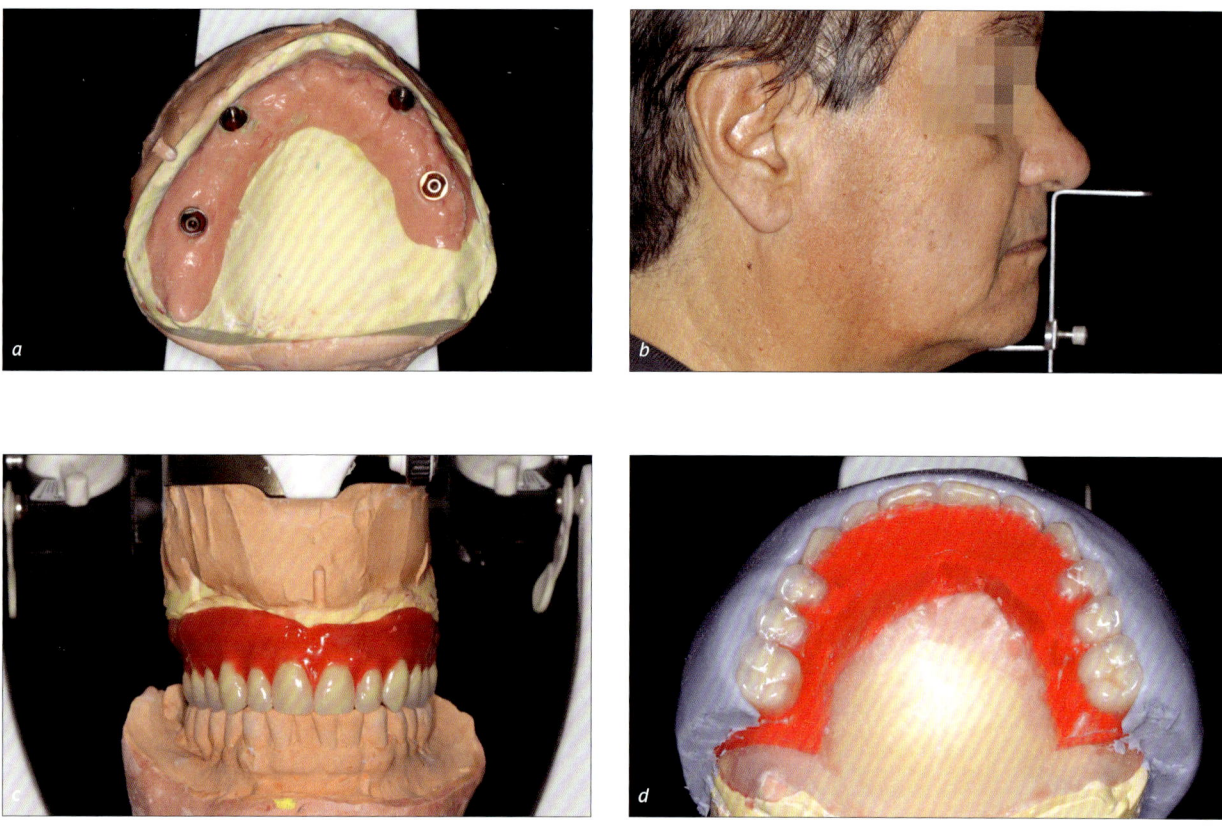

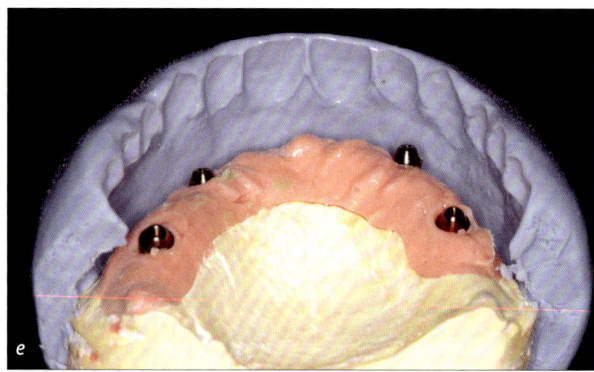

Figs 27a-e   Working model (a). Clinical VDO measurement (b). Trial set-up (c). Silicone index (d). Checking the space for the bar (e).

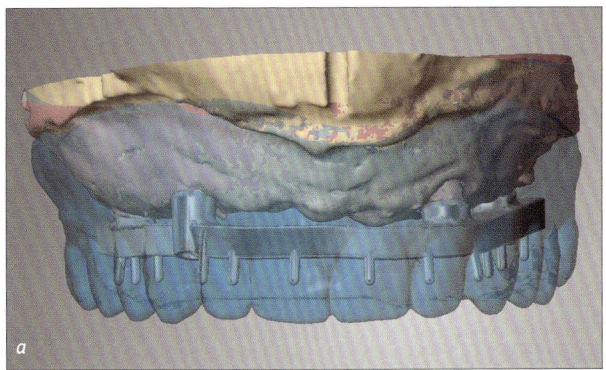
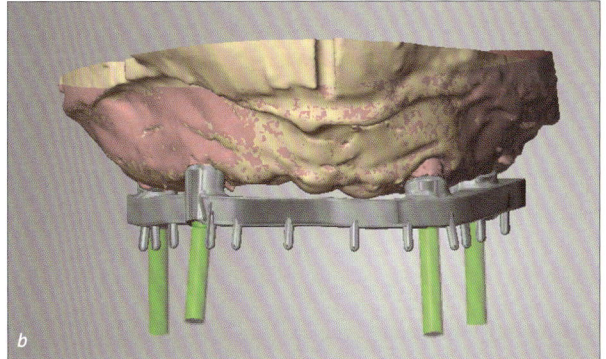
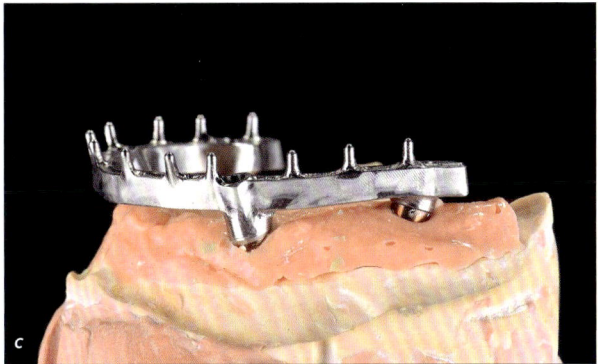

Figs 28a-c   Digital cast (a). CAD of the bar (b). Titanium bar (c).

The maxillary working model was scanned in an extraoral lab scanner (7 series, Dental Wings, Montreal, Canada) and a CAD/CAM-milled titanium bar was fabricated (Straumann Milling Center, Curitiba, Brazil) (Figs 28a-c).

A final wax try-in of the teeth on the titanium bar was performed and the denture was processed in the lab. A definitive hybrid maxillary full-arch fixed prosthesis was fitted (Figs 29a-d). Centric and lateral contacts were assessed to obtain uniform occlusal contacts distributed over the entire arch. Screw access holes were sealed with PTFE tape and composite resin. A convex mucosal contact surface facilitates the use of dental floss. The extension of the buccal flange was just sufficient to prevent the escape of air and phonetic difficulties, without compromising access for adequate oral hygiene at home (Fig 29e).

At delivery, some peri-implant marginal bone loss was observed, especially on the distal aspect of the tilted implants, which may have been caused by an inadequately balanced distribution of occlusal forces while the patient was using the provisional prosthesis without reinforcement from a metal framework. The patient was instructed in correct oral hygiene procedures and clinically followed every 3 months for 1 year. No significant additional bone loss or clinical complications were observed (Figs 30a-d). Peri-implant and periodontal indices were recorded at the one-year follow-up (Fig 31).

Discussion

Perfect harmony between the teeth, lips, and facial components is the goal of every prosthodontic treatment, whether performed in a conventional or digital workflow. In anterior restorations and extensive rehabilitations of complete arches, treatment planning must be guided by the face to obtain adequate esthetic and functional results (Spear and Kokich 2007; Calamia and coworkers 2011; Giannuzzi and Motlagh 2015).

A great challenge when rehabilitating patients with complete or anterior partial edentulism has been to relate the face to a definitive cast and fabricate wax patterns in harmony with the face. In the digital workflow, the challenge remains the same, but now these facial references need to be transferred to the virtual cast in the planning software. Complex rehabilitations are commonly associated with out-of-balance esthetics and occlusal conditions that present unreliable occlusal references and require correction.

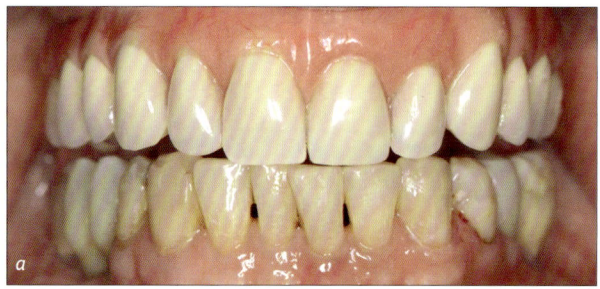
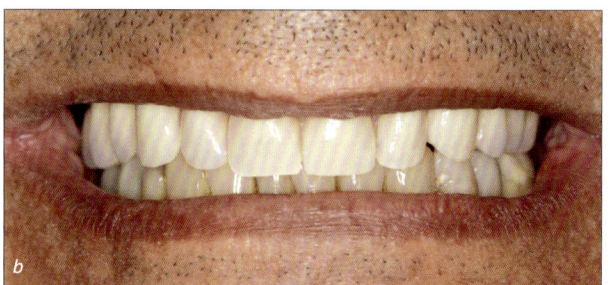
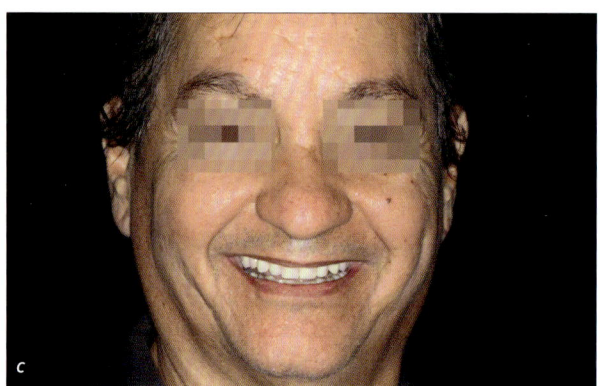
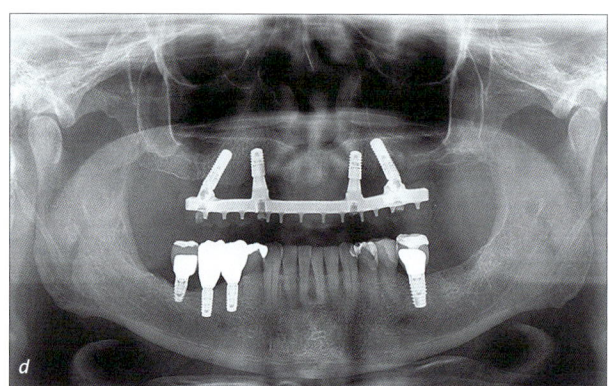
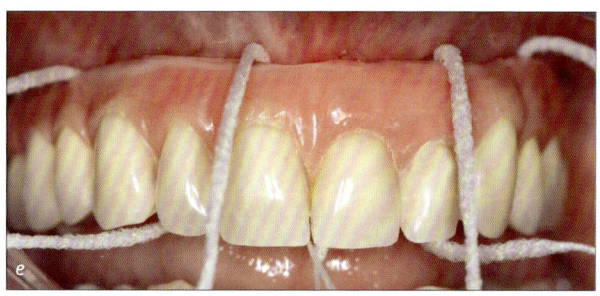

Figs 29a-e   Final restorations. Intraoral view (a). Smile (b). Facial view (c). Radiograph (d). Access for home oral hygiene (e).

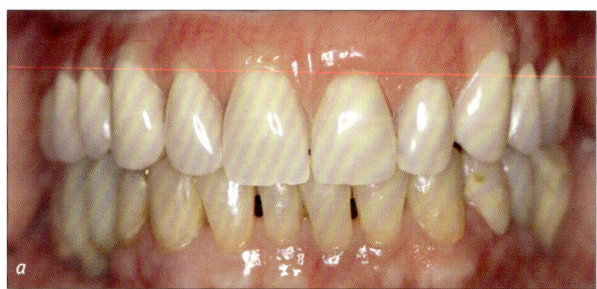
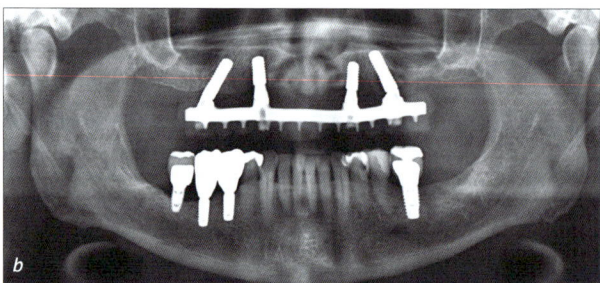
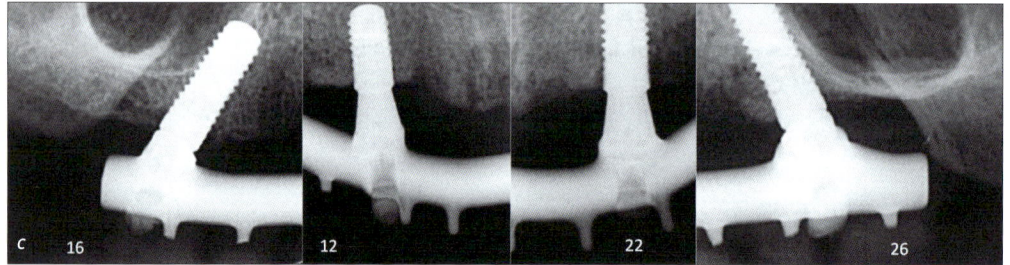
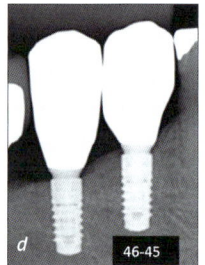

Figs 30a-d   1-year follow-up. Clinical view (a). Panoramic radiograph (a). Periapical radiographs of teeth 16, 12, 22, and 26 (c). Periapical radiograph of teeth 45 and 46 (d).

Examples of such situations may include patients with partial edentulism where the extraction of all remaining teeth is indicated. This is a challenging situation, because as long as the compromised teeth have not been extracted, the clinical evaluation of the teeth for the new dental prostheses may be difficult or even impossible. The use of digital resources may be the only way to visualize the future dental set-up before the extractions are performed. This virtual waxing must be guided by facial references and must be in harmony with the smile, making a facial approach to planning essential (Coachman and coworkers 2017).

Various authors have reported on different clinical surgical and prosthodontic solutions assisted by digital technology (Stapleton and coworkers 2014; Lanis and coworkers 2015a, Lewis and coworkers 2015; Arunyanak and coworkers 2016; Charette and coworkers 2016). The 3D facial scan has been successfully integrated into the CAD/CAM workflow for partial and full-arch rehabilitations (Joda and Gallucci 2015; Harris and coworkers 2017; Hassan and coworkers 2017) and for esthetic restorations (Lin and coworkers 2017). A recent consensus statement (Hämmerle and coworkers 2015) recommends:

- As guided surgery may add precision to flapless surgery, it can have its implications in geriatric patients and individuals with compromised medical conditions.
- Digital technology can provide technical, clinical, and procedural benefits.
- Where available, multiple patient-related data sets (e.g., CBCT, intraoral and laboratory scans, virtual planning for implants and restorations) should ideally be integrated to maximize their synergistic diagnostic value.

Further scientific validation and large-scale clinical studies on digital treatment modalities are still needed to understand the impact of this promising technology for modifying well-established conventional protocols (Joda and coworkers 2017a).

The treatment planning of the presented case included both digital and conventional workflows at different clinical stages, seeking to leverage the benefits of each.

Recording a comprehensive case history, clinical examinations, respect for biological principles, and a thorough knowledge of the relevant esthetic and functional parameters remain the keys to the success of the digital workflow, just as with conventional workflows.

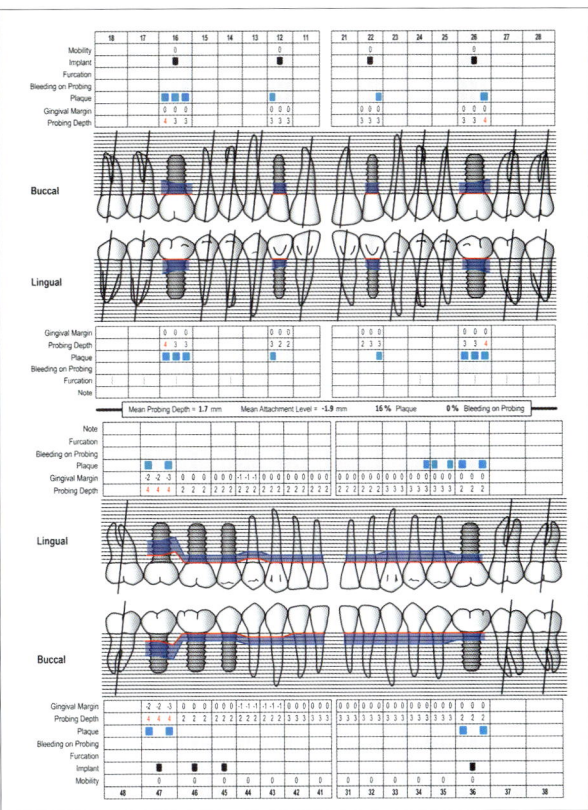

Fig 31   Peri-implant and periodontal indices at the one-year follow-up.

Acknowledgments

Implant planning
Dr. Christian Coachman, Francis Coachman, and Guillermo Manzano – DSD Planning Center, Madrid, Spain

Surgical procedures
Dr. Claudia Riquelme, Fabio Luiz Munhoz, and Tiago Rebelo da Costa – School of Dentistry, University of São Paulo, São Paulo, Brazil

Restorative procedures
Dr. Dalva Cruz Laganá, Yolanda Natali Raico-Gallardo, Rosely Cordon, and Nataly Zambrana – School of Dentistry, University of São Paulo, São Paulo, Brazil

Laboratory procedures
Straumann Group Digital Center – Curitiba, Brazil
Schayder Dental Studio – São Paulo, Brazil

13.13   Rehabilitating a Maxillofacial Defect with Transplanted Free Vascularized Fibula Segments and a Full-Arch Fixed Dental Prosthesis

G. Raghoebar, R. Schepers, A. Vissink, M. Witjes

A 43-year-old male patient was referred to the department of Oral and Maxillofacial Surgery, University Medical Center Groningen, Netherlands for secondary reconstruction of the maxilla. Twelve years previously, a hemimaxillectomy had been performed elsewhere because of a maxillary osteosarcoma. The resulting defect had been reconstructed using a deep circumflex iliac-artery flap and radial forearm flap. The patient had then been rehabilitated with a tooth-supported prosthesis.

The patient was referred to our department because the retaining three upper molars had a poor prognosis, having become mobile due to periodontal disease and overloading (Figs 1 and 2). The patient complained of a lack of retention and stability of his maxillary denture. He was in good general health, did not take any regular medication, and did not smoke. He was offered a reconstruction with a free vascularized osseous flap and an implant-supported maxillary overdenture and gave his written informed consent.

The proposed treatment was divided into four phases. The first phase consisted of 3D virtual pre-planning of the fibula resection and implant positions for the desired reconstruction. The second phase consisted of prefabrication of the fibula flap by guided implant insertion, digital implant registration, and application of a skin graft around the implants. During the third phase, the implant-supported maxillary overdenture and the surgical guide for the fibula were manufactured. The fourth and final phase included the reconstructive surgery of the maxillary bony defect with the free vascularized fibula flap and the overdenture in the proper occlusion and position in the maxilla.

Phase 1: Virtual planning
3D virtual treatment planning began with a cone-beam computer tomography (CBCT) scan of the maxillofacial region, with the patient wearing the denture (i-CAT; Imaging Sciences International, Hatfield, PA. USA). A high-resolution CT angiography scan of the lower legs was also acquired (Somatom Definition Dual Source; Siemens Healthineers, Forchheim, Germany). In addition, a digital subtraction arteriogram (DSA) of the lower leg was made with a 0.6 mm collimation and a 30f kernel (medium smooth). All images were stored in uncompressed DICOM format. The scans of the maxillofacial region and fibula were imported into ProPlan CMF 1.3 (Synthes, Solothurn, Switzerland; and Materialise, Leuven, Belgium) to plan the reconstruction of the jaw defect in a virtual environment. The 3D models of the jaw defect and the fibula were created, and the fibula was virtually cut and planned to fit in the defect.

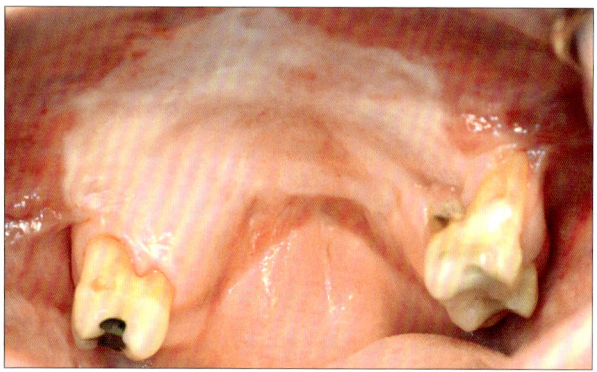

Fig 1   Clinical view of the maxillary defect at the time of referral to our department. The three retaining teeth were mobile and exhibited mucosal recession due to periodontal disease.

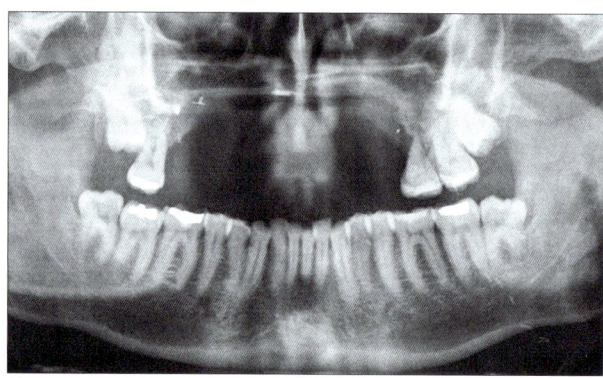

Fig 2   Panoramic radiograph revealing bone resorption around the retentive molars. Two impacted molars are also visible.

To plan the antagonist dentition and the implants, the virtual reconstruction file was converted to Simplant Pro 2011 (Materialise). The antagonist denture was scanned separately by CBCT (120 kV, 5 mA, 0.3 voxel size) and imported into the planning file as a 3D object. To create an optimal dental setup, virtual teeth were positioned on the antagonist dentition setup in the proper occlusion using the denture as a model. Virtual implants (Nobel Speedy, diameter 4.0 mm, length 10–13 mm; Nobel Biocare, Göteborg, Sweden) were planned in the optimal position to support the virtual antagonist dentition, creating a total reconstructive plan of fibula graft and implants (Fig 3a). A multidisciplinary team (maxillofacial surgeon, plastic surgeon, maxillofacial prosthodontist) judged the reconstructive plan to be clinically feasible. After all members of the multidisciplinary team had agreed, the file was converted to ProPlan CMF 1.3 to design the guides.

The implants were assigned to the appropriate fibula segments and digitally relocated to their original position before virtual cutting (Fig 3b). This step results in implant positions in the pre-cut fibula in the best planned position for optimal denture retention after cutting. On the original fibula, a drilling guide was designed virtually using 3-matic 7.0 (Materialise) to facilitate guided drilling and guided tapping of the implants in the fibula (Nobel guide; Nobel Biocare). Finally, the surgical guide for implant placement was 3D-printed in polyamide and sterilized with gamma radiation to be used intraoperatively (Fig 4).

Phase 2: Prefabrication of the fibula

During the first surgical step, implants were placed in the fibula and covered with a skin graft (Figs 4 to 8). First, the anterior plane of the fibula was exposed. Sharp edges, which had already been noticed during the planning phase, were trimmed to create a flat surface for implant placement with adequate bony margins. After trimming the top of the fibula, the surgical template was positioned and secured to the exposed fibula with miniscrews (KLS Martin, Tuttlingen, Germany) (Fig 4). The surgical template contained metal cylinders to hold removable sleeves of different diameters matching the diameters of the drill used to prepare the implant sites, according to the recommendations of the manufacturer. After drilling the holes, the surgical template was removed and screw tapping of the implant sites was performed. Six implants were inserted with a minimum torque of 35 Ncm (Fig 5). Next, an intraoperative optical scan of the implants with scanning abutments (Dentsply Sirona, York, PA, USA) was obtained with the Lava Chairside Oral Scanner C.O.S. (3M ESPE, St. Paul, MI, USA) to register the exact position and angulations (Fig 6). To check whether the intraoral scan was sufficiently accurate for

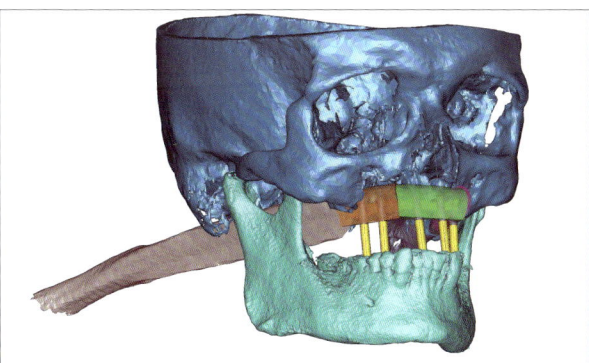

Fig 3a   Maxillary defect virtually reconstructed with a segmented fibula and implants.

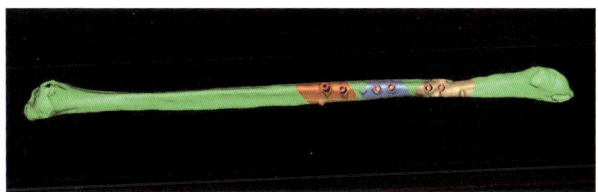

Fig 3b   Implants assigned to the appropriate fibula segments and digitally relocated to their original position before virtual cutting.

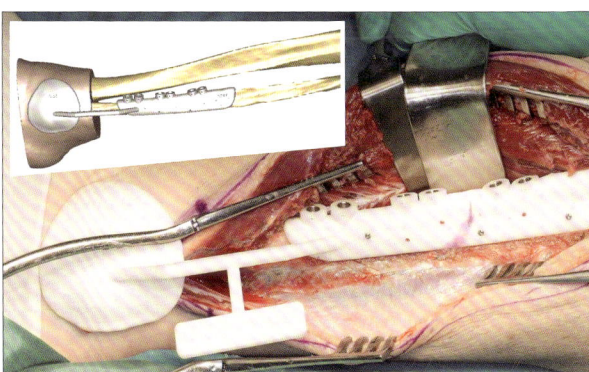

Fig 4   3D-printed surgical guide on the ventral rim of the fibula and attached to the bone of the fibula with miniscrews.

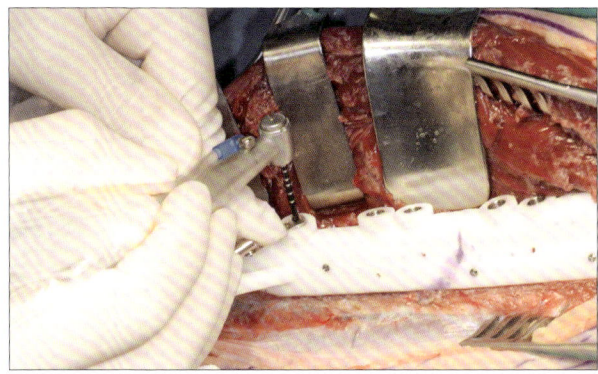

Fig 5   Implant sites in the fibula drilled in the predetermined direction using metal inserts placed in the drilling guide.

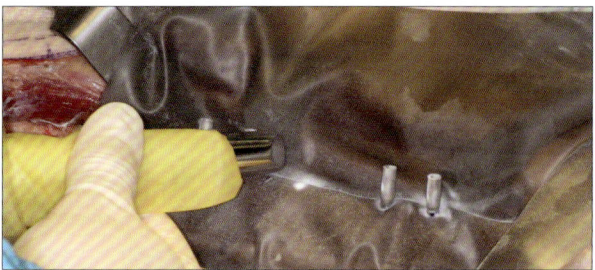

Fig 6   Intraoperative optical scan of the implants and scanning abutments in the fibula.

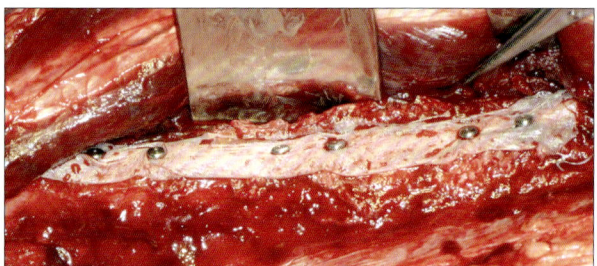

Fig 7   Split-thickness skin graft on top of the area in which the implants in the fibula were inserted.

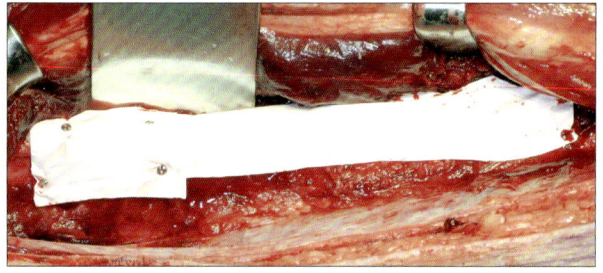

Fig 8   Gore-Tex patch attached on top of the skin graft (cf. Fig 7).

the fabrication of a titanium bar and as a fail-safe precaution, the position of the implants was also registered by taking impressions using impression posts and a conventional soft polyether impression paste (Impregum, 3M ESPE). The fibula in which the implants were placed was covered with a split-thickness skin graft (Fig 7) and the skin graft was covered by a matching Gore-Tex patch (W.L. Gore and Associates, Flagstaff, AZ, USA) (Fig 8). After primary wound closure, the implants and the split skin grafts were left to heal for six weeks.

Phase 3: Fabrication of the maxillary overdenture and surgical guide for the fibula

The optical scan of the scan abutments and of the final implant positions was imported into the ProPlan CMF 1.3 software and manually matched with the original fibula reconstruction planning. In this way, a superimposed fusion model was created that showed the accurate position of the implants. After updating the virtual 3D plan with the real implant positions in the fibula (Fig 9), the retentive bar for the maxillary overdenture was virtually designed on the implants (Fig 10). The designed bar was converted to the STL file format and milled from titanium (Fig 11).

A 3D-planned wafer was designed to transfer the position of the implants to the antagonist dentition of the patient (Fig 12). This wafer represents the space that the prosthesis occupies after the reconstruction; consequently, the wafer can be printed and used as a cast positioner (Fig 13). The wafer is also needed to transform the digital plan into a plaster model for conventional denture fabrication (Fig 14).

The surgical guide of the fibula was planned according to the (adjusted) virtual treatment plan, printed, and sterilized using gamma irradiation.

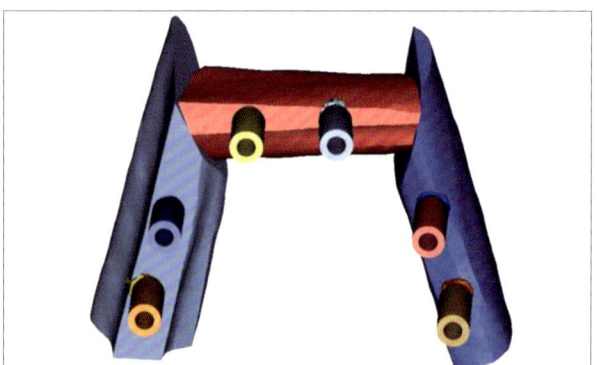

Fig 9   Planned implant positions replaced by real positions according to the scan to update the 3D plan.

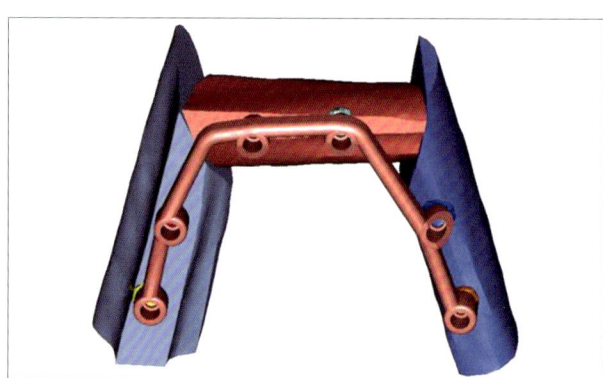

Fig 10   Virtually designed bar on the implants.

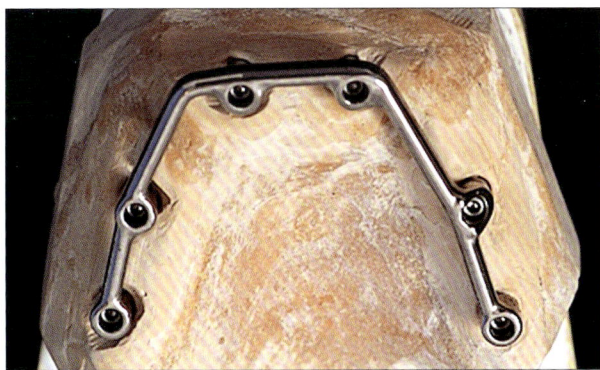

Fig 11   Bar design converted to STL file format and milled from titanium.

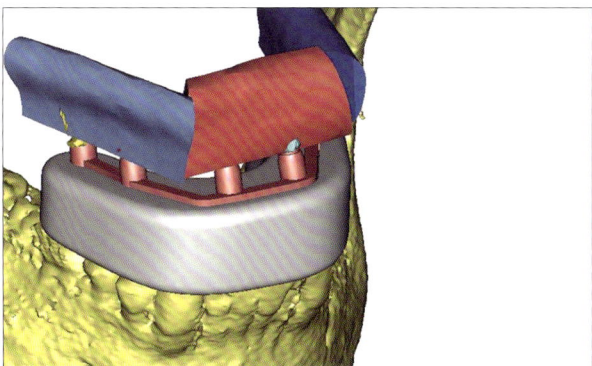

Fig 12   3D model of the maxillary reconstruction with a positioning wafer on top of the mandibular dentition.

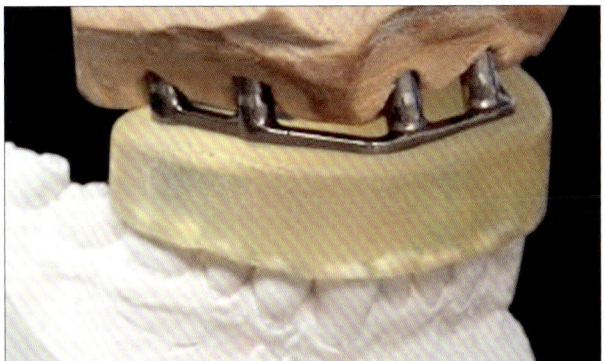

Fig 13   CAD/CAM titanium bar in the articulator to facilitate the fabrication of the maxillary implant-supported overdenture.

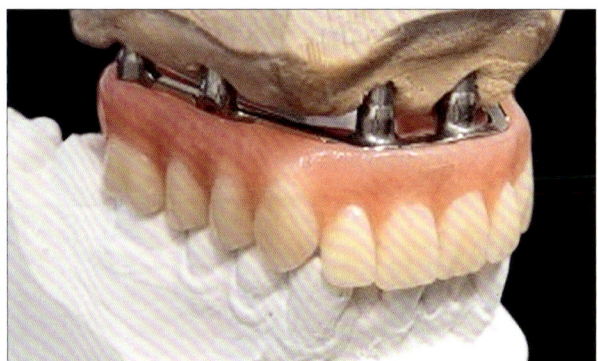

Fig 14   Fabrication of the implant-supported maxillary overdenture.

Phase 4: Surgical reconstruction of the maxillary defect

The second surgical step was planned at least six weeks after the prefabrication procedure to give the implants time to osseointegrate. The fibula with the implants was exposed, while the vascular supply of the fibula stayed intact (Fig 15). The surgical guide was secured on the implants (Fig 16) and the osteotomies were performed using a reciprocating saw with a 35-mm blade, guided by the sleeves in the surgical guide (Aesculap microspeed uni; Aesculap, Center Valley, PA, USA). After the osteotomies, the surgical guide was removed, the superstructure was screwed onto the implants (Fig 17), and the denture was secured to the bar with clips (Fig 18). Until this moment, the blood circulation of the graft remained intact to minimize the duration of flap ischemia.

Once the maxillary defect was exposed, the fibula was released as a free graft (Fig 19). To ensure a highly accurate fit of the graft in the oral defect, the intraoral defect edges are optimized as needed, based on the planned outcome and surgical guides (Fig 20). After preparation of the recipient site, the fibula was transplanted into the maxillary defect. The graft was guided by the positioning splint placed in occlusion and fixed using osteosynthesis plates and monocortical screws (KLS Martin). The implant-supported maxillary overdenture was placed on the bar (Fig 21).

Finally, the fibular artery and veins were connected to the blood vessels in the neck and the fibular skin graft was sutured to the oral mucosa. The patient was discharged after eleven days.

The clinical and radiographic follow-up revealed stable conditions of the peri-implant soft and hard tissues (Figs 22 to 24). The patient was pleased with the esthetic outcome and function provided by his implant-supported denture. The patient was referred back to the referring department for follow-up and professional maintenance.

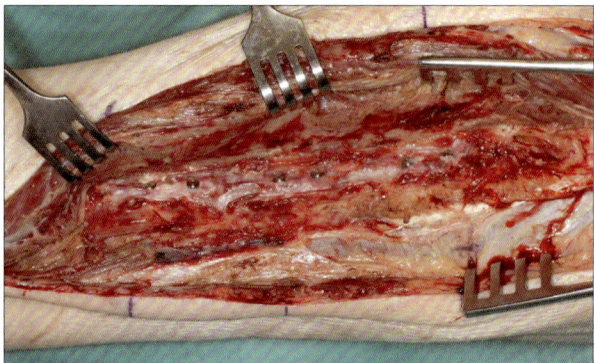

Fig 15   Exposed implants in the fibula.

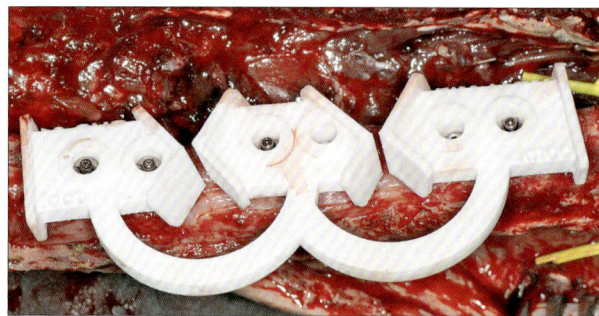

Fig 16   Virtually planned surgical guide for the fibula secured in place on the implants.

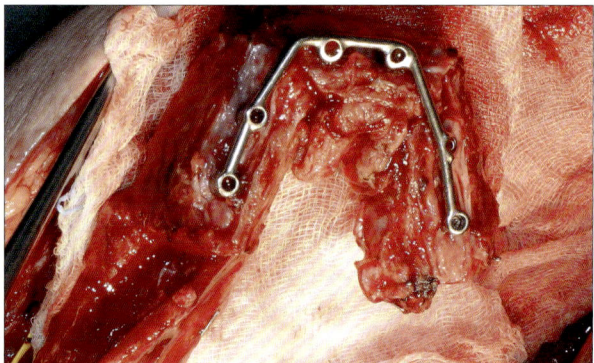

Fig 17   Titanium bar secured to the implants in the osteotomized fibula.

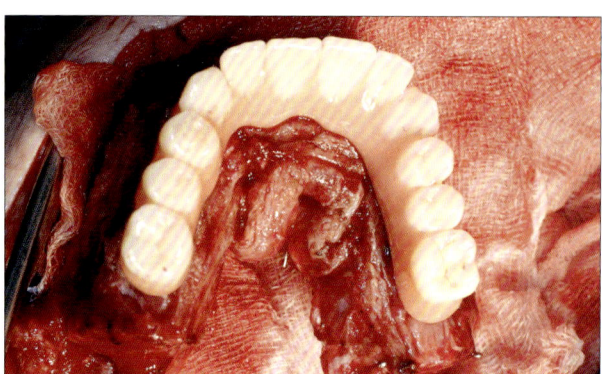

Fig 18   Denture attached to the bar with clips.

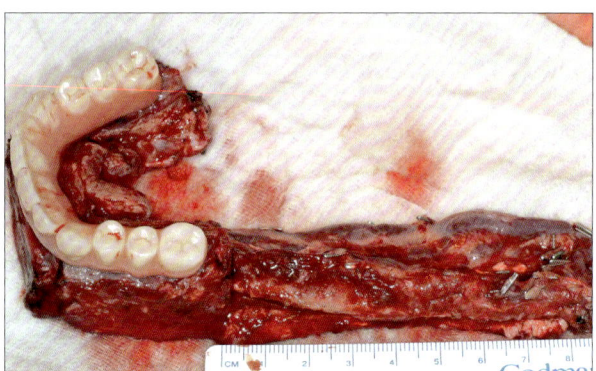

Fig 19   Fibula with the prosthesis raised as a free graft.

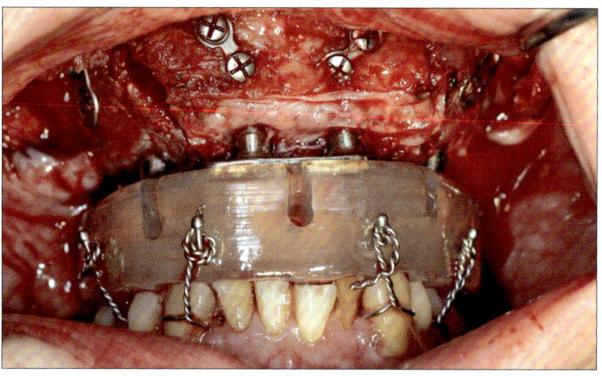

Fig 20   Fibula graft with the positioning splint in occlusion, attached to the remaining maxillary bone with osteosynthesis plates and monocortical screws.

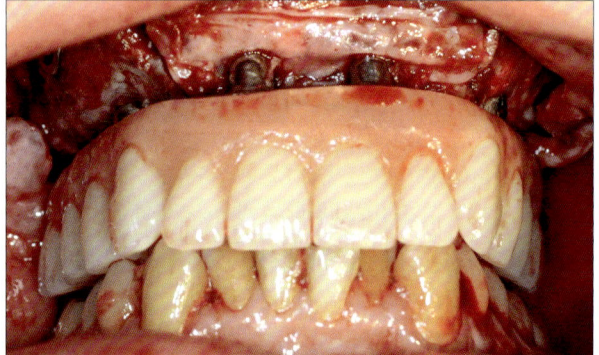

Fig 21   Implant-supported maxillary overdenture on the bar.

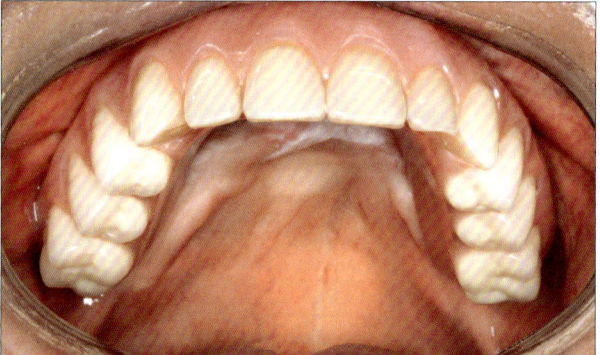

Fig 22   Clinical view of the implant-supported maxillary overdenture (1 year postoperatively).

G. Raghoebar, R. Schepers, A. Vissink, M. Witjes

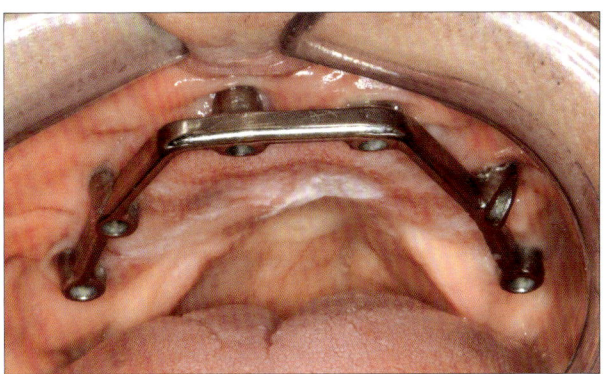

Fig 23   Clinical view of the implants and bar (1 year postoperatively).

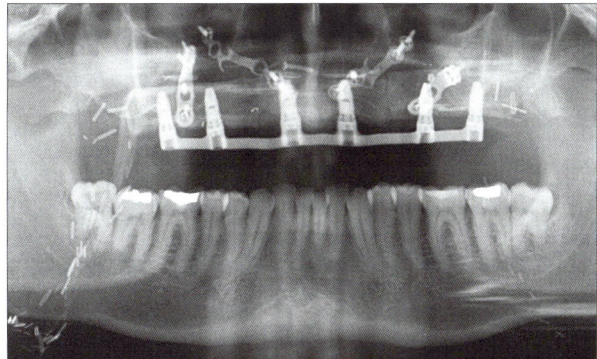

Fig 24   Panoramic radiograph showing the miniplates, implants, and retentive bar (1 year postoperatively).

Discussion

Digital planning and 3D printing to virtually plan and execute the reconstruction of maxillofacial defects with preconstructed fibula grafts pre-installed with dental implants are an accurate procedure (Schepers and coworkers 2016). It relies on preconstructed superstructures (denture or bridge) to guide the positioning of the graft in the defect according to the occlusion to achieve a favorable clinical outcome. The secondary reconstruction of maxillomandibular defects using preconstructed bone grafts of course implies that the patient must be willing to undergo at least two surgical procedures.

Major advantages of 3D planning in preconstructed fibula reconstructions include anatomical insight into the bony defect at the recipient site, the option of cutting and designing the fibula as preferred, and restoration of the dental occlusion. Planning backwards from the occlusion allows the optimal implant position in the bone flap to be achieved, ensuring that implant placement and prosthetic rehabilitation are not impaired by incorrect implant or bone positioning (Rohner and coworkers 2003).

Most of the laborious steps needed for analog preconstructed cases can be overcome by 3D planning; another benefit is the use of 3D-printed planned outcome models of the fibula graft. Thus, the recipient site can be prepared before harvesting the graft from the lower leg, which can reduce ischemic duration and safeguard the pedicle from damage due to manipulation of the graft on its way from and to the defect. Furthermore, the stable peri-implant soft-tissue layer created around the implants using a split-skin graft in the first surgical step is helpful in obtaining good peri-implant health.

In summary, for complex reconstructions, 3D virtual planning combined with 3D printed surgical guides might evolve to become the standard approach and treatment.

Acknowledgments

Prosthetic procedures
Dr. H. Reintsema – Department of Oral and Maxillofacial Surgery, University Hospital Groningen, Netherlands

Laboratory procedures
Gerrit van Dijk – Groningen, Netherlands

14 Technical and Clinical Recommendations

C. Evans, G. O. Gallucci, A. Tahmaseb

When looking at the introduction of digital workflows into dental practice, it is important to recognize that there will be a learning curve associated with the implementation of digital technology in a clinical setting. This learning curve involves both the technical and the clinical aspects.

Furthermore, technical developments and advances within this field progress rapidly, and a commitment to software and hardware upgrades will be essential for any clinician using digital workflows.

Technical considerations

The technical aspect of the learning curve is associated with an understanding of the different elements that make up the digital workflow, including the selection of an appropriate workflow for a given clinical situation. The selection of an open or closed workflow will determine the related devices, their file formats, and the software packages available. All stakeholders must be able to share and visualize the virtual treatment information to fully participate in the workflow. All components of the digital workflow must be software- and hardware-compatible in order for the members of the treatment team to access the files.

There are now materials, components, and laboratory workflows that can only be completed with the assistance of digital technology. Therefore, in selecting the technology for a digital workflow, the clinician must consider the advantages and disadvantages of each technical component.

Desirable features of digital impressions:

- Ability to export any digital impression file into any software package (open system)
- Ability to capture dental hard and soft tissues accurately over long spans
- An intraoral wand that is small enough to access all areas of the oral cavity
- Fast acquisition time and the ability to capture features in a moist environment
- Ability to capture true color
- Portability

Desirable features of CBCTs:

- Ability to minimize the patient's radiation exposure, consistent with the ALARA philosophy:
  - Variability in field of view
  - Low-exposure mode consistent with ALARA
  - Optimized scan mode
- Tools to compensate for patient movement to reduce motion artifacts
- Optimal voxel size to produce high-resolution images
- Optimal reconstruction software

Desirable features of planning software:

- Open software system
- Easy segmentation features allowing for manual modification
- Precise file-matching capabilities with the option for fine alignment
- Ability to communicate with CAD/CAM software
- Comprehensive tooth-shape library
- Ability to import multiple visible layers
- Comprehensive implant/abutment library
- Ability to export a surgical treatment plan
- Ability to design and export the file for a surgical guide
- Ability to allow a virtual prosthesis to be completed based on the planned implant position

Desirable features of CAD/CAM software:

- Open software system
- Ability to communicate with the planning software
- Extensive library of tooth shapes, fully customizable for clinical use
- Ability to receive surface-scan files from desktop or intraoral scanners
- Ability to integrate facial scans
- Ability to incorporate smile-design features in true color
- Unlimited design capabilities for all types of implant restorations, ranging from single crowns to complex fixed and removable complete edentulous solutions.
- A model builder for designing and fabricating 3D printed models
- Virtual articulation tools for occlusal analysis and planning
- Extensive library of prosthetic components
- Ability to export manufacturing files

Clinical considerations

Digital technology and its clinical use require an understanding of the clinical benefits that can be realized when such workflows are working optimally.

One of the more evident benefits of using a digital workflow is the possibility of acquiring very detailed preoperative information. This information is no longer static but allows for three-dimensional dynamic visualization of a case. Additionally, it allows us to preview the intended treatment plan in a virtual environment prior to the actual clinical intervention.

The ability of clinical and technical team members to interactively visualize detailed preoperative digital information, whether locally or remotely via a collaborative virtual environment, can bring many benefits to patient care. Multidisciplinary interaction to plan the final outcome, anticipating risks and managing potential complications, and the ability to accurately transfer the treatment plan to the clinical situation potentially reduces the overall treatment time and cost, providing predictable clinical outcomes.

But there are also some limitations inherent in the technology. Understanding these limitations and how to manage them will limit the risk of error in achieving an optimal outcome of the digital process. Additionally, at the time of writing, there is still a need for traditional analog technical processes, particularly when completing highly esthetic restorations. Future developments in the realm of materials may change this over time.

In addition to the above-mentioned technological and software improvements, it is obvious that the clinical hardware used will continuously improve. Advancements already realized have included more stable and more precisely fitting drilling guides, the elimination of tooling handles or consecutive guiding-sleeve sizes, which can prevent error multiplication and provide ways to enhance drill sequencing and localization.

Digital technologies are already part of modern medicine in general and of dentistry in particular, and they are becoming inseparable from our everyday practice.

As this book has shown throughout, digital implant dentistry is reshaping implant dentistry.

15   References

References have been listed in the order of (1) the first or only author's last name and (2) the year of publication. Identical short references are distinguished in the text by lowercase letters, which if used are given in parentheses at the end of the respective entry in this list of references.

Starting with this Volume 11 of the ITI Treatment Guide, Digital Object Identifier (DOI) names have been added to the individual references wherever they were available with reasonable effort, to allow readers to check the respective references quickly. For more information, refer to https://www.doi.org.

When entering a DOI name in the search field on that site, make sure not to enter the leading "doi:" or the trailing period. You may also access a reference by pointing your browser to https://doi.org/‹DOI name›, where ‹DOI name› should be replaced with the actual DOI name without the leading "doi:" or the trailing period (e.g., "10.1000/xyz123").

Abdulmakeed AA, Lim KG, Narhi TO, Cooper LF. Complete-arch implant supported monolithic zirconia fixed dental prostheses: A systematic review. J Prosthet Dent. **2016** Jun; 115(6): 672–677.e1. doi: 10.1016/j.prosdent.2015.08.025. Epub 2016 Jan 23.

Abduo J, Lyons K, Bennani V, Waddell N, Swain M. Fit of screw retained fixed implant frameworks fabricated by different methods: a systematic review. Int J Prosthodont. **2011** May–Jun; 24(3): 207–220.

Abduo J, Lyons K. Rationale for the use of CAD-CAM technology in implant prosthodontics. Int J Dent. **2013**; 2013:768121. doi: 10.1155/2013/768121. Epub 2013 Apr 16.

Abduo J. Fit of CAD/CAM implant frameworks: a comprehensive review. J Oral Implantol. **2014** Dec; 40(6): 758–766. doi: 10.1563/AAID-JOI-D-12-00117.

Abrahamsson I, Berglundh T, Glantz PO, Lindhe J. The mucosal attachment at different abutments. An experimental study in dogs. J Clin Periodontol. **1998** Sep; 25(9): 721–727.

Abrahamsson I, Cardaropoli G. Peri-implant hard and soft tissue integration to dental implants made of titanium and gold. Clin Oral Implants Res. **2007** Jun; 18(3): 269–274. Epub 2007 Feb 13.

[Academy of Prosthodontics, The]. The Glossary of Prosthodontic Terms; Ninth Edition (GPT9). J Prosthet Dent. **2017** May; 117(5S): e1–e105. doi: 10.1016/j.prosdent.2016.12.001.

Aghaloo TL, Moy PK: Which hard tissue augmentation techniques are the most successful in furnishing bony support for implant placement? Int J Oral Maxillofac Implants. **2007**; 22 Suppl: 49–70. Review. Erratum in: Int J Oral Maxillofac Implants. 2008 Jan–Feb; 23(1): 56.

Ahlers MO, Bernhardt O, Jakstat HA, Kordaß B, Türp JC, Schindler HJ, Hugger A. Motion analysis of the mandible: guidelines for standardized analysis of computer-assisted recording of condylar movements. Int J Comput Dent. **2015**; 18(3): 201–223.

Ahmadi RS, Sayar F, Rakhshan V, Iranpour B, Jahanbani J, Toumaj A, Akhoondi N. Clinical and histomorphometric assessment of lateral alveolar ridge augmentation using a corticocancellous freeze-dried allograft bone block. J Oral Implantol. **2017** Jun; 43(3): 202–210. doi: 10.1563/aaid-joi-D-16-00042. Epub 2017 Mar 22.

Alharbi N, Wismeijer D, Osman RB. Additive manufacturing techniques in prosthodontics: where do we currently stand? A critical review. Int J Prosthodont. **2017** Sep–Oct; 30(5): 474–484. doi: 10.11607/ijp.5079. Epub 2017 Jul 27.

Almasri R, Drago CJ, Siegel SC, Hardigan PC. Volumetric misfit in CAD/CAM and cast implant frameworks: a university laboratory study. J Prosthodont. **2011** Jun; 20(4): 267–274. doi: 10.1111/j.1532-849X.2011.00709.x. Epub 2011 Apr 14.

Amin S, Weber HP, Finkelman M, El Rafie K, Kudara Y, Papaspyridakos P. Digital vs. conventional full-arch implant impressions: a comparative study. Clin Oral Implants Res. **2017** Nov; 28(11): 1360–1367. doi: 10.1111/clr.12994. Epub 2016 Dec 31.

Andriessen FS, Rijkens DR, van der Meers WJ, Wismeijer DW. Applicability and accuracy of an intraoral scanner for scanning multiple implants in edentulous mandibles: a pilot study. J Prosthet Dent. **2014** Mar; 111(3): 186–194. doi: 10.1016/j.prosdent.2013.07.010. Epub 2013 Nov 8.

Antanasova M, Jevnikar P. Bonding of dental ceramics to titanium: processing and conditioning aspects. Current Oral Health Reports. **2016**. doi: 10.1007/s40496-016-0107-x.

Arısan V, Bölükbaşi N, Öksüz L. Computer-assisted flapless implant placement reduces the incidence of surgery-related bacteremia. Clin Oral Investig. **2013** Dec; 17(9): 1985 – 1993. doi: 10.1007/s00784-012-0886-y. Epub 2012 Dec 6.

Artopoulos A, Buytaert JA, Dirckx JJ, Coward TJ. Comparison of the accuracy of digital stereophotogrammetry and projection moiré profilometry for three-dimensional imaging of the face. Int J Oral Maxillofac Surg. **2014** May; 43(5): 654 – 662. doi: 10.1016/j.ijom.2013.10.005. Epub 2013 Nov 10.

Arunyanak SP, Harris BT, Grant GT, Morton D, Lin WS. Digital approach to planning computer-guided surgery and immediate provisionalization in a partially edentulous patient. J Prosthet Dent. **2016** Jul; 116(1): 8 – 14. doi: 10.1016/j.prosdent.2015.11.023. Epub 2016 Feb 9.

Adeyemo WL, Akadiri OA. A systematic review of the diagnostic role of ultrasonography in maxillofacial fractures. Int J Oral Maxillofac Surg. **2011** Jul; 40(7): 655 – 661. doi: 10.1016/j.ijom.2011.02.001. Epub 2011 Mar 5.

Becker W, Goldstein M, Becker BE, Sennerby L, Kois D, Hujoel P. Minimally invasive flapless implant placement: follow-up results from a multicenter study. J Periodontol. **2009** Feb; 80(2): 347 – 352. doi: 10.1902/jop.2009.080286.

Bellanova L, Paul L, Docquier PL. Surgical guides (patient-specific instruments) for pediatric tibial bone sarcoma resection and allograft reconstruction. Sarcoma. **2013**; 2013:787653. doi: 10.1155/2013/787653. Epub 2013 Mar 4.

Beretta M, Cicciu M, Poli PP, Rancitelli D, Bassi G, Grossi GB, Maiorana C. A retrospective evaluation of 192 implants placed in augmented bone: longÐterm followÐup study. J Oral Implantol. **2015** Dec; 41(6): 669 – 674. doi: 10.1563/aaid-joi-D-14-00123. Epub 2015 Feb 16.

Block MS, Emery RW, Lank K, Ryan J. Implant placement accuracy using dynamic navigation. Int J Oral Maxillofac Implants. **2017** Jan – Feb; 32(1): 92 – 99. doi: 10.11607/jomi.5004. Epub 2016 Sep 19.

Boas FE, Fleischmann D. CT artifacts: causes and reduction techniques. Imaging Med. **2012**; 4(2), 229 – 240.

Bornstein MM, Al-Nawas B, Kuchler U, Tahmaseb A. Consensus statements and recommended clinical procedures regarding contemporary surgical and radiographic techniques in implant dentistry. Int J Oral Maxillofac Implants. **2014**; 29 Suppl: 78 – 82. doi: 10.11607/jomi.2013.g1.

Bower JL, Christensen CM. Disruptive technologies: catching the wave. Harvard Business Review. **1995** Jan – Feb; 73(1); 43 – 53.

Brodala N. ITI Flapless surgery and its effect on dental implant outcomes. Int J Oral Maxillofac Implants. **2009**; 24 Suppl: 118 – 125.

Burke P. Serial stereophotogrammetric measurements of the soft tissues of the face. A case of a girl with mild facial asymmetry from 3 weeks to 10 years of age. Br Dent J. 1983 Dec 10; 155(11): 373 – 379.

Buser D, Chappuis V, Bornstein MM, Wittneben JG, Frei M, Belser UC. Long-term stability of contour augmentation with early implant placement following single tooth extraction in the esthetic zone: a prospective, cross-sectional study in 41 patients with a 5- to 9-year follow-up. J Periodontol. **2013** Nov; 84(11): 1517 – 1527. doi: 10.1902/jop.2013.120635. Epub 2013 Jan 24. (**a**)

Buser D, Chappuis V, Kuchler U, Bornstein MM, Wittneben JG, Buser R, Cavusoglu Y, Belser UC. Long-term stabilty of early implant placement with contour augmentation. J Dent Res. **2013** Dez; 92(12 Suppl): 176S – 182S. doi: 10.1177/0022034513504949. (**b**)

Bush K, Antonyshyn O. Three-dimensional facial anthropometry using a laser surface scanner: validation of the technique. Plast Reconstr Surg. **1996** Aug; 98(2): 226 – 235.

Buzayan M, Baug MR, Yunus N. Evaluation of accuracy of complete-arch multiple-unit abutment-level dental implant impressions using different impression and splinting materials. Int J Oral Maxillofac Implants. **2013** Nov – Dec; 28(6): 1512 – 1520. doi: 10.11607/jomi.2958.

Calamia JR, Levine JB, Lipp M, Cisneros G, Wolff MS. Smile Design and treatment planning with the help of a comprehensive esthetic evaluation form. Dent Clin North Am. **2011** Apr; 55(2): 187 – 209, vii. doi: 10.1016/j.cden.2011.01.012.

Carames J, Tovar Suinaga L, Yu YC, Pérez A, Kang M. Clinical advantages and limitations of monolithic zirconia restorations full arch implant supported reconstruction: case series. Int J Dent. **2015**; 2015:392496. doi: 10.1155/2015/392496. Epub 2015 Jun 1.

Carlsson GE: Dental occlusion: modern concepts and their application in implant prosthodontics. Odontology. **2009** Jan; 97(1): 8 – 17. doi: 10.1007/s10266-008-0096-x. Epub 2009 Jan 29.

Case CS. Some principles governing the development of facial contours in the practice of orthodontia. Columbia Dental Congress. **1893**; 2: 727.

Cassetta M, Giansanti M, Di Mambro A, Calasso S, Barbato E. Accuracy of two stereolithographic surgical templates: a retrospective study. Clin Implant Dent Relat Res. **2013** Jun; 15(3): 448 – 459. doi: 10.1111/j.1708-8208.2011.00369.x. Epub 2011 Jul 11.

Chan HL, Sinjab K, Chung MP, Chiang YC, Wang HL, Giannobile WV, Kripfgans OD. Non-invasive evaluation of facial crestal bone with ultrasonography. PLoS One. **2017** Feb 8; 12(2): e0171237. doi: 10.1371/journal.pone.0171237.

Charette JR, Goldberg J, Harris BT, Morton D, Llop DR, Lin WS. Cone beam computed tomography imaging as a primary diagnostic tool for computer-guided surgery and CAD-CAM interim removable and fixed dental prostheses. J Prosthet Dent. **2016** Aug; 116(2): 157 – 165. doi: 10.1016/j.prosdent.2016.02.004. Epub 2016 Apr 14.

Charette JR, Goldberg J, Harris BT, Morton D, Llop DR, Lin WS. Cone beam computed tomography imaging as a primary diagnostic tool for computer-guided surgery and CAD/CAM interim removable and fixed dental prostheses. J Prosthet Dent. **2016** Aug; 116(2): 157 – 165. doi: 10.1016/j.prosdent.2016.02.004. Epub 2016 Apr 14.

Chiapasco M, Zaniboni M. Clinical outcomes of GBR procedures to correct peri-implant dehiscences and fenestrations: a systematic review. Clin Oral Implants Res. **2009** Sep; 20 Suppl 4: 113 – 123. doi: 10.1111/j.1600-0501.2009.01781.x.

Chung S, McCullagh A, Irinakis T. Immediate loading in the maxillary arch: evidence-based guidelines to improve success rates: a review. J Oral Implantol. **2011** Oct; 37(5): 610 – 621. doi: 10.1563/AAID-D-JOI-10-00058.1.

Ciocca L, Fantini M, De Crescenzio F, Corinaldesi G, Scotti R. Direct metal laser sintering (DMLS) of a customized titanium mesh for prosthetically guided bone regeneration of atrophic maxillary arches. Med Biol Eng Comput. **2011** Nov; 49(11): 1347 – 1352. doi: 10.1007/s11517-011-0813-4. Epub 2011 Jul 21.

Coachman C, Paravina RD. Digitally enhanced esthetic dentistry—from treatment planning to quality control. J Esthet Restor Dent. **2016** Mar; 28 Suppl 1: S3 – 4. doi: 10.1111/jerd.12205.

Coachman C, Calamita MA, Coachman FG, Coachman RG, Sesma N. Facially generated and cephalometric guided 3D digital design for complete mouth implant rehabilitation: A clinical report. J Prosthet Dent. **2017** May; 117(5): 577 – 586. doi: 10.1016/j.prosdent.2016.09.005. Epub 2016 Nov 9.

D'Apuzzo N. Overview of 3D surface digitization technologies in Europe. In: Corner BD, Li P, Tocheri M, editors. Three-dimensional image capture and applications VII. Proc SPIE 6056. San Jose, Calif.: **2006**.

D'haese J, Ackhurst J, Wismeijer D, De Bruyn H, Tahmaseb A. (2017) Current state of the art of computer-guided implant surgery. Periodontol 2000. **2017** Feb; 73(1): 121 – 133. doi: 10.1111/prd.12175.

Davis DM, Packer ME, Watson RM. Maintenance requirements of implant-supported fixed prostheses opposed by implant-supported fixed prostheses, natural teeth, or complete dentures: a 5-year retrospective study. Int J Prosthodont **2003** Sep – Oct; 16: 521 – 523.

Dawood A, Marti Marti B, Sauret-Jackson V, Darwood A. 3D printing in dentistry. Br Dent J. **2015** Dec; 219(11): 521 – 529. doi: 10.1038/sj.bdj.2015.914.

De Bruyn H, Raes S, Ostman PO, Cosyn J. Immediate loading in partially and completely edentulous jaws: a review of the literature with clinical guidelines. Periodontol 2000. **2014** Oct; 66(1): 153 – 187. doi: 10.1111/prd.12040.

de Farias TP, Dias FL, Galvao MS, Boasquevisque E, Pastl AC, Albuquerque Sousa B. Use of prototyping in preoperative planning for patients with head and neck tumors. Head Neck. **2014** Dec; 36(12): 1773 – 1782. doi: 10.1002/hed.23540. Epub 2014 Jan 29.

De Marco AC, Jardini MA, Lima LP. Revascularization of autogenous block grafts with or without an e-PTFE membrane. Int J Oral Maxillofac Implants. **2005** Nov – Dec; 20(6): 867 – 874.

De Santis E, Lang NP, Favero G, Beolchini M, Morelli F, Botticelli D. Healing at mandibular block-grafted sites. An experimental study in dogs. Clin Oral Implants Res. **2015** May; 26(6): 516 – 522. doi: 10.1111/clr.12434. Epub 2014 Jun 12.

Deli R, Galantucci LM, Laino A, D'Alessio R, Di Gioia E, Savastano C, Lavecchia F, Percoco G. Three-dimensional methodology for photogrammetric acquisition of the soft tissues of the face: a new clinical-instrumental protocol. Prog Orthod. **2013** Sep 20; 14: 32. doi: 10.1186/2196-1042-14-32.

Bona AD, Pecho OE, Alessandretti R. Zirconia as a Dental Biomaterial. Materials (Basel). **2015** Aug 4; 8(8): 4978 – 4991. doi: 10.3390/ma8084978.

Di Giacomo GA, Cury PR, de Araujo NS, Sendyk WR, Sendyk CL. Clinical application of stereolithographic surgical guides for implant placement: preliminary results. J Periodontol. **2005** Apr; 76(4): 503 – 507.

Di Giacomo GA, da Silva JV, da Silva AM, Paschoal GH, Cury PR, Szarf G. Accuracy and complications of computer-designed selective laser sintering surgical guides for flapless dental implant placement and immediate de nitive prosthesis installation. J Periodontol. **2012** Apr; 83(4): 410 – 419. doi: 10.1902/jop.2011.110115. Epub 2011 Aug 5.

Dierens M, Collaert B, Deschepper E, Browaeys H, Klinge B, De Bruyn H. Patient-centered outcome of immediately loaded implants in the rehabilitation of fully edentulous jaws. Clin Oral Implants Res. **2009** Oct; 20(10): 1070 – 1077. doi: 10.1111/j.1600-0501.2009.01741.x. Epub 2009 Aug 30.

Eliasson A, Wennerberg A, Johansson A, Ortorp A, Jemt T. The precision of fit of milled titanium implant frameworks (I-Bridge) in the edentulous jaw. Clin Implant Dent Relat Res. **2010** Jun 1; 12(2): 81 – 90. doi: 10.1111/j.1708-8208.2008.00131.x. Epub 2008 Dec 3..

Ender A, Mehl A. Full arch scans: conventional versus digital impressions—an in-vitro study. Int J Comput Dent. **2011**; 14(1): 11 – 21.

Ersoy AE, Turkyilmaz I, Ozan O, McGlumphy EA. Reliability of implant placement with stereolithographic surgical guides generated from computed tomography: clinical data from 94 implants. J Periodontol. **2008** Aug; 79(8): 1339 – 1345. doi: 10.1902/jop.2008.080059.

Esposito M, Grusovin MG, Felice P, Karatzopoulos G, Worthington HV, Coulthard P. Interventions for replacing missing teeth: horizontal and vertical bone augmentation techniques for dental implant treatment. Cochrane Database Syst Rev. **2009** Oct 7; (4):CD003607. doi: 10.1002/14651858.CD003607.pub4.

Farman AG. Applying DICOM to dentistry.; J Digit Imaging. **2005** Mar; 18(1): 23 – 27. doi: 10.1007/s10278-004-1029-z. Epub 2004 Nov 25.

Ferrari M, Vicji A, Zarone F. Zirconia abutments and restorations: From Laboratory to clinical investigations. Dent Mater. **2015** Mar; 31(3): e63 – 76. doi: 10.1016/j.dental.2014.11.015. Epub 2015 Jan 7.

Figliuzzi M, Mangano FG, Fortunato L, De Fazio R, Macchi A, Iezzi G, Piattelli A, Mangano C. Vertical ridge augmentation of the atrophic posterior mandible with custom-made, computer-aided design/computer-aided manufacturing porous hydroxyapatite scaffolds. J Craniofac Surg. **2013** May; 24(3): 856 – 859. doi: 10.1097/SCS.0b013e31827ca3a7.

Flügge TV, Att W, Metzger MC, Nelson K. Precision of dental implant digitization using intraoral scanners. Int J Prosthodont. **2016** May – Jun; 29(3): 277 – 283. doi: 10.11607/ijp.4417.

Flügge T, Derksen W, Te Poel J, Hassan B, Nelson K, Wismeijer D. Registration of cone beam computed tomography data and intraoral surface scans - A prerequisite for guided implant surgery with CAD/CAM drilling guides. Clin Oral Implants Res. **2017** Sep; 28(9): 1113 – 1118. doi: 10.1111/clr.12925. Epub 2016 Jul 20.

Fokas G, Vaughn VM, Scarfe WC, Bornstein MM. Accuracy of linear measurements on CBCT images related to presurgical implant treatment planning: a systematic review. Clin Oral Implants Res. **2018** Oct; 29 Suppl 16: 393 – 415. doi: 10.1111/clr.13142.

Gallucci GO, Bernard JP, Bertosa M, Belser UC. Immediate loading with fixed screw-retained provisional restorations in edentulous jaws: the pickup technique. Int J Oral Maxillofac Implants. **2004** Jul – Aug; 19(4): 524 – 533.

Gallucci GO, Morton D, Weber HP. Int J Oral Maxillofac Implants. Loading protocols for dental implants in edentulous patients. **2009**; 24 Suppl: 132 – 146.

Gallucci GO, Benic GI, Eckert SE, Papaspyridakos P, Schimmel M, Schrott A, Weber HP. Consensus statements and clinical recommendations for implant loading protocols. Int J Oral Maxillofac Implants. **2014**; 29 Suppl: 287 – 290. doi: 10.11607/jomi.2013. g4.

Gallucci GO, Finelle G, Papadimitriou DE, Lee SJ. Innovative approach to computer-guided surgery and fixed provisionalization assisted by screw-retained transitional implants. Int J Oral Maxillofac Implants. **2015** Mar – Apr; 30(2): 403 – 410. doi: 10.11607/ jomi.3817.

Gärtner C, Kordaß B. The virtual articulator: development and evaluation. Int J Comput Dent. **2003** Jan; 6(1): 11 – 24.

Giannuzzi NJ, Motlagh SD. Full mouth rehabilitation determined by anterior tooth position. Dent Clin North Am. **2015** Jul; 59(3): 609 – 621. doi: 10.1016/j. cden.2015.03.004.

Gillot L, Noharet R, Cannas B. Guided surgery and presurgical prosthesis: preliminary results of 33 fully edentulous maxillae treated in accordance with the NobelGuide protocol. Clin Implant Dent Relat Res. **2010** May; 12 Suppl 1: e104 – e113. doi: 10.1111/j.1708-8208.2010.00236.x. Epub 2010 Apr 23.

Gimenez-Gonzalez B, Hassan B, Özcan M, Pradíes G. An in vitro study of factors influencing the performance of digital intraoral impressions operating on active wavefront sampling technology with multiple implants in the edentulous maxilla. J Prosthodont. **2017** Dec; 26(8): 650 – 655. doi: 10.1111/jopr.12457. Epub 2016 Mar 2.

Gross MD. Occlusion in implant dentistry. A review of the literature of prosthetic determinants and current concepts. Aust Dent J. **2008** Jun; 53 Suppl 1: S60 – S68. doi: 10.1111/j.1834-7819.2008.00043.x.

Guerrero ME, Jacobs R, Loubele M, Schutyser F, Suetens P, Steenberghe D. State-of-the-art on cone beam CT imaging for preoperative planning of implant placement. Clin Oral Investig. **2006** Mar; 10(1): 1 – 7. Epub 2006 Feb 16.

Guess PC, Att W, Strub JR. Zirconia in fixed implant prosthodontics. Clin Implant Dent Relat Res. **2012** Oct; 14(5): 633 – 645. doi: 10.1111/j.1708-8208.2010.00317.x. Epub 2010 Dec 22.

Hajeer MY, Millett DT, Ayoub AF, Siebert JP. Applications of 3D imaging in orthodontics: part I. J Orthod. **2004** Mar; 31(1): 62 – 70.

Hamalian TA, Nasr E, Chidiac JJ. Impression materials in fixed prosthodontics: influence of choice on clinical procedure. J Prosthodont. **2011** Feb; 20(2): 153 – 160. doi: 10.1111/j.1532-849X.2010.00673.x. Epub 2011 Feb 1.

Hämmerle CHF, Cordaro L, van Assche N, Benic GI, Bornstein M, Gamper F, et al. Digital technologies to support planning, treatment and fabrication processes and outcome assessments in implant dentistry. Summary and consensus statements. The 4th EAO consensus conference 2015. Clin Oral Implants Res. **2015** Sep; 26 Suppl 11: 97 – 101. doi: 10.1111/ clr.12648.

Harris BT, Montero D, Grant GT, Morton D, Llop DR, Lin WS. Creation of a 3-dimensional virtual dental patient for computer-guided surgery and CAD-CAM interim complete removable and fixed dental prostheses: A clinical report. J Prosthet Dent. **2017** Feb; 117(2): 197 – 204. doi: 10.1016/j.prosdent.2016.06.012. Epub 2016 Sep 22.

Hassan B, Nijkamp P, Verheij H, Tairie J, Vink C, van der Stelt P, van Beek H. Precision of identifying cephalometric landmarks with cone beam computed tomography in vivo. Eur J Orthod. **2013** Feb; 35(1): 38 – 44. doi: 10.1093/ejo/cjr050. Epub 2011 Mar 29.

Hassan B, Gimenez Gonzalez B, Tahmaseb A, Greven M, Wismeijer D. A digital approach integrating facial scanning in a CAD-CAM workflow for complete-mouth implant-supported rehabilitation of patients with edentulism: A pilot clinical study. J Prosthet Dent. **2017** Apr; 117(4): 486 – 492. doi: 10.1016/j.prosdent.2016.07.033. Epub 2016 Oct 27.

Hebel KS, Gajjar RC. Cement-retained versus screw-retained implant restorations: achieving optimal occlusion and esthetics in implant dentistry. J Prosthet Dent. **1997** Jan; 77(1): 28 – 35.

Holst S, Blatz MB, Bergler M, Goellner M, Wichmann M. Influence of impression material and time on the 3 dimensional accuracy of implant impressions. Quintessence Int. **2007** Jan; 38(1): 67 – 73.

Horner K, Islam M, Flygare L, Tsiklakis K, Whaites E. Basic principles for use of dental cone beam computed tomography: consensus guidelines of the European Academy of Dental and Maxillofacial Radiology. Dentomaxillofac Radiol. 2009 May; 38(4): 187 – 195. doi: 10.1259/dmfr/74941012.

Huang H, Chai J, Tong X, Wu HT. Leveraging motion capture and 3D scanning for high-fidelity facial performance acquisition. ACM Trans Graph. **2011** Jul; 30(4): 74:1 – 74:10.

International Organization for Standardization. ISO 12836:2012: Dentistry — Digitizing devices for CAD/CAM systems for indirect dental restorations — Test methods for assessing accuracy. Geneva: ISO; **2012**.

International Organisation for Standardization. ISO 12836:2015: Dentistry — Digitizing devices for CAD/CAM systems for indirect dental restorations — Test methods for assessing accuracy. Geneva: ISO; **2015**.

Ismail SF, Moss JP, Hennessy R. Three-dimensional assessment of the effects of extraction and non-extraction orthodontic treatment on the face. Am J Orthod Dentofacial Orthop. **2002** Mar; 121(3): 244 – 256.

Jacobs R, Salmon B, Codari M, Hassan B, Bornstein MM. Cone beam computed tomography in implant dentistry: recommendations for clinical use. BMC Oral Health. **2018** May 15; 18(1): 88. doi: 10.1186/s12903-018-0523-5.

Jaffin RA, Kumar A, Berman CL. Immediate loading of dental implants in the completely edentulous maxilla: a clinical report. Send to
Int J Oral Maxillofac Implants. **2004** Sep – Oct; 19(5): 721 – 730.

Jemt T: Three dimensional distortion of gold allot castings and welded titanium framework. Measurements of precision of fit between complete implant prostheses and the master casts in routine edentulous situations. J Oral Rehabil. **1995** Aug; 22(8): 557 – 564.

Jemt T, Bäck T, Petersson A. Precision of CNC-milled titanium frameworks for implant treatment in the edentulous jaw. Int J Prosthodont. **1999** May – Jun; 12(3): 209 – 215.

Joda T, Brägger U. Complete digital workflow for the production of implant-supported single-unit monolithic crowns. Clin Oral Implants Res. **2014** Nov; 25(11): 1304 – 1306. doi: 10.1111/clr.12270. Epub 2013 Oct 8.

Joda T, Brägger U. Digital vs. conventional implant prosthetic workflows: A cost/time analysis. Clin Oral Implants Res. **2015** Dec; 26(12): 1430 – 1435. doi: 10.1111/clr.12476. Epub 2014 Sep 2. (**a**)

Joda T, Gallucci GO. The virtual patient in dental medicine. Clin Oral Implants Res. **2015** Jun; 26(6): 725 – 726. doi: 10.1111/clr.12379. Epub 2014 Mar 26. (**b**)

Joda T, Brägger U. Time-efficiency analysis comparing digital and conventional workflows for implant crowns: A prospective clinical crossover trial. Int J Oral Maxillofac Implants. **2015** Sep – Oct; 30(5):1047 – 1053. doi: 10.11607/jomi.3963. (**c**)

Joda T, Brägger U. Time-efficiency analysis of the treatment with monolithic implant crowns in a digital workflow: A randomized controlled trial. Clin Oral Implants Res. **2016** Nov; 27(11): 1401 – 1406. doi: 10.1111/clr.12753. Epub 2016 Jan 6.

Joda T, Ferrari M, Gallucci GO, Wittneben JG, Brägger U. Digital technology in fixed implant prosthodontics. Periodontol 2000. **2017** Feb; 73(1): 178 – 192. doi: 10.1111/prd.12164. (**a**)

Joda T, Ferrari M, Brägger U. Monolithic implant-supported lithium disilicate (LS2) crowns in a complete digital workflow: A prospective clinical trial with a 2-year follow-up. Clin Implant Dent Relat Res. **2017** Jun; 19(3): 505 – 511. doi: 10.1111/cid.12472. Epub 2017 Jan 16. (**b**)

Jokstad A. Computer-assisted technologies used in oral rehabilitation and the clinical documentation of alleged advantages—a systematic review. J Oral Rehabil. **2017** Apr; 44(4): 261 – 290. doi: 10.1111/joor.12483. Epub 2017 Feb 27.

Jung RE, Schneider D, Ganeles J, Wismeijer D, Zwahlen M, Hämmerle CH, Tahmaseb A. Computer technology applications in surgical implant dentistry: s systematic review. Int J Oral Maxillofac Implants. **2009**; 24 (Suppl): 92–109.

Jung RE, Fenner N, Hämmerle CH, Zitzmann NU. LongÐterm outcome of implants placed with guided bone regeneration (GBR) using resorbable and nonÐresorbable membranes after 12–14 years. Clin Oral Implants Res. **2013** Oct; 24(10): 1065–1073. doi: 10.1111/j.1600-0501.2012.02522.x. Epub 2012 Jun 15.

Kapos T, Evans C. CAD/CAM technology for implant abutments, crowns, and superstructures. Int J Oral Maxillofac Implants. **2014**; 29 Suppl: 117–136. doi: 10.11607/jomi.2014suppl.g2.3.

Karl M, Holst S. Strain development of screw-retained implant- supported fixed restorations: Procera implant bridge versus conventionally cast restorations. Int J Prosthodont. **2012** Mar–Apr; 25(2): 166–169.

Karl M, Taylor TD. Effect of cyclic loading on micromotion at the implant-abutment interface. Int J Oral Maxillofac Implants. **2016** Nov–Dec; 31(6): 1292–1297. doi: 10.11607/jomi.5116.

Kau CH, Richmond S, Incrapera A, English J, Xia JJ. Three-dimensional surface acquisition systems for the study of facial morphology and their application to maxillofacial surgery. Int J Med Robot. **2007** Jun; 3(2): 97–110.

Kirsch C, Ender A, Attin T, Mehl. Trueness of four different milling procedures used in dental CAD/CAM systems Clin Oral Investig. **2017** Mar; 21(2): 551–558. doi: 10.1007/s00784-016-1916-y. Epub 2016 Jul 28.

Klammert U, Vorndran E, Reuther T, Müller FA, Zorn K, Gbureck U. Low temperature fabrication of magnesium phosphate cement scaffolds by 3D powder printing. J Mater Sci Mater Med. **2010** Nov; 21(11): 2947–2953. doi: 10.1007/s10856-010-4148-8. Epub 2010 Aug 26.

Klotz MW, Taylor TD, Goldberg AJ. Wear at the titanium-zirconia implant-abutment interface: a pilot study. Int J Oral Maxillofac Implants. **2011** Sep–Oct; 26(5): 970–975.

Kökat AM, Akça K. Fabrication of a screw-retained fixed provisional prosthesis supported by dental implants. J Prosthet Dent. **2004** Mar; 91(3): 293–297.

Koop R, Vercruyssen M, Vermeulen K, Quirynen M. Tolerance within the sleeve inserts of different surgical guides for guided implant surgery. Clin Oral Implants Res. **2013** Jun; 24(6): 630–634. doi: 10.1111/j.1600-0501.2012.02436.x. Epub 2012 Mar 13.

Koralakunte PR, Aljanakh M: The role of virtual articulator in prosthetic and restorative dentistry. J Clin Diagn Res. **2014** Jul; 8(7): ZE25–28. doi: 10.7860/JCDR/2014/8929.4648. Epub 2014 Jul 20.

Kordaß B, Gärtner C, Söhnel A, Bisler A, Voss G, Bockholt U, Seipel S: The virtual articulator in dentistry: concept and development. Dent Clin North Am. **2002** Jul; 46(3): 493–506, vi.

Lam WY, Hsung RT, Choi WW, Luk HW, Pow EH: A 2-part facebow for CAD-CAM dentistry. J Prosthet Dent. **2016** Dec; 116(6): 843–847. doi: 10.1016/j.prosdent.2016.05.013. Epub 2016 Jul 28.

Laney WF, N Broggini, D Buser, DL Cochran, LT Garcia WV Giannobile, E Hjorting-Hansen, TD Taylor: Glossary of Oral and Maxillofacial Implants. Quintessence Publishing, **2017**.

Lanis A, Padial-Molina M, Gamil R, Alvarez del Canto O. Computer-guided implant surgery and immediate loading with a modifiable radiographic template in a patient with partial edentulism: A clinical report. J Prosthet Dent. **2015** Sep; 114(3): 328–334. doi: 10.1016/j.prosdent.2015.03.012. Epub 2015 May 23. (**b**)

Lanis A, Álvarez del Canto O. The combination of digital surface scanners and cone beam computed tomography technology for guided implant surgery using 3Shape implant studio software: a case history report. Int J Prosthodont. **2015** Mar–Apr; 28(2): 169–178. (b)

Lanis A, Llorens P, Alvarez del Canto O. Selecting the appropriate digital planning pathway for computer-guided implant surgery. Int J Comp Dent. **2017**; 20(1): 75–85.

Lazarides A, Erdmann D, Powers D, Eward W. Custom facial reconstruction for osteosarcoma of the jaw. J Oral Maxillofac Surg. **2014** Nov; 72(11): 2375.e1–10. doi: 10.1016/j.joms.2014.07.018. Epub 2014 Jul 25.

Le M, Papia E, Larsson C. The clinical success of tooth- and implant supported zirconia-based fixed dental prostheses. A systematic review. J Oral Rehabil. **2015** Jun; 42(6): 467–480. doi: 10.1111/joor.12272. Epub 2015 Jan 10.

Lee SJ, Macarthur RX 4th, Gallucci GO. An evaluation of student and clinician perception of digital and conventional implant impressions. J Prosthet Dent. **2013** Nov; 110(5): 420–423. doi: 10.1016/j.prosdent.2013.06.012. Epub 2013 Aug 30.

Lee HG, Kim YD. Volumetric stability of autogenous bone graft with mandibular body bone: ConeÐbeam computed tomography and threeÐdimensional reconstruction analysis. J Korean Assoc Oral Maxillofac Surg. **2015** Oct; 41(5): 232–239. doi: 10.5125/jkaoms.2015.41.5.232. Epub 2015 Oct 20.

Lee JS, Hong JM, Jung JW, Shim JH, Oh JH, Cho DW. 3D printing of composite tissue with complex shape applied to ear regeneration. Biofabrication. **2014** Jun; 6(2): 024103. doi: 10.1088/1758-5082/6/2/024103. Epub 2014 Jan 24.

Lee M, Wu BM. Recent advances in 3D printing of tissue engineering scaffolds. Methods Mol Biol. **2012**; 868: 257–267. doi: 10.1007/978-1-61779-764-4_15.

Lehman H, Casap N. Rapid-prototype titanium bone forms for vertical alveolar augmentation using bone morphogenetic protein-2: design and treatment planning objectives. Int J Oral Maxillofac Implants. **2014** Mar–Apr; 29(2):e259–264. doi: 10.11607/jomi.te62.

Leighton Y, Carvajal JC. Protocolo protésico de carga inmediata en mandíbula y maxilares desdentados utilizando una cubeta multifuncional ("Protocol [for] immediately loaded prostheses in edentulous jaws using a multifunctional tray"). Int J Odontostomat. **2013**; 7(2): 299–304. doi: 10.4067/S0718-381X2013000200021.

Leighton Fuentealba Y, Carvajal Herrera JC. Immediately loaded prosthesis in edentulous jaws using a multifunctional tray protocol. Int J Odontostomat [online], **2013**; 7(2): 299–304. doi: 10.4067/S0718-381X2013000200021.

Leticia S, Antonio BM, Ana CD. Impact of abutment material on peri-implant soft tissue color. An in vitro study. Clin Oral Investig. **2017** Sep; 21(7): 2221–2233. doi: 10.1007/s00784-016-2015-9. Epub 2016 Nov 22.

Lewis SG, Llamas D, Avera S. The UCLA abutment: a four-year review. J Prosthet Dent. **1992** Apr; 67(4): 509–515.

Lewis RC, Harris BT, Sarno R, Morton D, Llop DR, Lin WS. Maxillary and mandibular immediately loaded implant-supported interim complete fixed dental prostheses on immediately placed dental implants with a digital approach: a clinical report. J Prosthet Dent. **2015** Sep; 114(3): 315–322. doi: 10.1016/j.prosdent.2015.03.021. Epub 2015 Jun 3.

Li H, Adams B, Guibas LJ, Pauly M. Robust single-view geometry and motion reconstruction. ACM Trans Graph. **2009** Dec; 28(5): 175:1–175:10.

Li J, Hsu Y, Luo E, Khadka A, Hu J. Computer-aided design and manufacturing and rapid prototyped nanoscale hydroxyapatite/polyamide (n-HA/PA) construction for condylar defect caused by mandibular angle ostectomy. Aesthetic Plast Surg. **2011** Aug; 35(4): 636–640. doi: 10.1007/s00266-010-9602-y. Epub 2010 Oct 23.

Liang X, Jacobs R, Hassan B, Li L, Pauwels R, Corpas L, Souza PC, Martens W, Shahbazian M, Alonso A, Lambrichts I. A comparative evaluation of cone beam computed tomography (CBCT) and multi-slice CT (MSCT). Part I: On subjective image quality. Eur J Radiol. **2010** Aug; 75(2): 265–269. doi: 10.1016/j.ejrad.2009.03.042. Epub 2009 May 1. (**a**)

Liang X, Lambrichts I, Sun Y, Denis K, Hassan B, Li L, Pauwels R, Jacobs R. A comparative evaluation of cone beam computed tomography (CBCT) and multi-slice CT (MSCT). Part II: On 3D model accuracy. Eur J Radiol. **2010** Aug; 75(2): 270–274. doi: 10.1016/j.ejrad.2009.04.016. Epub 2009 May 6. (**b**)

Lin GH, Chan HL, Bashutski JD, Oh TJ, Wang HL. The effect of flapless surgery on implant survival and marginal bone level: a systematic review and meta-analysis. J Periodontol. **2014** May; 85(5): e91–e103. doi: 10.1902/jop.2013.130481. Epub 2013 Oct 23.

Lin WS, Harris BT, Phasuk K, Llop DR, Morton D. Integrating a facial scan, virtual smile design, and 3D virtual patient for treatment with CAD-CAM ceramic veneers: A clinical report. J Prosthet Dent. **2018** Feb; 119(2): 200–205. doi: 10.1016/j.prosdent.2017.03.007. Epub 2017 Jun 13.

Linkevicius T, Apse P. Influence of abutment material on stability of peri-implant tissues: a systematic review. Int J Oral Maxillofac Implants. **2008** May–Jun; 23(3): 449–456.

Linkevicius T, Vaitelis J. The effect of zirconia or titanium as abutment material on soft peri-implant tissues: a systematic review and meta-analysis. Clin Oral Implants Res. **2015** Sep; 26 Suppl 11: 139 – 147. doi: 10.1111/clr.12631. Epub 2015 Jun 13.

Löe H, Silness J. Periodontal disease in pregnancy. Acta Odontologica Scandinavica. **1963** Dec; 21: 533 – 551.

Lops D, Stellini E, Sbricoli L, Cea N, Romeo E, Bressan E. Influence of abutment material on peri-implant soft tissues in anterior areas with thin gingival biotype: a multicentric prospective study. Clin Oral Implants Res. **2017** Oct; 28(10): 1263 – 1268. doi: 10.1111/clr.12952. Epub 2016 Oct 3.

Lorenzana ER, Allen EP. The single-incision palatal harvest technique: a strategy for esthetics and patient comfort. Int J Periodontics Restorative Dent. **2000** Jun; 20(3): 297 – 305.

Loubele M, Bogaerts R, Van Dijck E, Pauwels R, Vanheusden S, Suetens P, Marchal G, Sanderink G, Jacobs R. Comparison between effective radiation dose of CBCT and MSCT scanners for dentomaxillofacial applications. Eur J Radiol. **2009** Sep; 71(3): 461 – 468. doi: 10.1016/j.ejrad.2008.06.002. Epub 2008 Jul 18.

Lübbers HT, Medinger L, Kruse A, Grätz KW, Matthews F. Precision and accuracy of the 3dMD photogrammetric system in craniomaxillofacial application. J Craniofac Surg. **2010** May; 21(3): 763 – 767. doi: 10.1097/SCS.0b013e3181d841f7.

Maal TJ, Plooij JM, Rangel FA, Mollemans W, Schutyser FA, Bergé SJ. The accuracy of matching three-dimensional photographs with skin surfaces derived from cone-beam computed tomography. Int J Oral Maxillofac Surg. **2008** Jul; 37(7): 641 – 646. doi: 10.1016/j.ijom.2008.04.012. Epub 2008 Jun 9.

Maestre-Ferrín L, Romero-Millán J, Peñarrocha-Oltra D, Peñarrocha-Diago MA. Virtual articulator for the analysis of dental occlusion: An update. Med Oral Patol Oral Cir Bucal. **2012** Jan 1; 17(1): e160 – 163.

Maló P, Rangert B, Nobre M. All-on-4 immediate-function concept with Brånemark System implants for completely edentulous maxillae: a 1-year retrospective clinical study. Clin Implant Dent Relat Res. **2005**; 7 Suppl 1: S88 – S94.

Maló P, de Araújo Nobre M, Borges J, Almeida R. Retrievable metal ceramic implant-supported fixed prostheses with milled titanium frameworks and all-ceramic crowns: retrospective clinical study with up to 10 years of follow-up. J Prosthodont. **2012** Jun; 21(4): 256 – 264. doi: 10.1111/j.1532-849X.2011.00824.x. Epub 2012 Feb 19.

Mangano F, Zecca P, Pozzi-Taubert S, Macchi A, Ricci M, Luongo G, Mangano C. Maxillary sinus augmentation using computer-aided design/computer-aided manufacturing (CAD/CAM) technology. Int J Med Robot. **2013** Sep; 9(3): 331 – 338. doi: 10.1002/rcs.1460. Epub 2012 Sep 7.

Mansoor A, Bagci U, Foster B, Xu Z, Papadakis GZ, Folio LR, Udupa JK, Mollura DJ. Segmentation and image analysis of abnormal lungs at CT: current approaches, challenges, and future trends. Radiographics. **2015** Jul – Aug; 35(4): 1056 – 1076. doi: 10.1148/rg.2015140232.

Matta RE, Bergauer B, Adler W, Wichmann M, Nickenig HJ. The impact of the fabrication method on the three-dimensional accuracy of an implant surgery template. J Craniomaxillofac Surg. **2017** Jun; 45(6): 804 – 808. doi: 10.1016/j.jcms.2017.02.015. Epub 2017 Feb 20.

Maveli TC, Suprono MS, Kattadiyil MT, Goodacre CJ, Bahjri K: In vitro comparison of the maxillary occlusal plane orientation obtained with five facebow systems. J Prosthet Dent. **2015** Oct; 114(4): 566 – 573. doi: 10.1016/j.prosdent.2015.02.030. Epub 2015 Jun 30.

Mertens C, Löwenheim H, Hoffmann J. Image data based reconstruction of the midface using a patient-specific implant in combination with a vascularized osteomyocutaneous scapular flap. J Craniomaxillofac Surg. **2013** Apr; 41(3): 219 – 225. doi: 10.1016/j.jcms.2012.09.003. Epub 2012 Oct 13.

Misch C, Bidez MW. Occlusal considerations for implants-supported prostheses: implant-protected occlusion. In: Misch C, editor. Dental Implant Prosthetics. San Louis: Elsevier Mosby; **2005**. 472 – 510.

Miyanaji H, Zhang S, Lassell A, Ali Zandinejad A, Yang L: Optimal process parameters for 3D printing of porcelain structures. Procedia Manufacturing. **2016**; 5: 870 – 887. doi: 10.1016/j.promfg.2016.08.074.

Modabber A, Gerressen M, Stiller MB, Noroozi N, Füglein A, Hölzle F, Riediger D, Ghassemi A. Computer-assisted mandibular reconstruction with vascularized iliac crest bone graft. Aesthetic Plast Surg. **2012** Jun; 36(3): 653 – 659. doi: 10.1007/s00266-012-9877-2. Epub 2012 Mar 7.

Mora MA, Chenin DL, Arce RM. Software tools and surgical guides in dental-implant-guided surgery. Dent Clin North Am. **2014** Jul; 58(3): 597 – 626. doi: 10.1016/j.cden.2014.04.001.

Moss JP, Linney AD, Lowey MN. The use of three-dimensional techniques in facial esthetics. Semin Orthod. **1995** Jun; 1(2): 94 – 104.

Nakamura K, Kanno T, Milleding P, Örtengren U. Zirconia as dental implant abutment material: a systematic review. Int J Prosthodont. **2010** Jul – Aug; 23(4): 299 – 309.

Neumeister A, Schulz L, Glodecki C. Investigations on the accuracy of 3D-printed drill guides for dental implantology. Int J Comput Dent. **2017**; 20(1): 35 – 51.

Nkenke E, Zachow S, Benz M, Maier T, Veit K, Kramer M, Benz S, Häusler G, Neukam FW, Lell M. Fusion of computed tomography data and optical 3D images of the dentition for streak artefact correction in the simulation of orthognathic surgery. Dentomaxillofac Radiol. **2004** Jul; 33(4): 226 – 232.

Ortorp A, Jemt T. Clinical experiences of CNC-milled titanium frameworks supported by implants in the edentulous jaw: 1-year prospective study. Clin Implant Dent Relat Res. **2000**; 2(1): 2 – 9.

Ortorp A, Jemt T. CNC-milled titanium frameworks supported by implants in the edentulous jaw: a 10-year comparative clinical study. Clin Implant Dent Relat Res. **2012** Mar; 14(1): 88 – 99. doi: 10.1111/j.1708-8208.2009.00232.x. Epub 2009 Aug 17.

Paniz, G, Stellini E, Meneghello R, Cerard Ai, Gobbato EA, Bressan E. The precision of fit of cast and milled full-arch implant-supported restorations. Int J Oral Maxillofac Implants. **2013** May – Jun; 28(3): 687 – 693. doi: 10.11607/jomi.2990.

Papaspyridakos P, Mokti M, Chen CJ, Benic GI, Gallucci GO, Chronopoulos V. Implant and prosthodontic survival rates with implant fixed complete dental prostheses in the edentulous mandible after at least 5 years: a systematic review. Clin Implant Dent Relat Res. **2014** Oct; 16(5): 705 – 717. doi: 10.1111/cid.12036. Epub 2013 Jan 11.

Papaspyridakos P, Gallucci GO, Chen CJ, Hanssen S, Naert I, Vandenberghe B. Digital versus conventional implant impressions for edentulous patients: accuracy outcomes. Clin Oral Implants Res. **2016** Apr; 27(4): 465 – 472. doi: 10.1111/clr.12567. Epub 2015 Feb 13.

Papaspyridakos P, Rajput N, Kudara Y, Weber HP. Digital workflow for fixed implant rehabilitation of an extremely atrophic edentulous mandible in three appointments. J Esthet Restor Dent. **2017** May 6; 29(3): 178 – 188. doi: 10.1111/jerd.12290. Epub 2017 Mar 18.

Papaspyridakos P, Kang K, DeFuria C, Amin S, Kudara Y, Weber HP. Digital workflow in full-arch implant rehabilitation with segmented minimally veneered monolithic zirconia fixed dental prostheses: 2-year clinical follow-up. J Esthet Restor Dent. **2018** Jan; 30(1): 5 – 13. doi: 10.1111/jerd.12323. Epub 2017 Aug 9.

Peñarrocha-Oltra D, Agustín-Panadero R, Bagán L, Giménez B, Peñarrocha M. Impression of multiple implants using photogrammetry: description of technique and case presentation. Med Oral Patol Oral Cir Bucal. **2014** Jul; 19(4): e366 – e371.

Pettersson A, Kero T, Gillot L, Cannas B, Fäldt J, Söderberg R, Näsström K. Accuracy of CAD/CAM-guided surgical template implant surgery on human cadavers: Part I. J Prosthet Dent. **2010** Jun; 103(6): 334 – 342. doi: 10.1016/S0022-3913(10)60072-8.

Pettersson A, Komiyama A, Hultin M, Näsström K, Klinge B. Accuracy of virtually planned and template guided implant surgery on edentate patients. Clin Implant Dent Relat Res. **2012** Aug; 14(4): 527 – 537. doi: 10.1111/j.1708-8208.2010.00285.x. Epub 2010 May 11.

Pjetursson BE, Asgeirsson AG, Zwahlen M, Sailer I. Improvements in implant dentistry over the last decade: comparison of survival and complication rates in older and newer publications. Int J Oral Maxillofac Implants. **2014**; 29 Suppl: 308 – 324. doi: 10.11607/jomi.2014suppl.g5.2.

Plaster U. Mastering the occlusal plane. Inside Dental Technology. **2014** Jan; 5(1).

Pruksakorn D, Chantarapanich N, Arpornchayanon O, Leerapun T, Sitthiseripratip K, Vatanapatimakul N. Rapid-prototype endoprosthesis for palliative reconstruction of an upper extremity after resection of bone metastasis. Int J Comput Assist Radiol Surg. **2015** Mar; 10(3): 343 – 350. doi: 10.1007/s11548-014-1072-2. Epub 2014 May 20.

Purcell BA, McGlumphy EA, Yilmaz B, Holloway JA, Beck FM. Anteroposterior spread and cantilever length in mandibular metal-resin implant-fixed complete dental prostheses: a 7- to 9-year analysis. Int J Prosthodont. **2015** Sep – Oct; 28(5): 512 – 518. doi: 10.11607/ijp.4172.

Raico Gallardo YN, da Silva-Olivio IRT, Mukai E, Morimoto S, Sesma N, Cordaro L. Accuracy comparison of guided surgery for dental implants according to the tissue of support: a systematic review and meta-analysis. Clin Oral Implants Res. **2017** May; 28(5): 602 – 612. doi: 10.1111/clr.12841. Epub 2016 Apr 8.

Rangel FA, Maal TJ, Bergé SJ, van Vlijmen OJ, Plooij JM, Schutyser F, Kuijpers-Jagtman AM. Integration of digital dental casts in 3-dimensional facial photographs. Am J Orthod Dentofacial Orthop. **2008** Dec; 134(6): 820 – 826. doi: 10.1016/j.ajodo.2007.11.026.

Rangel FA, Maal TJ, Bronkhorst EM, Breuning KH, Schols JG, Bergé SJ, Kuijpers-Jagtman AM. Accuracy and reliability of a novel method for fusion of digital dental casts and cone beam computed tomography scans. PLoS One. **2013**; 8(3): e59130. doi: 10.1371/journal.pone.0059130. Epub 2013 Mar 20.

Ras F, Habets LL, van Ginkel FC, Prahl-Andersen B. Method for quantifying facial asymmetry in three dimensions using stereophotogrammetry. Angle Orthod. **1995**; 65(3): 233 – 239.

Rasia-dal Polo M, Poli PP, Rancitelli D, Beretta M, Maiorana C. Alveolar ridge reconstruction with titanium meshes: a systematic review of the literature. Med Oral Patol Oral Cir Bucal. **2014** Nov 1; 19(6): e639 – e646. doi: 10.4317/medoral.19998.

Rohner D, Jaquiery C, Kunz C, Bucher P, Maas H, Hammer B Maxillofacial recon- struction with prefabricated osseous free flaps: a 3-year experience with 24 patients. Plast Reconstr Surg. **2003** Sep; 112(3): 748 – 757.

Rompen E, Domken O, Degidi M, Pontes AE, Piattelli A. The effect of material characteristics, of surface topography and of implant components and connections on soft tissue integration: a literature review. Clin Oral Implants Res. **2006** Oct; 17 Suppl 2: 55 – 67.

Rosati R, De Menezes M, Rossetti A, Sforza C, Ferrario VF. Digital dental cast placement in 3-dimensional, full-face reconstruction: a technical evaluation. Am J Orthod Dentofacial Orthop. **2010** Jul; 138(1): 84 – 88. doi: 10.1016/j.ajodo.2009.10.035.

Sanz-Sánchez, Sanz-Martín, Figuero E, Sanz M. Clinical efficacy of immediate implant loading protocols compared to conventional loading depending on the type of the restoration: a systematic review. Clin Oral Implants Res. **2015** Aug; 26(8): 964 – 982. doi: 10.1111/clr.12428. Epub 2014 Jun 11.

Sanz-Sánchez I, Sanz-Martín I, Carrillo de Albornoz A, Figuero E, Sanz M. Biological effect of the abutment material on the stability of peri-implant marginal bone levels: a systematic review and meta-analysis. Clin Oral Implants Res. **2018** Oct; 29 Suppl 18: 124 – 144. doi: 10.1111/clr.13293. Epub 2018 Jun 15.

Schepers RH, Kraeima J, Vissink A, Lahoda LU, Roodenburg JL, Reintsema H, Raghoebar GM, Witjes MJ. Accuracy of secondary maxillofacial reconstruction with prefabricated fibula grafts using 3D planning and guided reconstruction. J Craniomaxillofac Surg. **2016** Apr; 44(4): 392 – 399. doi: 10.1016/j.jcms.2015.12.008. Epub 2016 Jan 6.

Schlee M, Rothamel D. Ridge augmentation using customized allogenic bone blocks: proof of concept and histological findings. Implant Dent. **2013** Jun; 22(3): 212 – 2088. doi: 10.1097/ID.0b013e3182885fa1.

Schrott A, Riggi-Heiniger M, Maruo K, Gallucci GO. Implant loading protocols for partially edentulous patients with extended edentulous sites—a systematic review and meta-analysis. Int J Oral Maxillofac Implants. **2014**; 29 Suppl: 239 – 255. doi: 10.11607/jomi.2014suppl.g4.2.

Shah N, Bansal N, Logani A. Recent advances in imaging technologies in dentistry. World J Radiol. **2014** Oct 28; 6(10): 794 – 807. doi: 10.4329/wjr.v6.i10.794.

Shi JY, Zhang XM, Qiao SC, Qian SJ, Mo JJ, Lai HC. Hardware complications and failure of three-unit zirconia-based and porcelain-fused-metal implant-supported fixed dental prostheses: a retrospective cohort study with up to 8 years. Clin Oral Implants Res. **2017** May; 28(5): 571–575. doi: 10.1111/clr.12836. Epub 2016 Mar 16.

Shillingburg HT, Hobo S, Whitsett LD: Fundamentals of fixed prosthodontics. Quintessence Publishing Co: 2nd ed. **1981**.

Silva NRFA, Sailer I, Zhang Y, Coelho PG, Guess PC, Zembic A, Kohal RJ. Performance of Zironia for Dental Healthcare. Materials (Basel). **2010** Feb; 3(2): 863–896. doi: 10.3390/ma3020863.

Simion M, Fontana F. Autogenous and xenogeneic bone grafts for the bone regeneration. A literature review. Minerva Stomatol. **2004** May; 53(5): 191–206.

Solaberrieta E, Etxaniz O, Mínguez R, Muniozguren J, Arias A. Design of a virtual articulator for the simulation and analysis of mandibular movements in dental CAD/CAM. Proceedings of the 19th CIRP Design Conference—Competitive Design. Cranfield University: **2009**.

Solaberrieta E, Arias A, Barrenetxea L, Etxaniz O, Mínguez R, Muniozguren J. A virtual dental prosthesis design method using a virtual articulator. Proceedings of the 11th International Design Conference, Dubrovnik, Croatia, May 17–20, **2010**. 443–452.

Solaberrieta E, Mínguez R, Barrenetxea L, Etxaniz O. Direct transfer of the position of digitized casts to a virtual articulator. J Prosthet Dent. **2013** Jun; 109(6): 411–414. doi: 10.1016/S0022-3913(13)60330-3.

Spear FM, Kokich VG. A multidisciplinary approach to esthetic dentistry. Dent Clin North Am. **2007**; 51: 487–505, x–xi.

Stapleton BM, Lin WS, Ntounis A, Harris BT, Morton D. Application of digital diagnostic impression, virtual planning, and computer-guided implant surgery for a CAD/CAM-fabricated, implant-supported fixed dental prosthesis: a clinical report. J Prosthet Dent. **2014** Sep; 112(3): 402–408. doi: 10.1016/j.prosdent.2014.03.019. Epub 2014 May 13.

Stieglitz LH, Gerber N, Schmid T, Mordasini P, Fichtner J, Fung C, Murek M, Weber S, Raabe A, Beck J. Intraoperative fabrication of patient-specific moulded implants for skull reconstruction: single-centre experience of 28 cases. Acta Neurochir (Wien). **2014** Apr; 156(4): 793–803. doi: 10.1007/s00701-013-1977-5. Epub 2014 Jan 18.

Svanborg P, Stenport V, Eliasson A. Fit of cobalt-chromium implant frameworks before and after ceramic veneering in comparison with CNC-milled titanium frameworks. Clin Exp Dent Res. **2015** Oct 26; 1(2): 49–56. doi: 10.1002/cre2.9.

Tahmaseb A, van de Weijden JJ, Mercelis P, De Clerck R, Wismeijer D. Parameters of passive fit using a new technique to mill implant- supported superstructures: an in vitro study of a novel three-dimensional force measurement-misfit method. Int J Oral Maxillofac Implants. **2010** Mar–Apr; 25(2): 247–257.

Tahmaseb A, De Clerck R, Eckert S, Wismeijer D. Reference-based digital concept to restore partially edentulous patients following an immediate loading protocol: a pilot study. Int J Oral Maxillofac Implants. **2011** Jul–Aug; 26(4): 707–717.

Tahmaseb A, De Clerck R, Aartman I, Wismeijer D. Digital protocol for reference-based guided surgery and immediate loading: a prospective clinical study. Int J Oral Maxillofac Implants. **2012** Sep–Oct; 27(5): 1258–1270.

Tahmaseb A, Wismeijer D, Coucke W, Derksen W. Computer technology applications in surgical implant dentistry: a systematic review. Int J Oral Maxillofac Implants. **2014**; 29 Suppl: 25–42. doi: 10.11607/jomi.2014suppl.g1.2.

Tahmaseb A, Wu V, Wismeijer D, Coucke W, Evans C. The accuracy of static computerÐaided implant surgery: a systematic review and metaÐanalysis. Clin Oral Implants Res. **2018** Oct; 29 Suppl 16: 416–435. doi: 10.1111/clr.13346.

Takasaki H. Moiré topography. Appl Opt. **1970** Jun 1; 9(6): 1467–1472. doi: 10.1364/AO.9.001467.

Tanner JM, Weiner JS. The reliability of the photogrammetric method of anthropometry, with a description of a miniature camera technique. Am J Phys Anthropol. **1949** Jun; 7(2): 145–186.

Tarnow DP, Emtiaz S, Classi A. Immediate loading of threaded implants at stage 1 surgery in edentulous arches: ten consecutive case reports with 1- to 5-year data. Int J Oral Maxillofac Implants. **1997** May – Jun; 12(3): 319 – 324.

Tarnow DP, Cho SC, Wallace SS. The effect of inter-implant distance on the height of inter-implant bone crest. J Periodontol. **2000** Apr; 71(4): 546 – 549.

Thomé E, Lee HJ, Sartori IA, Trevisan RL, Luiz J, Tiossi R. A randomized controlled trial comparing interim acrylic prostheses with and without cast metal base for immediate loading of dental implants in the edentulous mandible. Clin Oral Implants Res. **2015** Dec; 26(12): 1414 – 1420. doi: 10.1111/clr.12470. Epub 2014 Sep 19.

Torabi K, Farjood E, Hamedani S. Rapid prototyping technologies and their applications in prosthodontics, a review of literature. J Dent (Shiraz). **2015** Mar; 16(1): 1 – 9.

Truninger TC, Stawarczyk B, Leutert CR, Sailer TR, Hämmerle CH, Sailer I. Bending moments of zirconia and titanium abutments with internal and external implant-abutment connections after aging and chewing simulation. Clin Oral Implants Res. **2012** Jan; 23(1): 12 – 18. doi: 10.1111/j.1600-0501.2010.02141.x. Epub 2011 Mar 28.

van der Meer WJ, Andriessen FS, Wismeijer D, Ren Y. Application of intra-oral dental scanners in the digital workflow of implantology. PLoS One. **2012**; 7(8): e43312. doi: 10.1371/journal.pone.0043312. Epub 2012 Aug 22.

Van Loon JAW. A new method for indicating normal and abnormal relations of the teeth to the facial lines. Dental Cosmos. **1915**; 57: 973 – 983,1093 – 1101,1229 – 1235.

Venet L, Perriat M, Mangano FG Fortin T. Horizontal ridge reconstruction of the anterior maxilla using customized allogeneic bone blocks with a minimally invasive technique—a case series. BMC Oral Health. **2017** Dec 8; 17(1): 146. doi: 10.1186/s12903-017-0423-0.

Venezia P, Torsello F, Cavalcanti R, D'Amato S. Retrospective analysis of 26 complete-arch implant-supported monolithic zirconia prostheses with feldspathic porcelain veneering limited to the facial surface. J Prosthet Dent. **2015** Oct; 114(4): 506 – 512. doi: 10.1016/j.prosdent.2015.02.010. Epub 2015 Jun 5.

Vigolo P, Givani A, Majzoub Z, Cordioli G. A 4-year prospective study to assess peri-implant hard and soft tissues adjacent to titanium versus gold-alloy abutments in cemented single implant crowns. J Prosthodont. **2006** Jul – Aug; 15(4): 250 – 256.

Waasdorp JA, Reynolds MA. Allogeneic Block Grafts: A Systematic Review, Int J Oral Maxillofac Implants. **2010** May – Jun; 25(3): 525 – 531.

Wakasugi-Sato N, Kodama M, Matsuo K, Yamamoto N, Oda M, Ishikawa A, Tanaka T, Seta Y, Habu M, Kokuryo S, Ichimiya H, Miyamoto I, Kito S, Matsumoto-Takeda S, Wakasugi T, Yamashita Y, Yoshioka I, Takahashi T, Tominaga K, Morimoto Y. Advanced clinical usefulness of ultrasonography for diseases in oral and maxillofacial regions. Int J Dent. **2010**; 2010:639382. doi: 10.1155/2010/639382. Epub 2010 Apr 27.

Welander M, Abrahamsson I, Berglundh T. The mucosal barrier at implant abutments of different materials. Clin Oral Implants Res. **2008** Jul; 19(7): 635 – 641. doi: 10.1111/j.1600-0501.2008.01543.x. Epub 2008 May 19.

Wennerberg A, Carlsson GE, Jemt T. Influence of occlusal factors on treatment outcome: a study of 109 consecutive patients with mandibular implant-supported fixed prostheses opposing maxillary complete dentures. Int J Prosthodont. **2001** Nov – Dec; 14: 550 – 555.

Wesemann C, Muallah J, Mah J, Bumann A. Accuracy and efficiency of full-arch digitalization and 3D printing: A comparison between desktop model scanners, an intraoral scanner, a CBCT model scan, and stereolithographic 3D printing. Quintessence Int. **2017**; 48(1): 41 – 50. doi: 10.3290/j.qi.a37130.

Widmann G, Bale RJ. Accuracy in computer-aided implant surgery—a review. Int J Oral Maxillofac Implants. **2006** Mar – Apr; 21(2): 305 – 313.

Widmann G, Stoffner R, Schullian P, Widmann R, Keiler M, Zangerl A, Puelacher W, Bale RJ. Comparison of the accuracy of invasive and noninvasive registration methods for image guided oral implant surgery. Int J Oral Maxillofac Implants. **2010** May – Jun; 25(3): 491 – 498.

Wismeijer D, Mans R, van Genuchten M, Reijers HA. Patients' preferences when comparing analogue implant impressions using a polyether impression material versus digital impressions (intraoral scan) of dental implants. Clin Oral Implants Res. **2014** Oct; 25(10): 1113 – 1118. doi: 10.1111/clr.12234. Epub 2013 Aug 14.

Wong KV, Hernandez A. A review of additive manufacturing. International Scholarly Research Network, Mechanical Engineering. **2012:** Article ID 208760, 10 pages. doi:10.5402/2012/208760.

Zembic A, Bösch A, Jung RE, Hämmerle CH, Sailer I. Five-year results of a randomised controlled clinical trial comparing zirconia and titanium abutments supporting single implant crowns in canine and posterior regions. Clin Oral Implants Res. **2013** Apr; 24(4): 384 – 390. doi: 10.1111/clr.12044. Epub 2012 Oct 2.

Zhang L, Snavely N, Curless B, Seitz SM. Spacetime faces: high resolution capture for modeling and animation. ACM Trans Graph. **2003** Aug; 23(3): 548 – 558.

Zhou LB, Shang HT, He LS, Bo B, Liu GC, Liu YP, Zhao JL. Accurate reconstruction of discontinuous mandible using a reverse engineering/computer-aided design/ rapid prototyping technique: a preliminary clinical study. J Oral Maxillofac Surg. **2010** Sep; 68(9): 2115 – 2121. doi: 10.1016/j.joms.2009.09.033. Epub 2010 Jun 12.

Zitzmann NU, Kovaltschuk I, Lenherr P, Dedem P, Joda T. Dental students' perceptions of digital and conventional impression techniques: a randomized controlled trial. J Dent Educ. **2017** Oct; 81(10): 1227 – 1232. doi: 10.21815/JDE.017.081.